AF856537

EFFECT OF ACUTE ISCHAEMIA ON MYOCARDIAL FUNCTION

M. F. OLIVER
M.D., F.R.C.P.Lond., F.R.C.P.Ed.
Reader in Medicine, University of Edinburgh
Consultant Physician, Royal Infirmary, Edinburgh

D. G. JULIAN
M.A., M.D., F.R.C.P.Lond., F.R.C.P.Ed., F.R.A.C.P.
Senior Lecturer in Medicine, University of Edinburgh
Consultant Physician, Royal Infirmary, Edinburgh

K. W. DONALD
D.S.C., Q.P., M.A., M.D., D.Sc., F.R.C.P.Lond., F.R.S.E.
Professor of Medicine, University of Edinburgh
Consultant Physician, Royal Infirmary, Edinburgh

EFFECT OF ACUTE ISCHAEMIA ON MYOCARDIAL FUNCTION

Proceedings of the
Seventh Pfizer International Symposium
held in Edinburgh from 29-31 May 1972

Edited by

M. F. OLIVER

D. G. JULIAN

K. W. DONALD

The Williams & Wilkins Company
Baltimore

© LONGMAN GROUP LIMITED, 1972

All rights reserved. No part of this publication may be reproduced, stored in a retrieval system, or transmitted in any form or by any means, electronic, mechanical, photocopying, recording or otherwise, without the prior permission of the publishers (Churchill Livingstone, Teviot Place, Edinburgh)

ISBN 0 443 01015 3

PRINTED IN GREAT BRITAIN

PREFACE

OUR purpose in selecting the theme of acute myocardial ischaemia for the Seventh International Pfizer Symposium was twofold. First, knowledge of the effects of acute ischaemia on myocardial metabolism, electrophysiology and contractility has been accumulating rapidly in the last five years but there has been little opportunity for investigators working in different disciplines to meet together and discuss this subject in depth. Second, and no less important, there is a need to integrate and report as a whole much of the work which has recently and will shortly be published in specialized journals. It is hoped that this book will achieve this purpose.

It may be a surprise to the clinical cardiologist to realize how ill understood are so many of the basic mechanisms related to, for example, angina or ventricular fibrillation. But, on reflection, this will seem less unexpected if it is remembered that it has only recently been possible to measure changes in myocardial blood flow and action potential in the intact contracting heart, to estimate myocardial enzyme and amine concentration, to record the events leading to the onset of ventricular fibrillations, to measure substrate exchange across the myocardium, to determine what influences the requirements for myocardial nutrients and to analyse myocardial contractility. Many questions, currently unanswerable, are raised throughout this book and so a further aim should be achieved. This is the catalysis, provocation and reassembly of ideas so that more work on myocardial ischaemia will result.

K. W. DONALD
M. F. OLIVER
D. G. JULIAN

ACKNOWLEDGMENTS

WE want particularly to thank the Executive Committee and the Trustees of the Pfizer Foundation for making this Symposium possible, and the Dean of the Post-Graduate Board for Medicine, University of Edinburgh, Major General J. M. Matheson, O.B.E., M.D., F.R.C.P.Ed., F.R.C.S., for his invaluable support.

The rapporteurs for the sessions—Dr B. J. Kirby, Dr I. Nimmo, Dr S. R. Reuben, Dr R. Riemersma, Dr R. A. Strange and Dr C. W. Vellani—were assiduous in their help with the preparation of the manuscripts and we are most grateful to them. Mrs Eva Riemersma gave much valuable time to the references and index and Miss S. Bucher, Miss R. Dodd, Miss I. Johnston, Mrs J. Rodger, Miss M. Sharp, Mrs C. Winney were greatly appreciated for their secretarial assistance.

Finally, we wish to thank all those, including the publishers, who have made it possible to produce this book in such a short time.

LIST OF PARTICIPANTS

ALLISON, S. P. *General Hospital, Nottingham.*

BARRATT, A. M. *Department of Pharmacology, School of Medicine, University of Leeds, Leeds, LS2 9NL.*

BURGES, R. *Pharmacology Research Group, Pfizer Ltd., Sandwich, Kent.*

CARLSON, L. A. *Department of Geriatrics, University of Uppsala, Box 641, S—751 27, Uppsala, 1, Sweden.*

CONTI, C. R. *Department of Cardiology, Johns Hopkins Medical School, Baltimore, Maryland, U.S.A.*

DONALD, K. W. *Department of Medicine, University of Edinburgh, Royal Infirmary, Edinburgh, EH3 9YW.*

DURRER, D. *Department of Cardiology, Academisch Ziekenhuis, Cardiologische Kliniek, Eerste Helmersstraat 104, Amsterdam-Oud West, Netherlands.*

FISHER, R. B. *Department of Biochemistry, University of Edinburgh Medical School, Edinburgh, EH8 9AG.*

FITZGERALD, J. D. *Pharmacology Department, Imperial Chemical Industries Ltd., Pharmaceuticals Division, Mereside, Alderley Park, Macclesfield Cheshire, SK10 4TG.*

GUDBJARNASON, S. *Department of Chemistry, Science Institute, University of Iceland, 3 Dunhaga, Reykjavik, Iceland.*

HAN, J. *Department of Medicine, Albany Medical College of Union University, Albany, New York, 12208, U.S.A.*

HENDERSON, A. H. *Department of Cardiology, Welsh National School of Medicine, Heath Park, Cardiff, CF4 4XN.*

HERBACZYNSKA-CEDRO, K. *Medical Research Centre, Polish Academy of Sciences, Warsaw, Poland.*

JENNINGS, R. B. *Department of Pathology, Northwestern University, Ward Memorial Building, 303 E. Chicago Avenue, Chicago, Illinois, 60611, U.S.A.*

JULIAN, D. G. *Department of Cardiology, Royal Infirmary, Edinburgh, EH3 9YW.*

KAIJSER, L. *Department of Clinical Physiology, Karolinska Sjukhuset, S—104 01 Stockholm, 60, Sweden.*

KIRBY, B. J. *Department of Medicine, Royal Infirmary, Edinburgh, EH3 9YW.*

KITCHIN, A. H. *Department of Cardiology, Western General Hospital, Edinburgh, EH4 2XU.*

KURIEN, V. A. *29, Haynes Street, Manchester, Connecticut 06040, U.S.A.*

LASSERS, B. W. *Department of Medicine, Royal Infirmary, Edinburgh, EH3 9YW.*

LAWRIE, T. D. V. *Department of Cardiology, University of Glasgow, Royal Infirmary, Glasgow, C4.*

LIVESLEY, B. *Cardiac Department, King's College Hospital, Denmark Hill, London SE5 9RS.*

MANN, R. D. *Pfizer Europe, 55 rue du Moulin à Papier, 1160 Brussels, Belgium.*

MARQUIS, R. M. *Department of Cardiology, Royal Infirmary, Edinburgh, EH3 9YW.*

MASERI, A. *Fisiologia Clinica, Laboratorio del Consiglio Nazionale delle Ricerche, University of Pisa, Via Savi, 8, Pisa, Italy.*

MATTHEWS, M. B. *Department of Cardiology, Western General Hospital, Edinburgh, EH4 2XU.*

MJØS, O. D. *Institute for Experimental Medical Research, University of Oslo, Ulleval Hospital, Oslo, Norway.*

MUIR, A. L. *Department of Medicine, Royal Infirmary, Edinburgh, EH3 9YW.*

NIMMO, I. A. *Department of Biochemistry, University of Edinburgh Medical School, Edinburgh, EH8 9AG.*

NOBLE, M. I. M. *Charing Cross Hospital Medical School, Fulham Hospital, London, W6.*

O'BRIEN, J. A. *Department of Biochemistry, University of Edinburgh Medical School, Edinburgh, EH8 9AG.*

OLIVER, M. F. *Department of Cardiology, Royal Infirmary, Edinburgh, EH3 9YW.*

OPIE, L. *Department of Medicine, University of Cape Town Medical School, Observatory, Cape Town, South Africa.*

PARKER, J. O. *Etherington Hall, Queen's University, Kingston, Ontario, Canada.*

PARRATT, J. R. *Department of Pharmacology, University of Strathclyde, Royal College, George Street, Glasgow, C1.*

RANDLE, P. J. *Department of Biochemistry University of Bristol, Medical School, University Walk, Bristol, BS8 1TD.*

REUBEN, S. R. *Department of Cardiology, Royal Infirmary, Edinburgh, Edinburgh, EH3 9YW.*

REUTER, H. *Department of Pharmacology, University of Bern, Pharmakologisches Institut, 3000 Bern, Friedbuhlstrasse 49, Switzerland.*

RIEMERSMA, R. A. *Lipid Research Laboratory, Department of Clinical Chemistry, Royal Infirmary, Edinburgh, EH3 9YW.*

SHAHAB, L. *Deutsche Akademie der Wissenschaften zu Berlin, Institut für Kreislaufforschung, 115 Berlin-Buch, Lindenberger Weg, 70, German Democratic Republic.*

STRANGE, R. C. *Lipid Research Laboratory, Department of Clinical Chemistry, Royal Infirmary, Edinburgh, EH3 9YW.*

TAGGART, P. I. *Middlesex Hospital Medical School, Institute of Clinical Research, 32-48 Hanson Street, London, W1P 7DR.*

THOMAS, M. *Department of Medicine, Royal Postgraduate Medical School, Hammersmith Hospital, London, W12 0HS.*

TURNER, R. W. D. *Department of Cardiology, Western General Hospital, Edinburgh, EH4 2XU.*

VELLANI, C. W. *Department of Medicine, Royal Infirmary, Edinburgh, EH3 9YW.*

VERGROESEN, A. J. *Unilever Research, Olivier van Noortlaan 120, Vlaardingen, Netherlands.*

WALLACE, A. G. *Division of Cardiology, Duke University Medical Center, Department of Medicine, Cardiovascular Division, Durham, North Carolina 27710, U.S.A.*

WHITBY, L. G. *Department of Clinical Chemistry, Royal Infirmary, Edinburgh, EH3 9YW.*

CONTENTS

ISOLATED HEART PREPARATIONS

J. A. O'Brien

This paper is concerned with the problem of the measurement of the metabolic activity of the isolated rat heart and with the properties of the preparation in controlled hypoxia.

Changes occur in the properties of the isolated rat heart during the initial period of perfusion. Oxygen uptake,[1] the permeability to non-metabolized sugar in the absence of insulin,[2,3] lactate output and, in some circumstances, glucose uptake[4] decrease to constant rates. The period of change may be as short as 15 minutes in the case of oxygen consumption but as long as one hour for glucose uptake by hearts taken from fed rats. It is the practice in many laboratories to perfuse hearts for between 5 and 20 minutes before making any experimental measurements but change in properties may still occur subsequently. Estimates of the average metabolic rates over 30 minutes may therefore be misleading. Over short periods when a closed circuit system of recirculating perfusate is used a compromise must be struck between the difficulties of precisely measuring small changes in the amount of substrate and those of the interpretation of estimates made when the composition of the perfusate changes rapidly. The compromise favours the use of substrate concentrations high enough to make the rate of metabolism independent of changes in concentration. Such concentrations may be unphysiological.

Many of these problems can be overcome in a system of perfusion in which a substrate is infused steadily into recirculating perfusate whose volume is kept constant by withdrawal at a rate equal to infusion. An apparatus for this purpose has been described in detail by Fisher and O'Brien.[4] In this system the instantaneous rate of metabolism is given by the equation:

$$v = i\,(a - x) - P\frac{dx}{dt}$$

where v is the rate of substrate utilization, i is the rate of infusion, a is the concentration of the infused substrate, x is the concentration of substrate in the perfusate, P is the volume of recirculating perfusate and t is the time.

By the application of the above equation to perfusate collections made at regular short intervals (2 to 5 min) the uptake by hearts of glucose at physiological concentrations has been followed in detail and it has been shown that in the absence of insulin it decreases smoothly to an almost constant level and that, once this has happened, the perfusate concentration also moves in an exponential fashion to a constant level. In the presence of sufficient insulin, glucose uptake is constant from the beginning of perfusion, and perfusate glucose concentration reaches a steady state concentration in a relatively short time thereafter.

The decrease in glucose uptake rate in the absence of added insulin is probably due to the decrease in effective insulin in the perfusion system, since in the presence of adequate insulin there is no sign of any other cause of decrease. If this is right, then it takes 30 to 60 min after preliminary washout to bring insulin activity down to a negligible level.

With this system no arbitrary assumption has to be made about when the state of the heart becomes basal, and there is one other substantial advantage, namely, that there is no lower limit to the substrate concentration which can be used other than those imposed by analytical methods, so that the system can be used to study very rapidly turning over metabolites. Glucose metabolism has been studied over the range 0·02 mM to 10 mM (0·4 to 180 mg/100 ml). At the lowest concentration the rate of uptake by the heart each hour is equal to ten times the glucose content of recirculating perfusate.

The apparatus of Fisher and O'Brien has been adapted to allow controlled variation in the oxygen tension presented to the heart. Figure 1, 1 depicts the modification. Infusate is introduced into the lead carrying perfusate to the heart. Two perfusates are used, one equilibrated with 5 per cent CO_2 in oxygen, the other equilibrated with 5 per cent CO_2 in nitrogen. One of them is used for recirculation and the other for infusion. With variation of the infusion rate this allows any arterial oxygen tension to be established in the range 10 to 700 mmHg. The oxygen tension can be altered almost instantaneously by adjusting the infusion rate.

Flow-through oxygen electrodes are placed before and after the point of infusion. From the oxygen tensions determined at these points and the rate of infusion the coronary flow can be calculated.

A third electrode measures the oxygen tension of the effluent from the heart so that the oxygen consumption can be estimated. The arrangements for gaseous exchange in the apparatus are sufficient to re-equilibrate the recirculating perfusate in one passage.

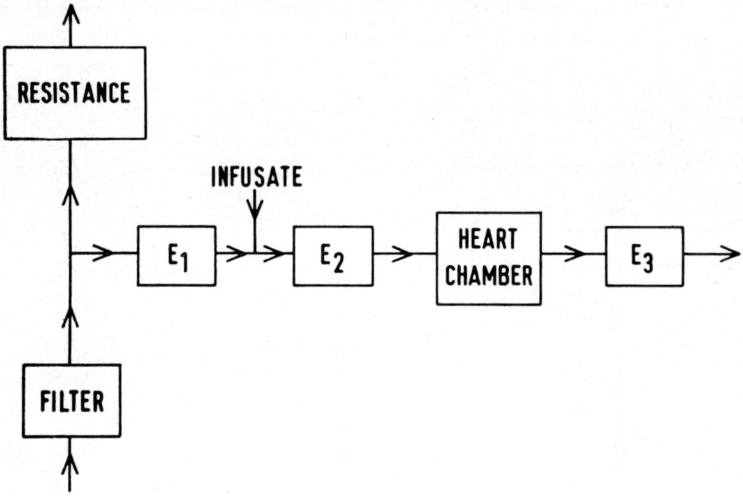

FIG. 1, 1. Diagram of the modification of the apparatus of Fisher and O'Brien[4] for the study of the hypoxic heart. E_1, E_2 and E_3 are oxygen electrodes.

Preliminary experiments have been made with this system on the effect of insulin and hypoxia on oxygen consumption and glucose utilization. The infusate glucose concentration was 4 mM and the steady state concentration was never less than 3 mM at which level glucose utilization by the aerobic heart is maximal. Insulin, when used, was present at 100 mU/ml or 2 mU/ml and the perfusion pressure was always 40 mmHg. The stability of the rates of oxygen consumption, coronary flow and glucose uptake at any one level of hypoxia was indicated by the constancy of the outputs from the oxygen electrodes and the analysis of the time-course of the perfusate glucose concentration.

Figure 1, 2 shows that even at arterial oxygen tensions much higher than physiological, the oxygen uptake is dependent on oxygen tension, but that it tends to decrease less sharply in the presence of insulin. Figure 1, 3 shows that in the presence of insulin oxygen uptake is sustained until the venous oxygen tension corresponds to a true anoxia, but that the decrease in oxygen uptake in the absence of insulin occurs long before the heart is truly anoxic.

The presumption is that the determining factor is the ability of the heart to oxidize glucose at a given oxygen tension. Preliminary experiments have shown that the oxygen uptake falls at least as much in the absence of glucose as in its presence and that insulin

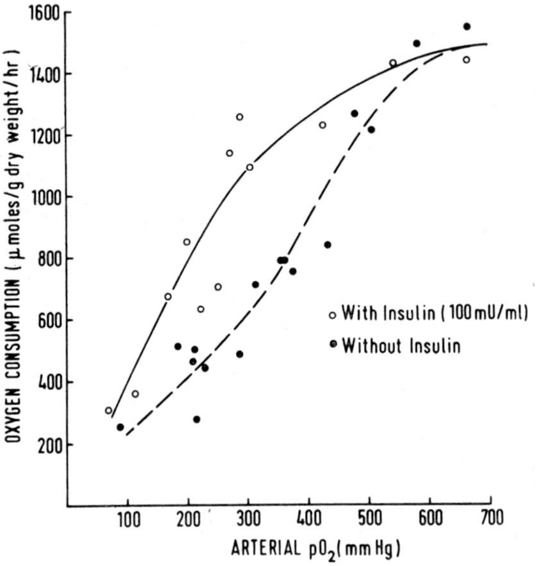

FIG. 1, 2. The relationship between arterial oxygen tension and oxygen consumption in the presence and absence of insulin. The data were obtained from 15 hearts.

does not then restore the oxygen uptake. The sustaining effect of insulin therefore seems to be due to an increase in the rate of oxidation of exogenous glucose. At the lower insulin concentration (2 mU/ml) the same sustaining effect is seen.

The effects of insulin and hypoxia on glucose utilization are shown in Figure 1, 4. Glucose uptake is stimulated by insulin at all degrees of hypoxia and is markedly increased when the oxygen tension of the effluent from the heart approaches zero. If the oxygen consumption equivalent to the complete oxidation of the glucose uptake of the heart is calculated, the increase in the equivalent oxygen consumption due to insulin is of the same order as the maximum difference in oxygen consumption sustained by insulin (Fig. 1, 3). This is consistent with the notion that insulin increases the rate of oxidation of exogenous glucose. It is implicit that the oxidation of endogenous substrate must limit oxygen consumption by the hypoxic heart in the absence of insulin.

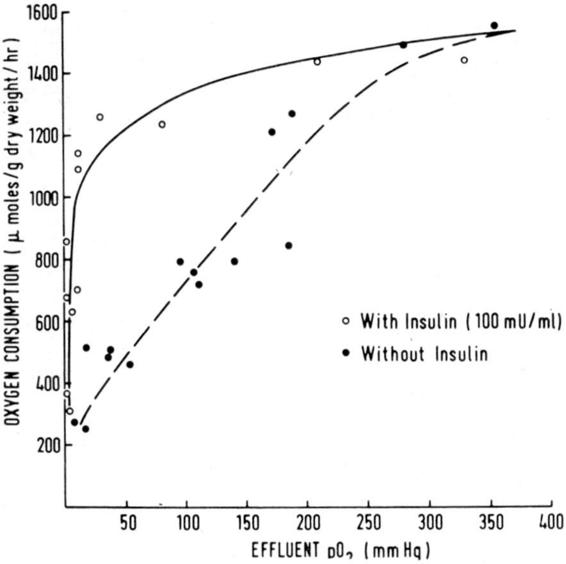

FIG. 1, 3. The relationship between the oxygen tension of the coronary effluent and oxygen consumption in the presence and absence of insulin. The data were obtained from 15 hearts.

The effects of insulin on oxygen consumption can be interpreted as being secondary to an increase in the cell permeability to glucose. Anoxia has also been shown to increase permeability to non-metabolized sugars.[5] The effects of hypoxia on the rates of glucose uptake are consistent with these observations, but they suggest that the effects of hypoxia and insulin are additive. Estimates of the parameters of glucose permeation from an analysis of the kinetics of the glucose utilization by the aerobic rat heart indicate that the maximum rate of permeation in the presence of insulin is approximately 0·45 mmoles/g dry weight/hour (Fisher and O'Brien, un-

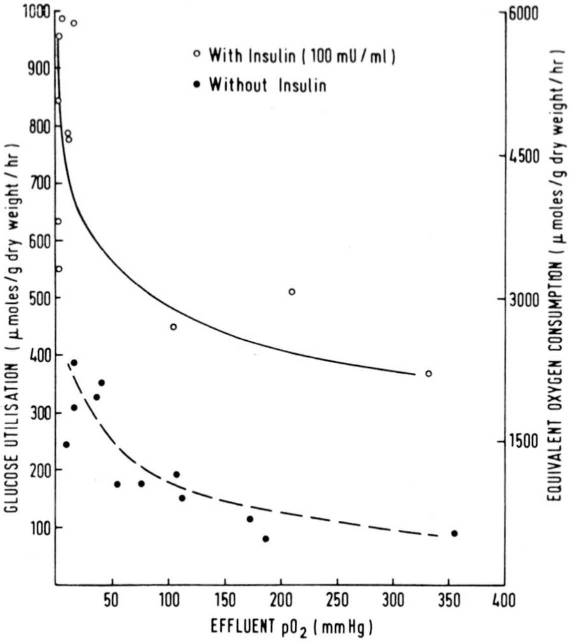

FIG. 1, 4. The relationship between the oxygen tension of the coronary effluent and glucose utilization and equivalent oxygen consumption in the presence and absence of insulin. The data were obtained from 15 hearts.

published observation). The rate of uptake of nearly 1 mmole/g dry weight/hour observed when the coronary effluent is almost totally depleted of oxygen can only be accounted for by an increase in permeability due to anoxia.

Acknowledgements

I am grateful to Professor R. B. Fisher for his valuable comments and to Miss P. Brown for her skilful technical assistance.

REFERENCES

1 FISHER, R. B. & WILLIAMSON, R. J. (1961). The oxygen uptake of the perfused rat heart. *Journal of Physiology* **158,** 86-101.

2 ZACHARIAH, P. (1961). Contractility and sugar permeability in the perfused rat heart. *Journal of Physiology* **158,** 59-72.

3 FISHER, R. B. & GILBERT, J. C. (1970). Kinetics of pentose permeation in the perfused rat heart. *Journal of Physiology* **210,** 287-295.

4 Fisher, R. B. & O'Brien, J. A. (1972). The effect of endogenous and added insulin on the time course of glucose uptake by the the isolated perfused rat heart. *Quarterly Journal of Experimental Physiology* **57,** 176-191.
5 Morgan, H. E., Cadenas, E.. Regen, D. M. & Park, C. R. (1961). Regulation of glucose uptake in muscle II. *Journal of Biological Chemistry* **236,** 262-268.

Discussion

Fisher. Your work suggests the effects of hypoxia are dependent upon the hormonal status of the heart which is difficult to determine in most systems. Would you agree with this?

O'Brien. Yes, I would.

Noble. Could you give us an idea of the mechanical performance of a heart set up like this?

O'Brien. Heart rate and oxygen consumption are constant at a particular oxygen tension.

Carlson. Does your perfusion medium contain fatty acids?

O'Brien. It does not.

Carlson. Two points of interest are the decrease in glucose uptake without insulin and the increased glucose uptake in the presence of hypoxia plus insulin. With regard to the first point, have you measured if there is release of insulin from your preparation, and could the decrease in glucose uptake be due to a decrease in the insulin content of the receptor, or would you rather think that it could be related to the rate of utilization of endogenous substrates?

O'Brien. The permeability of the perfused rat heart to non-metabolized sugars falls progressively over the period during which glucose uptake is falling. The basal level of permeability is achieved immediately in hearts from animals treated with anti-insulin serum. Both effects can be explained in terms of elution or destruction of insulin without involving endogenous substrates.

Carlson. Could the increased permeability for glucose during hypoxia be explained by an increase in binding of insulin under these conditions? Could the oxygen content influence the amount of insulin bound to membranes?

O'Brien. I do not think so, because hypoxia considerably increases glucose uptake by the insulin-free heart.

Randle. It is unlikely that the effects of anoxia are due to insulin because they are as marked in the heart from the alloxan diabetic animal as they are in the normal animal. We suggested a number of years ago that the effects of anoxia on glucose transport are due to alterations in adenine nucleotide concentrations. With regard to the maintenance of oxygen consumption with insulin and glucose, could this be due to the maintenance of adenine nucleotides? Dr Morgan and I, when we were studying the regulation of glycogen breakdown on the heart, found that in perfusions without external glucose there was a steady decline in the total adenine–nucleotide concentration in the tissue. I wonder whether insulin and glucose would tend to maintain the total adenine-nucleotide concentration. Have you done any measurements of ATP, ADP and AMP?

O'Brien. I have not measured adenine-nucleotide levels. But since oxygen consumption is stable whether or not insulin is present, it may be that glucose alone can maintain their levels.

Opie. It appears that for a given oxygen tension, in the presence of insulin, there is a higher uptake by the heart of oxygen and glucose. Does this mean that the contribution of glucose as fuel is really unchanged? Could insulin simply directly affect the oxygen uptake through unknown mechanisms?

O'Brien. My results do not show an increase by insulin of oxygen uptake by the aerobic heart and the maintenance of oxygen uptake by insulin at lower oxygen tensions requires the presence of glucose. So I do not think insulin directly stimulates oxygen uptake.

Opie. Supposing your mechanical work is the same with or without insulin during hypoxia, the oxygen uptake has increased relative to the mechanical work. This sort of data gave rise to the concept that fatty acids might be ‘ toxic ’ or ‘ bad ’ to the oxygen limited heart. Are we perhaps in a situation where we have to argue that insulin is bad for the oxygen-limited heart?

Randle. Is the work really the same, Dr O'Brien? This seems to me an absolutely crucial factor affecting the oxygen consumption of the heart. You have difference in oxygen consumption of four- or fivefold. How much glucagon was there in your insulin preparations? Glucagon is known to stimulate cardiac contraction.

O'Brien. I have used both soluble and crystalline insulin and obtained the same effects, but I do not know their relative glucagon content.

Vergroesen. Using a comparable kind of recirculating perfusion apparatus we made some observations which may complicate the issue even more. We measured the increase in prostaglandin (PG) concentration in the perfusion fluid due to endogenous PG biosynthesis in myocardial tissue. Even without the presence of precursors of fatty acids, such as arachidonic acid, quite appreciable amounts of PG are synthesized during the period of recirculation. Willebrands and Tasseron (*American Journal of Physiology* **215,** 1089-1095, 1968) studied the interaction between insulin and PG on glucose and fatty acid metabolism in the heart. They demonstrated a clear influence of PG under some conditions resulting in a preference of the heart to metabolize fatty acids instead of glucose. Do you have any idea to what extent increasing PG concentration in the perfusion fluid can have influenced your result?

O'Brien. In my system of perfusion, any substance produced by the heart at a constant rate will reach a constant concentration in the perfusate. If this is true of prostaglandin formation, any effect of prostaglandins would also be constant after the initial period of perfusion.

Burges. I have been doing a considerable amount of work in this area with a somewhat less sophisticated perfusion apparatus. There are several points I would like to make. The first is that the mechanical performance of the heart is of critical importance as has been mentioned. Some preliminary experiments using fasted hearts suggest that insulin does cause a positive inotropic effect in a Langendorff perfused heart. This could explain a considerable amount of this increased oxygen consumption. The second point is the nutritional state of the hearts and the problem of fatty acid utilization. Using fasted hearts, one finds that a fairly lengthy preperfusion of insulin leads to a fairly steady rise in glucose utilization rate which suggests that the heart is switching from utilization of endogenous lipids to utilization of glucose.

Fisher. Several speakers have referred to increases in oxygen consumption produced by insulin in this system but we are not talking about increases in oxygen uptake but about failure of oxygen uptake to fall when the oxygen tension is reduced.

Henderson. Previous work has shown that insulin enhances mechanical performance in the perfused rat heart when this is oxygen-limited, and I imagine that this was likely to have been so in the present experiments. I am intrigued that insulin apparently increases oxygen extraction under these circumstances. I wonder whether its effect is due solely to increasing glycolytic energy supply, or whether it might not also influence contractile performance more directly by altering cation exchange across the cell membrane—a sort of coupled effect on excitation—contraction coupling.

Opie. In the Langendorff system, the systolic pressure is fixed by the perfusion pressure. Hence heart rate is the major determinant of oxygen consumption. It should be easy to count the heart rate during insulin addition and see whether there is a fourfold difference to account for the difference in oxygen uptake. If the heart rate is the same, then uncoupling of metabolism must be considered to explain the insulin effect.

Randle. We have developed a method for measuring glycolytic rate in a drip-through perfusion system which obviates the difficulties Dr O'Brien has been talking about. We use glucose labelled with tritium in the 5 position and measure the production of tritiated water in the perfusate on a minute-to-minute basis. One has to measure the specific activity of the hexose monophosphates in the heart because it is not necessarily the same as that of the glucose in the medium.

METHODS OF INDUCING MYOCARDIAL ISCHAEMIA

M. F. Oliver

Introduction

No existing model adequately reproduces the metabolic and electrophysiological changes which occur in human myocardial ischaemia. This is not surprising if one considers the complexity of the condition with which we are confronted.

Coronary atherosclerosis is a slowly occlusive process which progresses over many years with sudden crises resulting in abrupt interference with blood flow. This process includes the formation of platelet-fibrin thrombi with release of such substances as adenosine diphosphate, histamine and serotonin; the deposition of cholesterol in the subintimal region; extensive changes in collagen structure with endothelial thickening; and variable degrees of hypoxia of the arterial wall. The extent of arterial narrowing has also to be taken into account because this, together with the speed of the occlusive process, has a considerable influence in determining the formation of coronary collateral vessels. Techniques in which the coronary artery is acutely ligated or constricted, or occluded from within, cannot be expected to reproduce many of these conditions.

The majority of patients with symptoms of ischaemic heart disease have more than one coronary artery with atherosclerotic narrowing. Yet it is rare for models of myocardial ischaemia to incorporate methods of reducing flow in more than one artery.

The state of the recipient myocardium is critical in determining its response to occluded flow. In most experimental situations it is healthy. But the human myocardium is exposed transiently over a number of years to episodes of reduced flow and oxygenation, and develops variable degrees of patchy fibrosis and local metabolic changes such as triglyceride infiltration, local loss of catecholamines and, perhaps, of cations, and impaired contractility.

Myocardial ischaemia

The development of ischaemia in the myocardium results from any serious disturbance of the equilibrium between oxygen demand and oxygen supply.

Oxygen demand is determined by the heart rate, the contractile state of the myocardium and left ventricular wall tension, which in its turn is determined by left ventricular pressure and volume. In most experimental models, these indices are normal before occlusion of coronary flow but they are probably not so in man.

Oxygen supply is determined by the extent of arterial oxygen extraction and by coronary blood flow; this is dependent on the balance between aortic diastolic filling pressure and coronary vascular resistance. Induced hypoxia does not mimic myocardial ischaemia since the consequences of reduced flow are not taken into account. This can lead to a reduction of energy substrates and reduced removal of metabolites. There are important regional differences in myocardial flow and, for example, when there is myocardial ischaemia, flow to the subendocardial regions is reduced to a greater extent than in the subepicardial regions. Experimental conditions for inducing myocardial ischaemia seldom produce selective alteration in regional flow or provide for alterations in coronary vascular resistance in parts of the coronary circulation not directly affected by experimental procedure.

Myocardial ischaemia should not be thought of as a static situation. There are many influences which determine myocardial function in the ischaemic and infarcting muscle. After ischaemia develops, myocardial perfusion will be influenced, for example, by the balance between collateral flow and wall tension, the spread of thrombus formation into vessels not directly occluded, and the release of vasoactive compounds, such as adenosine and potassium ions, etc. Such interactions cannot be reproduced in anv controlled way in the experimental situation of coronary artery ligation or constriction.

Methods of producing myocardial ischaemia

Most experience has been derived from methods of producing myocardial infarction. These can be classified into those which lead to abrupt occlusion of a coronary artery and those which aim at gradual obstruction, and can be further classified into open chest, closed chest, and open followed by closed chest induction of ischaemia (Table 2, 1).

Ligation of a coronary artery will produce a different type of occlusion from that resulting from electrolysis. The former is likely to be quicker and the latter associated with the release of various factors which potentiate and antagonize intravascular coagulation. The use of a balloon catheter[1 2] for closed chest occlusion of a coronary artery is in our experience reasonably reliable but the

Table 2, 1. *Methods commonly used for inducing experimental myocardial ischaemia*

Open chest:	Ligation Electrical
Closed chest: Acute	— balloon catheter — electrolysis — radioopaque spheres — microsphere embolization — metallic mercury
Subacute	— helical wire — steel cylinders
Chronic	— induced atheroma
Open and closed chest:	Ameroid constrictors Balloon-cuffs Hydraulic constrictors

balloon may deflate and the position in which the balloon is placed, even under image intensification, is not always the same and depends to some extent upon the anatomy of the coronary arteries of the individual preparation. Electrolysis[3] from a catheter will, as stated above, produce intravascular thrombosis and this may not be very quick and certainly leads to extensive intimal damage. The introduction of radioopaque spheres[4] through a catheter placed in one or other coronary arteries has the disadvantage that no control can be obtained over these spheres once introduced. The use of plastic microspheres,[5] graded according to the size of the infarct required, is another method of inducing infarction but is more commonly used for studying myocardial flow (labelled with ^{131}I) or with the induction of cardiogenic shock. Metallic mercury also leads to cardiogenic shock.[6]

The speed with which acute occlusion is introduced may determine survival. In dogs, for example, ventricular fibrillation following abrupt occlusion of a coronary artery occurs either during a brief first phase of ectopic excitation lasting up to about 15 minutes or during a delayed third phase from about 5 to 7 hours to 4 days:[7] the intervening second phase of 15 min to 5 to 7 hours is relatively quiet. During the first phase local release of intracellular potassium and sympathetic nerve stimulation are important, while third phase arrhythmias are more products of the degenerating myocardium.

The introduction of a helical wire[8] from the end of a catheter can lead to slowly progressive thrombus formation and gradual occlusion of a coronary artery over many hours and the majority of dogs so treated survive several weeks. The release of steel cylinders[9] from a catheter has the same result.

Coronary atheroma can be produced in cebus monkeys[10] by feeding a high cholesterol, high saturated fat diet, and in dogs[11] by also suppressing thyroid activity; these systems take many months to become effective and are expensive and time-consuming. Furthermore, the lesions which result in the majority of species are not comparable to those obtained in man. Spontaneous atheroma, myocardial ischaemia and infarction occur in mini-pigs[12] and this species might prove a suitable model.

The use of an open chest preparation for the introduction of various systems which can be used later for occlusion of the coronary arteries may provide a more comparable model for myocardial ischaemia than any of those hitherto discussed. Of course, the very fact that an operation has to be done will lead to haemodynamic and metabolic changes which will not occur with closed chest preparations, but in a number of weeks after recovery from surgery a relatively stable situation is present. There are various methods that have been used for late occlusion of coronary arteries and those particularly favoured include Ameroid constrictors[13] placed round the coronary arteries; these constrictors act as a consequence of their hygroscopic nature, progressively swell and gradually occlude the coronary arteries. Balloon cuffs,[14] an adjustable hydraulic constrictor and loose ligatures have been used. The use of the adjustable hydraulic constrictor in association with pneumatic cuffs and electromagnetic flowmeters allows repeated and temporary occlusion of coronary arteries for a number of weeks,[15] and the measurement of the rate of appearance and regression of coronary collaterals and the effects of drugs on them. The subject of collateral circulation has recently been reviewed in detail.[16]

Advantages of different methods

The main advantages of the open-chest approach is that it becomes possible to occlude a coronary artery, either by ligation or some other method, at a precise and carefully chosen site and subsequently it is possible by the use of an ECG and surface electrode mapping to identify the area of ischaemia. Microelectrode probes can be introduced to the exposed myocardium to study electrophysiological changes related to the induced myocardial ischaemia. Blood can be sampled from local surface veins in the hope of giving more accurate information about metabolic changes from the area of ischaemia: this may be particularly valuable when ischaemia rather than infarction is studied. A number of reports have been made of changes which take place in the venous blood returning from infarcted areas but it is often difficult to know exactly from where this blood originates, particularly if a negative pressure is needed to obtain it. A further advantage of the open-chest approach is that biopsies can be obtained from the exposed myocardium.

The closed chest preparation also has a number of very considerable advantages. Minimal trauma is necessary to induce myocardial ischaemia or infarction and the very considerable haemodynamic changes which take place during thoracotomy are therefore avoided. Additionally, the metabolic consequences of tissue damage are minimized. Since the chest preparation is closed, epicardectomy will not be undertaken. The effect of epicardectomy is similar to that of stellate ganglionectomy or β-adrenergic blockade and induces an effective sympathectomy,[17 18] presumably rendering the myocardium less sensitive to external stimuli. No ligation of or interference with the small sympathetic nerves running along the arteries occurs and it is likely that the local concentration of catecholamines in the ischaemic myocardium will be different from that occurring when these small nerves have been interrupted.

The advantage of delaying induction of ischaemia several weeks after operation are obvious in that it is possible to do this in a conscious animal and in a situation where time has been allowed to pass for the development of collateral vessels.'[15]

Standardization of models of inducing ischaemia

When metabolic or electrophysiological studies are to be undertaken, it is important to consider a number of factors which could influence the measurements made. These include the species under study: thus dogs differ from primates in the ease with which arrhythmias can be induced. The breed may also be important since beagles, for example, appear to be appreciably less sensitive to the induction of ischaemia than mongrels: in our experience, greyhounds are particularly likely to develop arrhythmias and they have a larger and heavier heart per kg body weight than other dogs. The nutritional status of the animal must be taken into account: if derived from a random source, this is likely to be very variable and quite different from that obtained when animals are reared and prepared in special colonies. For metabolic studies, it is probably crucial that animals are on a controlled and stable metabolic regime before the procedures are undertaken. The sex of the animal may be important and it is better in metabolic studies to study one sex, preferably males. Again, an aging animal may present a number of different problems from a young and immature one.

Premedication and anaesthesia may be of critical importance and has not received enough attention. The induction of anaesthesia can often be traumatic to the animal. Premedication is an obvious way to overcome this but the choice and dose of drugs for premedication must be carefully considered. Similarly, the choice of anaesthetic agent is important. Inhalation anaesthetics have a number of different metabolic effects, such as catecholamine stimulation, compared with intravenous anaesthesia. Variation in the depth of anaesthesia is crucial if, for example, an attempt is being made to obtain a steady state for turnover studies or assessment of arrhythmias. Some indices are very sensitive to changes in the level of anaesthesia and it may be necessary to monitor the depth of anaesthesia for their interpretation. Again, the duration of anaesthesia may be important. Adequate ventilation with maintenance of arterial oxygen saturation can be crucial: monitoring of $P\text{O}_2$, $P\text{CO}_2$ and pH is necessary. The type of infusion which is used to maintain arterial and venous lines has to be taken into account since glucose or fructose infusions could alter some metabolic indices. Again, the use of anticoagulants must be considered and it should not be forgotten that heparin has a potent effect in inducing plasma lipolysis.

Finally, a greater effort should be made by investigators to declare in detail the nature of their experiments. Without consideration of these details, comparison of the results of experiments is often difficult. In Table 2, 2 an outline has been given of some of the information and measurements which should be included in each report.

Table 2, 2. *Data to be declared with all reports of induced myocardial ischaemia*

Species and breed	— random source
Nutrition	— colony reared
Sex	
Age	
Premedication	
Anaesthesia	— type and dose
	— adequacy of maintenance
	— duration
Method of occlusion	
Arteries occluded	
Site and size of ischaemia or infarction	
Ventilation	— arterial Po_2 and Pco_2
	— pH
Heart rate	
Blood pressure	
Incidence and time of occurrence of ventricular fibrillation	
Infusions	
Anticoagulants	

Summary

There is no experimental system of inducing myocardial ischaemia which mimics the situation in man, where there is extensive coronary atheroma and variable degrees of myocardial impairment. The commonly used methods for inducing myocardial ischaemia are described and criticized. Their advantages and disadvantages are considered. The choice of preparation should depend upon the purpose of the experiment. The lack of comparability of one preparation with another should be recognized. This will be reduced if the details of every procedure are declared in full: certain minimal standards for the reporting of results are suggested.

REFERENCES

1 Kurien, V. A., Yates, P. A. & Oliver, M. F. (1971). The role of free fatty acids in the production of ventricular arrhythmias after coronary artery occlusion. *European Journal of Clinical Investigation* **1,** 225-241.

2 Corday, E., Lang, T. W., Crexells, C. & Meerbaum, S. (1972). Intracoronary Balloon—A new model for induction of myocardial ischemia. *American Journal of Cardiology* **29,** 301.

3 SALAZAR, A. E. (1961). Experimental myocardial infarction. Induction of coronary thrombosis in the intact closed-chest dog. *Circulation Research* **9,** 1351-1356.
4 GENSINI, G. G., PALACIO, A., BUONANNO, C., KELLY, A. E. & MULLER, W. F. (1966). Superselective coronary occlusion under cinefluorographic control in experimental animals: technique and results (P). *Circulation* **34,** 108-109.
5 AGRESS, C. M., ROSENBERG, M. J., JACOBS, H. I., BINDER, M. J., SCHNEIDERMAN, A. & CLARK, W. G. (1952). Protracted shock in closed-chest dog following coronary embolization with graded microspheres. *American Journal of Physiology* **170,** 536-549.
6 LUNCH, S., MOGUILEVSKY, H. C., PIETRA, G., SHAFFER, A. B., HIRSCH, L. J. & FISHMAN, A. P. (1969). A reproducible model of cardiogenic shock in the dog. *Circulation* **39,** 205-218.
7 HARRIS, A. S. (1966). In *Mechanisms and Therapy of Cardiac Arrhythmias,* p. 239. Edited by L. S. Dreifus, W. Likoff & J. H. Moyer. New York and London: Grune & Stratton.
8 KORDENAT, R. K., KEZDI, P. & STANLEY, E. L. (1972). A new catheter technique for producing experimental coronary thrombosis and selective coronary visualization. *American Heart Journal* **83,** 360-364.
9 NAKHJAVAN, F. K., SHEDROVILZKY, H. & GOLDERG, H. (1968). Experimental myocardial infarction in dogs. *Circulation* **38,** 777-782.
10 WISSLER, R. W., FRAZIER, L. E., HUGHES, R. H. & RASMUSSEN, R. A. (1963). Atherogenesis in the monkey. *Nutrition Reviews* **21,** 150-152.
11 STEINER, A. & KENDALL, F. E. (1946). Atherosclerosis and arteriosclerosis in dogs following ingestion of cholesterol and thiouracil. *Archives of Pathology* **42,** 433-444.
12 ZUIGBE, F. T. (1965). In *Comparative Atherosclerosis,* p. 37. Edited by J. C. Roberts and R. Strauss. New York: Harper and Row.
13 LITVAK, H. A., SIDERIDES, L. E. & VINEBERG, A. M. (1957). The experimental production of coronary artery insufficiency and occlusion. *American Heart Journal* **53,** 505-518.
14 HOOD, W. B., JOUSON, J., KUMAR, R., KATAYAMA, I., NEIMAN, R. S. & NORMAN, J. C. (1970). Experimental myocardial infarction. I Production of left ventricular failure by gradual coronary occlusion in intact conscious dogs. *Cardiovascular Research* **4,** 73-83.
15 ELIOT, E. C., BLOOR, C. M., JONES, E. L., MITCHELL, W. B. & GREGG, D. E. (1971). Effect of controlled coronary occlusion on collateral circulation in conscious dogs. *American Journal of Physiology* **220,** 857-861.
16 SCHAPER, W. (1971). *The collateral circulation of the heart.* North-Holland Publishing Co.
17 KAYE, M. P. & RANDALL, W. C. (1970). Mechanism of decreased myocardial contractile force after epicardiectomy. *Cardiovascular Research* **5,** 154-159.
18 GEIS, W. P. & KAYE, M. P. (1972). In *Proceedings of National Conference on Research Animals in Medicine,* p. 52. Washington.

THE BABOON AS AN EXPERIMENTAL ANIMAL FOR THE PRODUCTION OF MYOCARDIAL INFARCTION: COMPARISON WITH THE MONGREL DOG

K. BRUYNEEL and L. H. OPIE

SIGNIFICANT differences exist between the baboon and the dog when used as an experimental animal for the production of coronary artery occlusion and acute myocardial infarction. The following comparative study is based on the study of about 70 baboons (*Papio ursinus,* the Cape Chacma baboon,[1]) and 60 mongrel dogs.

Anatomical differences

1. In dogs and baboons with matched body weight and sex, the ratio between the body weight and the total wet heart weight is about 25 per cent lower in the dog, indicating a relative cardiac hypertrophy in the dog. In the baboon the ratio of body weight/heart weight is close to man.[1] This hypertrophy of the dog heart is not limited to any specific part of the heart but there is proportional hypertrophy of the free wall of both ventricles, the ventricular septum, the atria, the atrial appendices, a segment of the pulmonary artery and of the aorta.

2. In the dog the left coronary artery almost always is the dominant artery and the circumflex artery is the major branch. The left coronary orifice is twice the size of the right coronary orifice and the free wall of the left ventricle is supplied by three to five (or more) diagonal branches of the anterior descending coronary artery, and descending branches of the circumflex artery. In the baboon, the left and right coronary artery provide a more balanced system with equal orifice sites. The anterior descending artery is the major branch of the left coronary artery and there is usually only one diagonal branch present as the ‘ third primary ’ coronary artery.[2]

3. In the baboon the major coronary vein draining the left ventricle does not run parallel to the whole length of the anterior descending coronary artery. Very often the areas supplied by the proximal and the distal halves of the anterior descending coronary artery have different venous drainages. The draining of the proximal area is by a vein running parallel to the anterior descending coronary artery in the great cardiac vein. The draining of the distal area is by a vein running diagonally from the apex directly towards the proximal part of the coronary sinus. In the dog each coronary and major branch artery is usually accompanied by two venae comitantes draining similar areas on either side of the artery.

4. The sympathetic and parasympathetic heart innervation of the baboon heart appears to resemble man in some respects and the dog in others.[3]

5. The bundle of His and the AV node are anatomically and physiologically closer to man in the baboon than in the dog.[4,5] The reaction to trauma to the conduction tissue in the baboon is also closer to man.

Differences relevant to experimental myocardial infarction

1. In the open-chest animal, ventricular arrhythmias developing in the first hour after coronary artery ligation, consistently progress to ventricular fibrillation in the baboon but seldom do so in the dog. In animals even farther removed from man such as the rabbit and rat, ventricular fibrillation is extremely rare even after major coronary artery ligation.

2. A lower heart rate (80 to 100 beats/min) can readily be achieved in the open-chest baboon in spite of the use of pentobarbitone. This could probably be due to the different response to premedication. The baboon responds readily to a tranquilizing drug, Sernylan (phencyclidine) and then requires only a very low dose of pentobarbitone. Even with the additional use of morphine in the dog, it is not usual to achieve slow heart rates in the dog when pentobarbitone is used.

3. In the dog a slow heart rate (when achieved) may hinder the development of myocardial infarction. This may be why pentobarbitone is a standard anaesthetic agent when myocardial infarction must be produced in the dog.

4. The blood pressure in the anaesthetized baboon is in the normal human range, whereas the dog anaesthetized with pentobarbitone is hypertensive.

5. The speed of maximal development of epicardial ST-segment elevation over the infarcting myocardium is more rapid in the baboon.

6. The infarcting area is bluer and more sharply defined in the baboon.

7. Ligation of only one coronary artery produces a uniform infarcting area in the baboon, even if a small vessel is chosen. To obtain the same size and severity of infarction in the dog, ligation of two or three coronary arteries is usually necessary unless a major artery such as the circumflex or the main anterior descending is ligated. Occasionally even ligation of the main anterior descending

artery in the mongrel dog is not followed by a clearly visible infarcting area.

8. The distal part of the ligated artery in the baboon remains empty after ligation while it is filled by retrograde flow in the dog. It seems that the collateral coronary blood flow in the infarcting myocardium is better developed in the dog than in the baboon. Schaper *et al.*[6] could demonstrate that experimental infarcts in dogs were always smaller than the perfusion area of the occluded coronary artery. Meesmann *et al.*[7] showed that the occurrence of ventricular fibrillation in dogs following ligation of a large coronary artery (anterior descending or circumflex) was dependent on the degree of collateral circulation. When well-developed, the collateral circulation in the dog prevented ventricular fibrillation in almost all the cases.

9. Infarcts of about 10 per cent of the total heart weight in baboons usually show a marked systolic ventricular bulging which is rarely seen in mongrel dogs with the same size of infarct (possibly because of the relative hypertrophy in the dog).

10. The critical size of infarct required to produce primary ventricular fibrillation can readily be defined in baboons. When the size of infarct is more than 14 per cent of the total heart weight, there is always ventricular fibrillation. Dogs frequently survive similar sized infarcts but the critical size of infarction is more difficult to measure since the infarcting area is not so clearly defined.

Electrophysiologic differences

When the beating dog heart with or without infarction is rapidly removed from the body, a mechanical or electrical stimulus can excite the endocardium or epicardium of the ventricles and atria to contract for about 15 to 20 min and 5 to 10 min respectively. No such phenomenon is found in the baboon after 3 to 4 min. It appears that the dog maintains an excitation–contraction reaction to mechanical stimuli for a longer period of ischaemia suggesting that the dog heart is better adapted to hypoxia.

Blood biochemistry

1. There is a significant difference in the plasma arterial K^+. In 37 mongrel dogs the initial arterial plasma K^+ was $4{\cdot}4 \pm 0{\cdot}1$ (SEM) mEq/litre in both females and in males. In the baboon the

initial arterial plasma K^+ was $4{\cdot}2 \pm 0{\cdot}2$ mEq/litre for 10 females and $3{\cdot}8 \pm 0{\cdot}1$ mEq/litre for 52 males.

2. The haemoglobin was about 14 g/100 ml in baboons and in healthy dogs but a large proportion of mongrel dogs showed a haemoglobin of 12 g/100 ml or less. Dogs appear to be more prone to intestinal parasites with consequent blood loss. Probably the diet of mongrel dogs is also inadequate.

3. The plasma calcium was 10 mg/100 ml in dogs and about 8·5 mg/100 ml in baboons, even though the plasma albumin was about 3 g/100 ml in baboons and 1·5 g/100 ml in dogs.

4. The initial arterial plasma free fatty acid concentrations in these anaesthetized animals were similar. The blood cholesterol was significantly lower in the baboon (dog: 198 ± 40, $n=12$; baboon $148 \pm 7{\cdot}5$, $n=28$; values in mg/100 ml; means $\pm$SD; $p<0{\cdot}025$); this difference may reflect dietary habits as baboons are normally vegetarian.

5. Plasma total protein, inorganic phosphate and fasting blood glucose were identical in baboons and dogs.

Closed-chest preparations

When a closed-chest preparation is desired then the dog offers definite advantages. The dog is spontaneously able to withstand apparently severe ventricular arrhythmias for hours and days after myocardial infarction. During the recovery process the dog is suitable for study in the awake unrestrained, unsedated state. With care, ventricular function studies can be performed in the slightly sedated dog. In contrast, it is very difficult to study the wild baboon without heavy sedation.

Conclusions

The baboon heart has the advantage of being closer to man. As a model of myocardial infarction, coronary artery ligation in the baboon consistently produces a severe infarction with a marked tendency to ventricular fibrillation. The mongrel dog model produces a less fatal infarction with many more arrhythmias and less tendency to spontaneous ventricular fibrillation.

ACKNOWLEDGMENTS

We thank the Chris Barnard Fund and also the Ethical Drug Association Foundation for financial support.

REFERENCES

1 Hill, W. C. O. (1965). In *The Baboon in Medical Research,* Vol. II p. 3. Edited by H. Vagtborg. Austin: University Texas Press.

2 Brink, A. J., Lewis, C. M., Bosman, A. R., Lochner, A. (1970). The baboon (*Papio ursinus*) heart (coronary blood supply, muscle function and metabolism). *Folia Primat* **13,** 11-22.

3 Randall, W. C., Armour, J. A., Randall, D. C. & Smith, O. A. (1971). Functional anatomy of the cardiac nerves in the baboon. *Anatomical Record* **170,** 183-198.

4 Pruitt, R. D., Watt, T. B. & Murao, S. (1965). Left axis deviation: its relation to experimentally induced lesion of the anterior left bundle branch system in canine and primate heart. *Annals of the New York Academy of Science* **127,** 204-223.

5 Truex, R. C. & Smythe, M. Q. (1965). Comparative morphology of the cardiac conduction tissue in animals. *Annals New York Academy Science* **127,** 19-33.

6 Schaper, W., Remeysen, P. & Xhonneux, R. (1969). The size of myocardial coronary artery ligation. *Zeitschrift für Kreislaufforschung* **58,** 904-909.

7 Meesmann, W., Schuls, F. W., Schley, G. & Adolphsen, P. (1970). Das Elektrokardiogram nach akuten experimentellen Koronar verschluss in Abhängigket von Spontakollateralen des Herzens. *Zeitschrift für Gesamte Experimentälen Medizines* **153,** 246-261.

Discussion

Han. We produce advanced coronary atherosclerosis in minipigs by feeding a high fat and high cholesterol diet. We found that production of myxoedema is not necessary when this diet is associated with praecordial irradiation. These pigs develop clinical and anatomical features similar to human coronary artery disease at 6 to 8 months from starting the diet. They develop ventricular arrhythmia and AV block and die suddenly of ventricular fibrillation in most cases. This appears to be a good model for the study of myocardial infarction.

Oliver. Irradiation not only produces quite extensive endothelial damage but also myocardial damage. Is there any enzyme loss from the myocardium in your preparation? Induced myxoedema is only necessary for atheroma production in the dog.

Han. Praecordial irradiation alone will not produce the features of myocardial infarction.

Carlson. A factor which might be important in metabolic studies in animals is the medical condition of the animal. I am thinking in particular of conditions such as clinically obvious diabetes and also glucose intolerance and obesity. There certainly are many other medical conditions we should consider in our experimental dogs.

Parratt. Dr Oliver mentioned that it is important to measure flow and metabolic changes in the ischaemic region. I think at the same time it is important to know what is happening in the so-called normal areas.

Jennings. I would like to re-emphasize some of the comments of Dr Oliver relative to the fact that we are really dealing with a multifactorial system whenever we do an experiment on acute ischaemia in either the open or closed-chest dog. Thus it is very important to frame precisely the question that you are attempting to answer and then use the model best suited to this purpose. Also, the limitations of the model employed should be kept in mind. A few examples will suffice. If one wishes to study the incidence of arrhythmias following occlusion in animals that are awake, then one must use a closed-chest preparation. If one is interested in keeping nerves intact, the artery should be occluded internally with, for example, the balloon catheter, because this spares the nerves on the surface of the vessel and on the epicardium. If, on the other hand, one wishes to perform direct studies of tissue metabolism *in vivo,* the open-chest dog is required. Here, sampling becomes a problem for not all parts of the heart are equally ischaemic. Consequently the sampling site must be chosen as a function of what kind of injury one wishes to study, severe ischaemia or mild ischaemia. I think that more precision in posing questions in this field will lead to much better experimentation.

Thomas. We don't know the mechanism of myocardial infarction in man nor indeed the pertinent mechanism during ischaemia and on that account it is rather difficult to design the analogous experiment. Even the apparently obvious difference between ischaemia and infarction may not be quite so clear. The most extreme experimental insult—tying a coronary artery—does not provide a distinct discrimination between infarction and ischaemia. Becker, Ferreira and I (*Cardiovasc. Res.*—in press) have studied the regional flow in the area of cyanosis following acute coronary ligation, and in the periphery of the cyanotic area the flow might be as high as 60 or 80 per cent of the control value so making the difference between infarction and ischaemia indistinct. This has very important implications in applying the principles developed from such techniques.

Kurien. A recent report shows that of those who die suddenly only 10 per cent have occlusion in a coronary artery. If they are dying without coronary artery occlusion, the model for study of sudden death and acute myocardial ischaemia may have to be changed. In fact patients are probably dying without infarction and from ischaemia.

Oliver. I think it is now clearly established that ventricular fibrillation occurs in patients who do not have infarction. There are a number of people now whose hearts have been successfully defibrillated and who have a normal ECG. It is not necessary to have infarction to die suddenly. This question of the extent of occlusion in relation to sudden death has been discussed for 15 or more years, and for those who say that there is no occlusion there is an equal number who say that this depends entirely on the precision with which you look for it.

MODELS FOR ELECTROPHYSIOLOGICAL STUDIES OF ISCHAEMIA

A. G. WALLACE

LIKE research in most areas of biology which relate to human disease, research in acute myocardial ischaemia would be facilitated by an animal preparation or model which satisfactorily simulates the human condition. I must hesitate at the outset of my remarks to indicate that while a number of animal preparations for the study of myocardial ischaemia and infarction do exist—probably none really simulates the condition in man very well. Much of what I will say is based upon experiments in animals in which one previously normal artery to the heart was occluded with an otherwise normal coronary circulation. Our colleagues in pathology tell us, however, that when a patient dies suddenly or as a consequence of a primary arrhythmia after recognized infarction, that the usual finding at *post mortem* examination is chronic diffuse obstructive disease of one or more coronary arteries without evidence of an acute obstruction which would correlate temporally with the clinical event. In addition we have little or no evidence that animals, and certainly anaesthetized animals, experience the intense pain or anxiety which patients suffer frequently with acute infarction. These experiences by the patient may and do indeed seem to contribute importantly to the initial clinical picture of infarction and very probably to certain of the earlier disturbances of cardiac rhythm. Finally, a great deal of work in the field of myocardial ischaemia has actually been based on studies of perfused hearts in which the oxygen content of the perfusate has been reduced (i.e. hypoxia) rather than reduced perfusion *per se*. There are good reasons to suspect that the consequences of hypoxic perfusion may differ importantly from a localized interruption of perfusion. In short, it is my judgement that considerable room must still be allowed for the possibility that events unique to diseased tissue and not yet adequately simulated by any animal model may influence the outcome of patients with ischaemic heart disease. These reservations are an expression of a general concern I have for the difficulty of simulating in animals a condition which mimics chronic disease in man.

All of us would agree, however, that at least two critical elements of any good experimental preparation are that the event to be studied should be predictable and that the preparation should permit instrumentation which allows valid measurements which give insight into the phenomenon being studied. It is against these two criteria of any good experiment that I would like to evaluate certain of the models which are representative of those used to study arrhythmias after experimental coronary occlusion and myocardial ischaemia.

Prior to 1950 most experiments dealing with acute myocardial infarction were performed in anaesthetized open chested animals and infarction was produced by acute ligation of a single coronary artery. When one of the coronary arteries was ligated at a proximal site ventricular fibrillation occurred in a majority of animals in 15 to 20 min. Ventricular fibrillation or sudden acute left ventricular failure produced a high mortality and this preparation was not very suitable for study. In 1950 Harris developed a preparation for the study of cardiac arrhythmias.[1] He was particularly interested in a preparation which had multiple ventricular extrasystoles and in which these occurred and persisted for 48 to 72 hours after coronary ligation. He developed a preparation which is still used widely today and is based on a two stage occlusion of a proximal coronary artery. The anterior descending coronary was identified and freed distal to the first septal perforating artery. Two ligatures were placed around the artery. With a 20 gauge needle lying adjacent to the coronary artery, the first ligature was tied and then the needle was removed. This produced a partial stenosis of the anterior descending. Thirty minutes later the second ligature was tied thus producing total obstruction. When the ligature was placed 2 to 3 cm distal to the origin of the left main coronary artery there was a relatively low acute mortality rate of approximately 20 per cent, and 80 per cent of the animals had multiple ventricular ectopic beats for a matter of hours. This preparation has been used widely to evaluate the effects of pharmacologic agents. It has been used by Harris and others to estimate potassium flux from ischaemic myocardium, to evaluate the catecholamine release from ischaemic myocardium and the protective influence of glucose, potassium and insulin solutions. It is still perhaps one of the best models for predictability of ventricular ectopic activity. One of the disadvantages of this preparation is that other types of arrhythmias seldom occur and it also has the obvious disadvantage that most interventions have to be evaluated either during or immediately after the operative intervention.

In 1960 Dr Vineberg and his colleagues adopted the principle of gradual occlusion of the coronary artery using Ameroid constrictors.[2] These constrictors are made of a metal sheath which contains casein. A small slit in the ameroid allows the instrument to be placed around a proximal coronary artery. The casein material had the property of swelling gradually when exposed to biological fluids and as the casein swelled it gradually occluded the coronary artery. This technique has been used extensively in the dog and in the mini-pig.[3] For some studies the mini-pig has advantages over the dog because the gross anatomy of the coronary arteries is more similar to man. The pig has a right dominant coronary artery which supplies the sinus and AV node in a very large percentage of animals. This is in contrast to the dog. When constrictors of appropriate size are selected, total occlusion of the coronary artery can be anticipated between the fourth and seventh day after its implantation in the majority of animals. In the pig continuous monitoring of the electrocardiogram reveals that when constrictors are placed around the anterior descending coronary artery there is approximately an 80 per cent mortality in otherwise untreated animals—most of this is attributable to ventricular ectopic activity leading to ventricular fibrillation. This particular model has been especially useful for the study of prophylactic antiarrhythmic agents and other potentially therapeutic interventions such as hyperbaric O_2;[3] but because the time of infarction is quite variable between the third and seventh day it does not lend itself well to acute electrophysiological studies.

In 1967 Chimoskey and Barger developed a device which is now widely used for a number of studies of coronary artery physiology.[4] A silistic implantable balloon is fixed to a nylon back and this unit is then wrapped around the coronary artery. The balloon cuff is connected to a piece of polyvinyl tubing which can then be brought out of the thorax and inflated at any desired time. Inflation occludes the coronary artery beneath the balloon. This technique has the advantage that more than one cuff can be placed, and the cuffs can be placed in any desired location. A second and major advantage is that the cuff can be inflated at any time after its insertion. A third and particularly important advantage for some studies is that the balloon can be deflated if one wishes to look only at repeated episodes of transient ischaemia. Of all the techniques currently in use this one gives the investigator the greatest degree of flexibility and control in a closed-chest awake preparation. In addition, another virtue of this preparation currently being explored is to occlude a coronary artery gradually several weeks after implanting the cuff, and to then wait 8 to 12 hours until infarction is well developed and arrhythmias are present. The animal can then be anaesthetized and the heart exposed for direct electrophysiological studies, or removed and prepared for other types of analyses—including microelectrode studies. We and others have found this approach useful for creating preparations of ischaemic or infarcted tissue which are then available for types of studies which cannot be performed in the intact animal.

A technique for producing coronary occlusion in the close-chested animal was first proposed in 1961 by Dr Salazar.[5] A catheter is passed fluoroscopically either into the anterior descending or circumflex branches of the left coronary artery or into the right coronary artery. Through this catheter a small teflon coated steel wire is passed. This wire is exposed for the last three millimetres and is positioned in the desired coronary artery. In the early 1950s it was demonstrated that when an artery was injured there was a loss of the normal potential difference which exists between the endothelial surface and the adventitia of the vessel. The endothelium of course is normally electronegative. It was subsequently demonstrated that when prosthetic material was placed in the circulation that the thrombogenicity of the material was related directly to its positive charge. Using these two principles Salazar demonstrated that when a small d.c. current was applied to the coronary artery that thrombosis could readily be induced. Between 100 and 400 μa of d.c. current induces a complete thrombosis of the involved coronary artery. As indicated above, the procedure does not require thoracotomy and indeed chronic catheters can be implanted and thrombosis induced in the awake animal. This technique produces coronary occlusion. The time of occlusion can be controlled and the site of occlusion can be relatively easily controlled. Its primary advantage is that it requires no thoracotomy. It again incorporates the useful principle of gradual occlusion. When the occlusions are suitably placed they lead to a high incidence of chaotic ventricular ectopic rhythms.

Lastly, I think we should at least briefly consider an atherosclerotic model of coronary artery disease. The major problem with all atherosclerotic models is that myocardial infarction is infrequent in its occurrence and even when it does occur it is not predictable in terms of its time of occurrence. Thus, while atherosclerotic models of coronary artery disease are potentially of considerable value in the study of the metabolism of the arterial wall they have not yet proved to be a suitable model for the study of either myocardial infarction or associated arrhythmias. Coronary atherosclerosis was produced by Sabiston and colleagues[6] in the dog by a combination of a high fat diet with either hypothyroidism or proximal aortic coarctation leading to hypertension. These animals readily developed xanthomatous degeneration of the coronary arteries with coronary obstruction and multiple myocardial scars. On the other hand frank infarction and arrhythmias were very unusual in this model. I illustrate it primarily to demonstrate again that the atherosclerotic models are not suitable for electrophysiological studies.

In summary a variety of models have been proposed to produce myocardial infarction for the purpose of electrophysiological studies. Some of these models involve acute studies in animals; some permit the chronic implantation of occlusive devices and some permit coronary occlusion without requiring thoracotomy. For acute studies the Harris model is still perhaps the most useful and for chronic studies the silistic balloon appears to be very desirable. A second consideration involves the type of species to be used. Most studies have been performed in the dog. The mini-pig is more difficult to work with because of its size, but the gross anatomy of their coronary arteries is more similar to man than the dog and the results of occlusion are more predictable. For producing infarction in predicted areas and for producing arrhythmias other than ventricular extra systoles the pig has proven to have some advantages. Atherosclerotic models are not at this time suitable for electrophysiologic study. All the models which I have discussed have a serious limitation in that it is difficult to know exactly where the infarct is to occur and to properly instrument the animal for sophisticated electrophysiologic study. I can summarize by saying that a number of models exist which are suitable for the study of the role of anti-arrhythmic agents in the prophylactic treatment of arrhythmias of specific types. On the other hand, at the present time models in the intact animal which permit sophisticated electrophysiological studies of the mechanisms of arrhythmias leave much to be desired and this certainly represents a fruitful area for future investigation.

REFERENCES

1 HARRIS, A. S. (1950). Delayed development of ventricular ectopic rhythms following experimental coronary occlusion. *Circulation* **1,** 1318-1328.
2 VINEBERG, A. (1960). Experimental gradual coronary artery constriction by ameroid constrictions. *Surgery* **47,** 765-771.
3 PETER, R. H. (1966). Effect of hyperbaric oxygenation on coronary artery occlusion in pigs. *Circulation Research* **18,** 89-96.
4 CHIMOSKEY, J. E. (1967). Temporary coronary occlusion in conscious dogs: collateral flow and electrocardiogram. *American Journal of Physiology* **212,** 1025-1032.
5 SALAZAR. A. E. (1961). Experimental myocardial infarction. Induction of coronary thrombosis in the intact closed-chest dog. *Circulation Research* **9,** 1351-1356.
6 SABISTON, D. C. (1961). Experimental production of canine coronary atherosclerosis. *Annals of Surgery* **153,** 13-22.

DISCUSSION

Durrer. I agree wth Dr Wallace that the human heart is a very complex organ. I think that everybody who wants to translate his findings from experimental animals to the human situation is bound to do something that may be called unscientific. I don't like pigs because they have no human heart. The specific conduction system is much more elaborate in the pig than in the human. In the human it is restricted to the subendocardial layer; in the pig it may even go up to the epicardium. I believe that the conduction system, which plays an important role in the genesis of arrhythmia, is very different from the human. The only animal we have found up to now which looks like the human heart is the dog heart. Have you found differences between pig hearts, human hearts and dog hearts in your studies of arrhythmias after occlusion?

Wallace. Yes, the main difference being that in the dog we have found it extremely difficult with any technique of coronary occlusion to produce arrhythmias which are similar to those which occur with posterior myocardial infarction in man. I know that Dr James (In 'Etiology of myocardial infarction', ed. by T. N. James and J. W. Keyes, Churchill, London, 1963) has worked with perfusions of the artery to the AV node in the dog and has been able to produce disturbances of AV conduction. In the pig there is a predominant right coronary artery, and this supplies both the SA and AV nodes in most animals.

Durrer. We have studied what happens when after half an hour of ischaemia you restore blood flow. We nearly always get ventricular fibrillation. Did you find that, too?

Wallace. We have not done any experiments with the restoration of blood flow. Epstein (*Circulation* (1972) **45,** 1273) has recently done a great deal of work using the dog in which he produced temporary occlusion of the coronary artery. When he opened the circulation, there was a very high incidence of ventricular ectopic beats.

Jennings. We have done many transient occlusions of the circumflex artery in the dog. Ventricular fibrillation occurring shortly after reflow is a common complication in this system. Sommers and I (*Archives of Internal Medicine* 1972, **129,** 780-789) recently reported on the effects of various therapies on this system. Using 20 min temporary occlusions the reflow VF rate was 55 per cent in controls. Oxygen tended to increase the rate and procainamide to reduce it, but neither effect was statistically significant. On the other hand, reserpine significantly reduced the incidence of VF but propranolol had no effect. Another feature of reflow VF is that it appears to be most common after 20 to 25 min of ischaemia and to have lower incidence after shorter periods of ischaemia as well as longer intervals, such as 45 min.

Wallace. We have been working with surgically denervated and pharmacologically denervated hearts by using 6-hydroxydopamine. Both these eradicate ventricular arrhythmias following coronary artery occlusion.

Jennings. Harris showed that there was a very high incidence of ventricular fibrillation when he acutely occluded the artery. I think it was over 75 per cent within 10 or 15 minutes. He then developed the two-stage procedure to reduce the incidence of ventricular fibrillation. In the first stage the degree of occlusion would be around 70 per cent after the needle was removed. After 30 min of partial occlusion he then acutely occluded the artery. Ventricular fibrillation seldom occurred after the second stage occlusion. Why do you think that was?

Wallace. I don't know, but an attractive idea is that collateral flow is developing during that period of partial stenosis.

Thomas. The cross-sectional area of an artery can be reduced to a considerable degree before the flow falls. We don't really know what the flow at this stage is; I know of no one who has used a flowmeter during the two-stage procedure.

Taggart. We have a small amount of data on human myocardial biopsies taken immediately at the end of a period of total coronary artery occlusion during the course of bypass surgery and second or subsequent biopsies, after 2 or 3 min of reflow when the aortic clamp is taken off. During this very short time of 2 to 3 min there is remarkable fall of intracellular potassium and again of intracellular sodium. The only explanation that we have is that during the process of total occlusion the extracellular space is not perfused. Extruded potassium might be expected to remain *in situ*, increasing in concentration in the ECF. Similarly, as sodium proceeds down its concentration gradient into the cell, ECF sodium diminishes. There may be a situation whereby as these chemical gradients increase further no shift is possible until on subsequent reflow the high extracellular potassium and low extracellular sodium are restored to something close to their original values.

Han. The increase in ventricular arrhythmias immediately after the release of coronary occlusion might be due to electrically unstable conditions in the myocardium associated with rapid changes in electrophysiological properties which are expected to occur with the reflow. That is to say that the temporal dispersion of recovery may be increased during any rapid change of refractory period because of change at different segments of the myocardium. Such an increase in non-uniformity of excitability may facilitate ventricular ectopic activity.

Opie. One of the major determinants thought to convert ischaemia to infarction is time. The longer the ischaemia the more often infarction develops in the Harris two-stage model. The question is: when did the ischaemia start—at the first stage or second stage? The 30 min of difference can be quite crucial in assessing whether it is ischaemia or infarction that has occurred.

Wallace. As I tried to indicate, the purpose of Dr Harris's experiments was to produce a preparation with arrhythmias for several days.

One of the things which has been puzzling for me as a physiologist has been the fact that when we look at normal muscle it is rare to find any automatic cells. Normal muscle seems to be characterized by the absence of automatic behaviour. Yet one of the very provocative experiments which I think Carmaliet (*Archive Internationale de Physiologie et de Biochemie* **73,** 171, 1966) did a number of years ago was to show that a left atrial appendage which demonstrated no evidence of spontaneous activity put in a solution for 4 hours that had zero potassium would depolarize. Then, when you restored the potassium it would take on automatic activity. Rapid changes in ion flux may do things to myocardial cells which most of us are not accustomed to seeing in stable preparations.

Jennings. I would like to make one thing clear relative to the difference between permanent and transient ischaemia in acute occlusions. In permanent ischaemia one has a reduction in flow to most of the myocardium supplied by the occluded vessel and a variable but so far unmeasured increase in collateral flow. In general, however, I am sure the flow still is reduced because cyanosis persists. In transient ischaemia, if the period of ischaemia is long enough to induce irreversible injury then an entirely different set of events occurs in the injured cells when the flow is restored. Now, one has cells which have been killed by the ischaemic process and are dying in the presence of restored arterial flow. The affected cells swell tremendously, accumulate incredible amounts of mitochondrial calcium phosphate and develop enormous contraction bands and other striking changes. It is not clear whether the reflow ventricular fibrillation is related to change in the cells which are irreversibly injured or in the surrounding cells. In permanent ischaemia of 60 min or more duration it seems likely that the arrhythmias originate from the reasonably well perfused, but ischaemic epicardial area.

Oliver. What is known about the speed of release of local catecholamines from the ischaemic area after acute occlusion? If this mostly occurs within 2 min, presumably the myocardial catecholamine concentration at 30 min in the Harris two-stage preparation will be completely different from that present 5 min or 15 min after occlusion. It has been shown that repeated inflation and occlusion during this half-hour period is associated under a graded decrease in the incidence of ventricular fibrillation and perhaps this is related to decreasing myocardial catecholamine concentration.

Shahab. In our experiments we have found that noradrenaline is released within a minute of coronary occlusion.

Kurien. In coronary artery occlusion experiments I could induce ventricular fibrillation on reflow only between 30 and 50 min after occlusion. After 1 to 1½ hours there was no arrhythmia—apparently because the ischaemic cells were dead. If one restored flow approximately 15 min after occlusion, no arrhythmia occurred. Therefore there seems to be a stage of ischaemia but not of complete death at which this phenomenon occurs. If cell death has taken place, there is no chance that sudden ionic changes and arrhythmia will not occur.

Taggart. In human atrial biopsies taken at various times after coronary artery occlusion during bypass surgery, the rate of disappearance of noradrenaline is very fast, dropping by about one third within the first 30 min, followed by a slow progressive loss. As has been shown in studies from Hammersmith Hospital on urine and from the London Hospital on blood, plasma concentrations of both noradrenaline and adrenaline rise to very high levels and persist. In the real-life situation you have a depleted myocardial noradrenaline with a high circulating concentration of both noradrenaline and adrenaline. I wonder to what extent this is reflected in the experimental preparations?

Wallace. Not at all as far as I know. The susceptibility to arrhythmias during catecholamine infusions in the stage of infarction has produced variable results. Some have found that catecholamines diminish the ventricular fibrillation threshold during coronary occlusion, but others have not been able to produce that result.

METHODS OF STUDYING REGIONAL MYOCARDIAL FLOW AND ALTERATIONS DURING ANGINA

A. Maseri

The study of the adaptations and reactions of the coronary circulation in acute ischaemia are of fundamental importance for the understanding of the sequence of events that, through metabolic alterations, leads to cell injury and death.

Animal studies have provided some basic elements for the understanding of the experimental ischaemia and infarction produced by the sudden occlusion of a single vessel.[1-3] However the sudden occlusion of a major coronary branch, as produced in animal models, seems rather remote from the pathogenesis of angina pectoris or of human myocardial infarction, because in man angina and infarction generally occur in the presence of slowly developing stenotic lesions, single or multiple, and of collaterals often in the absence of complete occlusions.[4-5] Hence the need to develop adequate methods for the study of both animal models and patients.

While pathological and electrocardiographic data indicate a patchy distribution of lesions in coronary artery disease in man, perfusion alterations in coronary patients have been sought using methods that measure total or average flow. Furthermore the presence of inhomogeneities of perfusion complicates or prevents the correct measurement of myocardial blood flow by the most commonly used methods in intact animal and in man. With outflow detection, often the accuracy of analytical techniques is not such to allow a precise determination of the low, prolonged tails of the curves observed in the presence of inhomogeneous perfusion.[6] With residue detection[7] and with potassium tracers fractionation methods,[8] perfusion inhomogeneities in zones seen with different counting efficiency cause errors in the estimate of flow, so that iso-efficiency counting systems are required. Furthermore, in the presence of gross non-homogeneous perfusion, the physiological significance of an average value of flow, or of total flow estimates, might be questionable because it can lead to erroneous conclusions when a reduced flow to one zone is compensated by an increased flow to another or when flow varies in opposite directions in adjacent zones.

Therefore, for the study of the adaptations of coronary circulation to coronary artery disease it is essential to use methods which can provide information on the behaviour of regional myocardial perfusion (Table 4, 1).

Table 4, 1 *Methods for the study of regional myocardial perfusion*

PRINCIPLES	TECHNIQUES	APPLICATIONS
Fractionation	chopped pieces of myocardium	(*sacrificed*) animal
Depot clearances	direct intramyocardial injection	*open-chest* animal and man
Regional dynamic imaging	intracoronary injection	*intact* animal or man

In animals that can be sacrificed, this can be achieved by determining the fractional distribution of tracers in chopped pieces of the myocardium.[9-11] In animals with exposed hearts or in man at open heart surgery, microinjections of radioactive gamma-emitting diffusible indicators allow the determination of local tissue clearances[12-13] but, obviously, in intact man neither of these techniques can be used. Therefore we developed a method which can be applied to patients undergoing diagnostic selective coronary arteriography. It is based on the use of a gamma camera computer system which allows us to determine the initial myocardial distribution of a gamma-emitting diffusible indicator and its regional washout curves following its intracoronary slug injection.[14-15]

Theoretical and methodological considerations

Fractionation. This method is based on the assumption that the indicator distribution to the myocardium (and its various regions) is proportional to flow and that this distribution is maintained up to the time the measurement is completed. Two possibilities exist: (1) the indicator does not recirculate (radioactive microspheres); (2) the indicator recirculates (potassium tracers, antipyrine), but tracer diffusion into the tissue and recirculation up to the time the measurements are taken should balance so that the basic condition, that regional concentration is proportional to flow, is met. Obviously if microspheres are of such a calibre (8 to 15 μm) that they are not concentrated near the axis of the stream[16] (while clustering is avoided), they should be the preferred type of indicator. In fact, their distribution is maintained indefinitely and, if tagged with different isotopes, several successive measurements are possible. Furthermore (and more important), they allow absolute quantitative measurements of the flow distribution when the injectate is correctly estimated.

The measurement of the injectate presents some technical problems because microspheres tend to stick to containers and syringes and two possible approaches exist: (1) the use of external counting systems to estimate the radioactivity in the syringe before and after the injection (with adequate calibration factors with the well counter); (2) the measurement of the injectate by the inverse use of the Stewart-Hamilton principle: if cardiac output is independently determined the determination of the primary arterial dilution curve of the tagged microspheres injected into the left atrium allows the correct calculation of the dose injected.

Depot clearance. This method is based on the intramyocardial microinjection of gamma emitting diffusible indicators and on the external recording of their washout curve, on the assumptions that the injection does not produce significant tissue trauma and that its removal is flow dependent. However these conditions are difficult to meet in practice because even a minute injection causes microvascular damage and because in the myocardium the flow pattern differs in the subendocardium (diastolic) and the subepicardium throughout the cycle.[17] Therefore for a given level of flow more indicator will be removed under steady flow than under intermittent perfusion with consequently slower apparent clearance values from the inner layers of myocardial wall. Furthermore, the information thus obtained is indeed applicable only to the very small tissue zone labelled by the indicator. These considerations also apply to the use of micro-electrodes implanted at different depths in the myocardial wall to record H_2 desaturation curves following intracoronary injection.[18]

Regional dynamic imaging. This method is the only one that can be applied to man outside the operating theatre. It is based on the intracoronary slug injection of a gamma-emitting diffusible indicator and on the recording of its regional myocardial initial (flow dependent) distribution and of its regional washout rates by a scintillation camera computer system. The problems involved in this technique have been recently discussed in detail.[15]

When myocardial scintigrams are recorded in 64×64 matrix form, the spatial resolution of the system in the plane perpendicular to the counter axis is practically determined by that of the scintillation camera (8 to 12 mm). On the planes parallel to the counter axis, the efficiency decreases with the depth inside the body because of the gamma radiation absorption in the tissues. Therefore, such a system permits the detection of inhomogeneities of perfusion on a plane perpendicular to the counter axis, as long as their size is wide enough in relation to the spatial resolution and extends enough in depth along the counter axis not to be obscured by the behaviour of the tracer in the remaining tissue included in the solid angle of the zone. A certain degree of ' cross over ' among zones is unavoidable and studies in multiple projections are useful. In particular perfusion gradients across the ventricular wall cannot be detected by this method.

The ideal indicator for the actual measurement of regional myocardial flow from the washout curves should have a number of characteristics: (1) a fat/myocardium partition coefficient close to 1 to avoid the problems of the ' tonometer effect ' of epicardial fat soluble indicators[2]; (2) absence of recirculation or possibility of subtraction of the contribution of recirculating indicator to the regional washout curves by the double injection method[19]; (3) gamma energies in the optimal range for the scintillation camera crystal and high resolution collimator (about 100 to 200 Kev); (4) short physical or biological half-life to allow high counting rates with low radiation exposure for patients. For the laboratories where cyclotron-produced isotopes are available, ^{123}I iodoantipyrine would be the ideal indicator because of its energy, half-life and partition coefficients. In fact, on the one hand, xenon, which has 80 Kev gammas and is eliminated at the alveolar level, would normally be a suitable isotope but cannot be used for actual flow measurements in man because of its high solubility in fat[7]: on the other hand, ^{125}I or ^{131}I iodoantipyrine do not have very suitable gamma energies (30 and 360 Kev respectively) but, most important, have very long biological and physical half-lives to allow more than one, or at most two injections.

For the semiquantitative evaluation of regional myocardial perfusion the requirements for the type of indicator are less critical. Although differences in regional perfusion cannot be assessed from xenon washout rates because the epicardial fat tonometer effect also influences the initial part of the curves,[7] they can reasonably be assessed from ^{125}I or ^{131}I iodoantipyrine initial regional washout rates since recirculation should not affect their initial slopes to a significantly different extent. Furthermore, the changes of regional distribution or myocardial perfusion can also be evaluated, following successive injections of xenon from the changes of its initial myocardial distribution and from the changes in initial regional washout rates. The possibility of using ^{133}Xe for this purpose is of practical interest because, since it is eliminated by the lungs, the dose of radioactivity injected can be considerably larger than for ^{125}I or ^{131}I iodoantipyrine (consequently with better counting statistics) and several successive injections are possible.

Experimental findings

Animal studies on myocardial flow transmural distribution. Under normal haemodynamic conditions, whereas depot clearance methods would suggest that flow to the subendocardium is lower than that to the subepicardium, fractionation methods indicate that flow is the same or even higher in the subendocardial regions. This difference is very likely related to the underestimate of subendocardial flow by depot clearance related to the intermittance of flow in this region.[18]

When coronary perfusion pressure is artificially lowered well below intraventricular pressure, subendocardial flow drops considerably with respect to subepicardial flow.[2-3] Accordingly, when an occlusion is produced in a single coronary branch, perfusion to the distal myocardium is greatly reduced especially to the subendocardium so that in this area the endo/epi ratio decreases to 0·6 to 0·8.[2]

Patient studies on regional myocardial perfusion during angina pectoris. The application of regional dynamic imaging has provided the demonstration that in patients with coronary artery disease regional differences of washout rates exist.[20] However, when xenon is used these differences can be related to the presence of zones of epicardial fat.[15] By using iodoantipyrine we were able to show that in an area of variable dimensions distally to a coronary occlusive or subocclusive lesion, flow at rest is reduced in respect to surrounding regions and that flow becomes uniform following nitroglycerin administration.[15 21] However, the potentialities of this method are best illustrated by two typical experimental studies that we carried out using ^{133}Xe to study regional perfusion changes during angina pectoris. We selected patients with an isolated subocclusive lesion of the anterior descending coronary artery or its

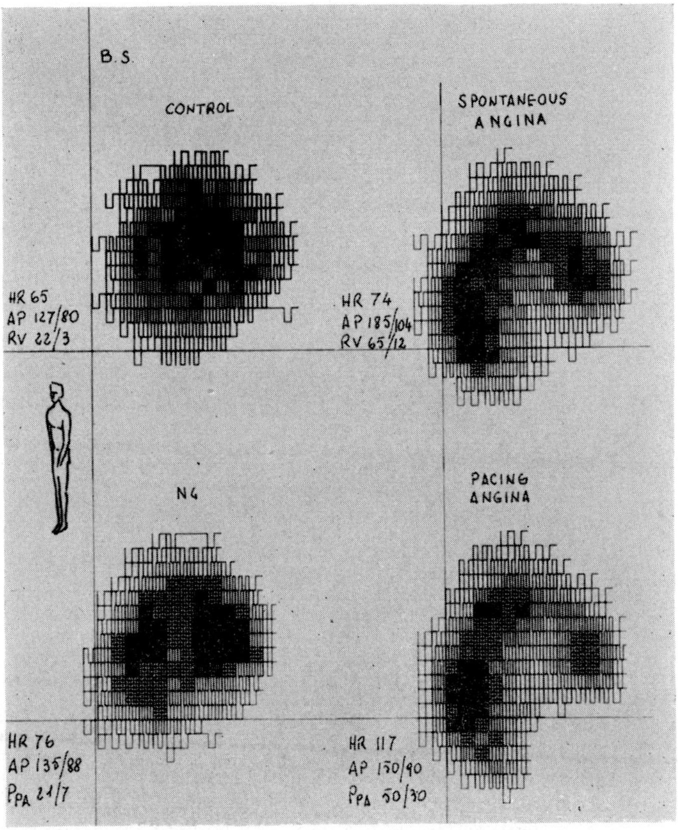

FIG. 4, 1. The initial distribution of the tracer in a patient with a subocclusive stenosis of the proximal anterior descending coronary artery. A marked deficit in the inferior and apical zone, both during spontaneous and pacing induced angina, are apparent, whereas following nitroglycerin the distribution appears relatively increased to the previously ischaemic zone. The alterations observed in spontaneous and pacing angina are very similar.

first main diagonal branch, and we studied them in the control state and during angina (spontaneous or induced by pacing) and following nitroglycerin administration. When the indicator was injected during angina, the initial scintigram demonstrates ventricular dilatation and a markedly reduced distribution of the indicator to the apical regions both during spontaneous and induced angina. These alterations of the initial tracer distribution disappear following nitroglycerin administration (Fig. 4, 1).[22] When angina is

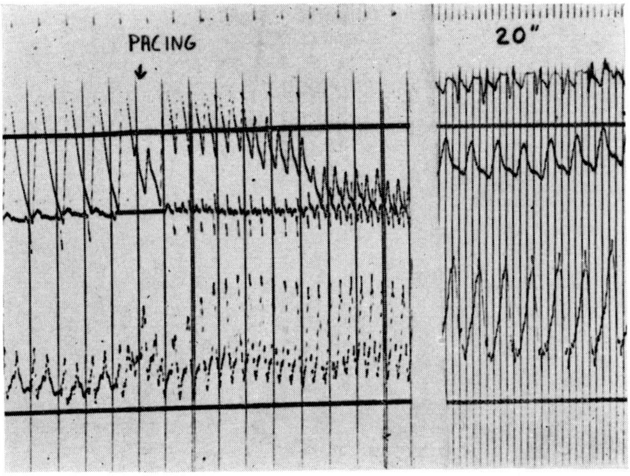

FIG. 4. 2. Original tracing of a patient in whom angina was induced by pacing after the intracoronary injection of ^{133}Xe. Timing 1 sec on the left, 0·1 sec in the centre and right panels. As soon as the heart rate is increased pulmonary 'wedge' pressure begins to rise and the T wave becomes negative; later on the wedge pressure is further increased ('a' and 'v' waves being fused because of the long P—R interval).

induced immediately following the intracoronary injection of the indicator so that the flow changes associated with angina do not affect the initial distribution but only the regional washout rates, the washout rate is dramatically reduced at the apex and this reduction spreads progressively to surrounding zones. The haemodynamic and ECG changes are illustrated in Figure 4, 2 and the simultaneous regional washout curves in Figure 4, 3.

Conclusions

In animals the application of the fraction method to the study of transmural distribution of perfusion has demonstrated that flow can be regulated by vasomotor control until coronary perfusion pressure falls below a critical level with respect to intraventricular pressure: then mechanical forces cannot any longer be compensated by further vasodilatation.

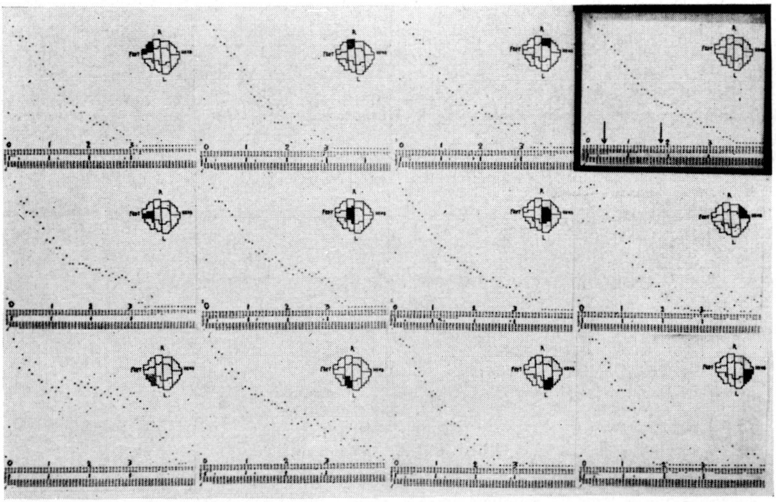

FIG. 4, 3. In the top right corner the precordial washout from the whole scintigram case of the study described in Figure 4, 2. The first arrow indicates the onset of pacing, the second the onset of pain. While the washout at the base continues unchanged, that from apex is markedly reduced soon after the onset of pacing. Subsequently the reduction of the washout rate spreads to surrounding zones.

The method of regional dynamic imaging, even applied on a semiquantitative basis for the study of perfusion alterations during angina, has provided more physiological information than any of the methods which (when correctly applied) would yield absolute measurements of total or of average flow. In fact it has allowed us to show that, in patients during angina, flow to the ischaemic zone is dramatically reduced and ischaemia progressively spreads to surrounding regions so that functional factors must play a significant role in the pathogenesis of the syndrome of acute coronary insufficiency in patients.

Further studies of the factors that control regional coronary perfusion pressure, local vasomotion and local mechanical forces are needed for achieving a better insight into this crucial problem.

REFERENCES

1 Khouri, E. M., Gregg, D. E., & Lowenshon, H. S. (1968). The flow in the major branches of the left coronary artery during experimental coronary insufficiency in the unanaesthetized dog. *Circulation Research* **23,** 99-109
2 Becker, L. C., Fortuin, N. J. & Pitt, B. (1971). Effect of ischaemia and antianginal drugs on the distribution of radioactive microspheres in the canine left ventricle. *Circulation Research* **28,** 263-269.
3 Buckberg, G. D., Fixler, D. E.. Archie, J. P. & Hoffman, J. E. (1972). Experimental subendocardial ischaemia in dogs with normal coronary arteries. *Circulation Research* **30,** 67-81.
4 Spain, D. M. & Brades, V. A. (1960). The relationship of coronary thrombosis to coronary atherosclerosis and ischaemic heart disease. *American Journal of Medical Science* **240,** 701-710.
5 Baroldi, G. & Scomazzoni, C. (1967). In *Coronary circulation in the normal and pathologic heart.* Government Printing Office A.F.I.P., American Registry of Pathology, Washington 20305, USA.
6 Klocke, F. J. & Wittenberg, S. M. (1972). In Symposium on *Myocardial Blood Flow in Man. Methods and Significance in myocardial disease.* Edited: A. Maseri. Minerva Medica—Torino. 121-136.
7 Maseri, A. (1972). In Symposium on *Myocardial Blood Flow in Man. Methods and Significance in Myocardial Disease.* Edited: A. Maseri. Minerva Medica—Torino. 145-156.
8 Donato, L., Maseri, A., Pesola, A. & Duce, T. (1972). In Symposium on *Myocardial Blood Flow in Man. Methods and Significance in Myocardial Disease.* Edited: A. Maseri. Minerva Medica—Torino. 183-192.
9 Love, W. D. & Burch, G. E. (1957). Differences in the rate of ^{86}Rb uptake by several regions of the myocardium of control dogs and dogs receiving l-norepinephrine or pitressin. *Journal of Clinical Investigation* **36,** 479-484.
10 Griggs, D. M. & Makamura, Y. (1968). Effect of coronary constriction on myocardial distribution of iodantipyrine-131-I. *American Journal of Physiology* **215,** 1082-1086.
11 Domenech, R. J., Hoffman, J. I. E., Noble, M. I. M., Saunders, K. B., Henson, J. R. & Subijanto, S. (1969). Total regional coronary blood flow measured by radioactive microspheres in conscious and anaesthetized dogs. *Circulation Research* **25,** 581-596.
12 Brandi, G., Fam, W. M. & McGregor, M. (1966). Estimation of coronary flow using intramyocardial injections of radioactive tracers (P). *Circulation* **34**^{III}, 64.
13 Honig, C. R., Harper, J. R. & Myers, W. W. (1967). In *Proc. Intern. Symposium Coronary Circulation Energetics Myocardium,* p. 31. Milan: Karger Basel.
14 Maseri, A., Mancini, P., L'Abbate, A. & Magini, G. (1971). Method for regional dynamic study of myocardial blood flow in man. *Journal of Nuclear Medicine* **15,** 54-57.
15 Maseri, A. & Mancini, P. (1972). In Symposium on *Myocardial Blood Flow in Man. Methods and Significances in Myocardial Disease.* Edited: A. Maseri. Minerva Medica—Torino.
16 Phibbs, R. H. & Wyler, F. N. (1967). Rheology of microspheres injected into circulation of rabbits. *Nature* **216,** 1339-1340.

17 AUKLAND, K. B., BOWER, B. & BERLINER, R. W. (1964). Measurement of local blood flow with hydrogen gas. *Circulation Research* **14,** 164-187.
18 KIRK, E. S., DOWNEY, J. M. & DOWNEY, H. F. (1972). In Symposium on *Myocardial Blood Flow in Man. Methods and Significance in Myocardial Disease.* Edited: A. Maseri. Minera Medica—Torino.
19 MASERI, A. Submitted for publication. *Journal of Applied Physiology.*
20 DWYER, E. M., DELL, R. B., CAMRON, P. J. (1971). Regional myocardial blood flow coronary artery disease. *Clinical Research* **19,** 311.
21 MASERI, A., MANCINI, P., L'ABBATE, A., BEDINI, A., PESOLA, A., & CONTINI, C., with the technical assistance of PISANI, P. Submitted for publication. *Circulation.*
22 L'ABBATE, A., MASERI, A., PESOLA, A. & MARZILLI, M. *Atti del 33 Congr. Soc. It. Cardiol.* Viareggio 1972 (in press).

DISCUSSION

Livesley. I was very interested in your slide (Fig. 1) which showed an area of reduced myocardial perfusion during the phase of spontaneous angina. It adds support to our working hypothesis that patients with myocardial ischaemia fall into one of three groups, namely: (1) those patients who have tachycardiac angina and in whom at a critically high heart rate there is inadequate myocardial blood supply because of coronary arterial obstruction; (2) those patients who develop bradycardiac angina, particularly at rest, and with it coronary arterial hypoperfusion (we have seen patients who have developed both angina at rest when the heart rate has fallen below, say, 55 per minute and also angina on effort when the heart rate has risen above 140 per minute); (3) those patients who develop spontaneous angina with no detectable change in heart rate.

I think we should be subgrouping patients with ischaemic heart disease in order to investigate them more adequately and I would like to know if your patients' heart rates fell during the hypoperfusive phase of spontaneous angina.

Maseri. In my opinion there are several types of angina. The patients we studied were a rather homogeneous group which, before being admitted to the gamma camera study, were paced so that we know at which level of pacing pain would appear. All these patients were admitted to our department because of severe angina induced by exercise and also occurring spontaneously but without an appreciable drop in heart rate. During the anginal attacks which occurred in the gamma camera studies we usually observed a progressive increase in arterial and wedge pressures.

Parratt. Dr Maseri has made a very important point concerning the measurement of flow in different parts of the ischaemic region, and also in the normal region, and I should like to describe a rather simpler experimental model (see Fig. 4, 4). Greyhounds were anaesthetized and ventilated. A catheter was placed in a branch of the left coronary artery under fluoroscopic control for the measurement of myocardial blood flow using a xenon clearance technique. Catheters were also positioned in the coronary sinus, right atrium,

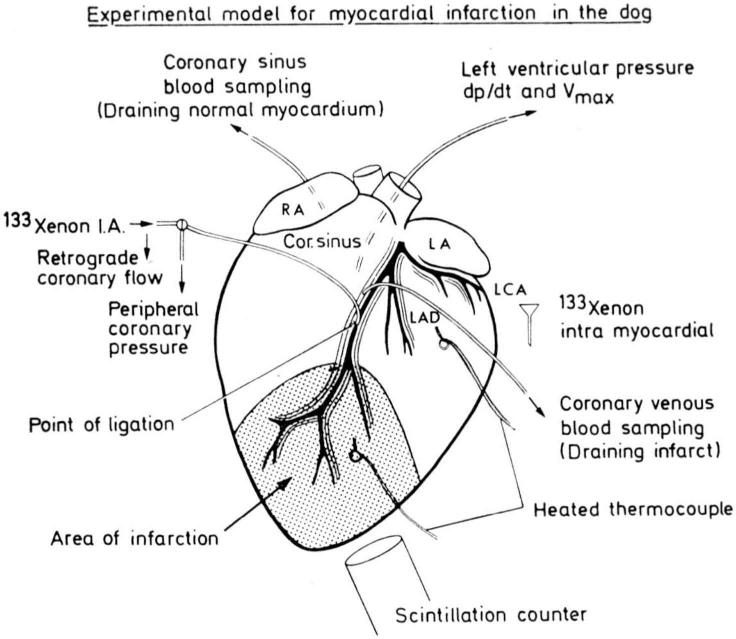

FIG. 4, 4.

left ventricle and descending aorta and were used for blood sampling and for pressure measurements. This gave basal prethoracotomy haemodynamic and metabolic values. After thoracotomy, the left anterior descending coronary artery was prepared for ligation. A catheter was placed in the vein adjacent to that artery so that blood could be sampled from the apical region. This blood was the same metabolically ($P\text{O}_2$, $P\text{CO}_2$, pH, lactate, etc) as that sampled from the coronary sinus. The artery was then ligated and blood sampled from the ischaemic area are described by Blair (*Circ. Res.* **9**, 333,

1961) and later used by Dr Thomas and Dr Opie. Flow in the normal myocardium was measured using three different methods. An electromagnetic flow-probe was placed around the circumflex artery to measure total flow to the normal region while local flow in the normal myocardium was measured using the heat clearance technique and by the local (intramyocardial) injection of xenon. Flow in the ischaemic region was assessed using heat clearance (which also enables comparison between deep and epicardial flows), by the clearance of radioactive xenon (injected into the artery catheterized distal to the point of ligation) and as backflow (retrograde flow) from the open arterial catheter. Using this technique we can therefore measure flow in both normal and ischaemic regions simultaneously and, by sampling blood from each region, measure regional myocardial oxygen consumption.

Taggart. Have you studied with your techniques the akinetic areas in the left ventricle that you see on coronary angiograms? If I understood you correctly, there wasn't a very good correlation with the degree of coronary narrowing. I am thinking of the problem involved in assessment for vein bypass surgery. Whereas in some people there is considerable amount of akinesis, there is an inbetween group of suspicious or uncertain looking ventricles. Does this technique throw any light on that?

Maseri. We are developing a method of evaluating simultaneously regional ventricular perfusion and contraction because I believe they are closely related. As to the second part of your question: we have observed reduced rates of perfusion to an area of variable dimensions beyond a subocclusive or an occlusive lesion. So far we have studied two patients after successful vein graft operations and have found that the perfusion was uniform following injection into the grafted anterior descending and into the main left coronary artery.

Muir. Can you tell us more about the discrimination you can get from the gamma camera and what are the effects of changing the left ventricular volume on the actual geometry of your counting?

Maseri. The resolution of the gamma camera with the standard 4000 holes collimator is about 1·2 cm. When the volume of the heart increases, the geometry of the counting cannot change much. With xenon there is about 50 per cent absorption by 5 cm perspex or water. Therefore since the ventricular displacement could be of the order of 1 cm it does not influence significantly the counting geometry, as we are only interested in a semiquantitative evaluation.

Wallace. I would like to ask you two questions which relate first to methodology and second to the interpretation which you gave of a decrease in flow during spontaneous and induced angina. The technical question relates to how this method applies to the measurement of flow into an area which has two potential sources of flow, the artery into which you injected the isotope and the collateral flow which may come from some other vessel. Secondly, would it not be an equally plausible interpretation of your result that during angina there is an increase in flow coming from collateral vessels rather than a decrease from the flow coming from the vessel into which you injected? I am still somewhat reluctant to accept the idea that episodes of angina occur because of a decrease in flow, rather than an increase in metabolic need relative to a rather fixed flow.

Maseri. First, any change in the amount of collateral flow would have had to come from the right coronary artery not from the circumflex because it also would have carried tagged blood, since only patients with a long main stem left coronary were selected so as to provide uniform mixing of the tracer with total left coronary flow. Second, we could not see collaterals from the right to the left in any of the patients. Third, when we produced angina after the intracoronary injection of the indicator so that the initial distribution of indicator was the same as in the control, the washout in the ischaemic area decreased dramatically. This can only mean that flow to these areas is proportionately reduced quite independently of where it came from. As to the last question I don't think that this reduction of flow to the ischaemic zone is necessarily the cause of angina but occurs simultaneously with angina. The initial condition is a disproportion between demand and supply, this leads probably to a vicious circle and to a dramatic reduction of flow.

Wallace. It could be that if the flow is decreased, this might be a consequence of dyskinesia in this area.

Maseri. It might be due to a steal phenomenon, to extramural mechanical obstruction to flow, or to local metabolic or nervous changes. Certainly, to invoke a steal phenomenon you must assume first a proximal obstruction on the vessel normally providing the collateral flow and second an increased flow in the muscle perfused by it. We selected patients who had an isolated lesion of anterior descending coronary artery or of its first main diagonal branch. Furthermore, significant increases of perfusion were observed in the left circumflex myocardial territory.

ULTRASTRUCTURAL CHANGES IN ACUTE MYOCARDIAL ISCHAEMIA

R. B. JENNINGS AND C. E. GANOTE

INTRODUCTION

SUDDEN occlusion of a major branch of a coronary artery in the experimental animal is followed by the sequence of events depicted in Figure 5, 1. The arterial blood flow through the obstructed vessel is reduced, and if the reduced flow provides inadequate oxygen to support aerobic respiration, the affected cells become *ischaemic*.[1] Ischaemia is manifest by a shift in intracellular respiration to the much less efficient anaerobic form; cellular energy levels decrease and become insufficient to provide either enough energy or the appropriate environment to maintain contraction and other specialized functions. Moreover, if the ischaemia is severe and prolonged, many of the affected cells die. The interval of time during which the ischaemic cells are viable, as determined by the fact that restoration of arterial flow results in restoration of function, is generally termed *reversible ischaemic injury*, while the injury is termed *irreversible* if restoration of arterial flow fails to prevent cell death. Irreversibly injured ischaemic cells eventually become *necrotic*, and the segmental area of obvious cell death in the portion of myocardium supplied by an occluded vessel is termed a *myocardial infarct*. Most of our efforts have been directed at the acute phase of ischaemic injury and particularly at learning what events occur during the shift to irreversibility (Fig. 5, 1).

The principal aim of this paper is to describe the sequential ultrastructural changes developing in previously healthy myocardial cells as a consequence of the sudden onset of ischaemia. The emphasis will be on the early effects of severe ischaemia induced by the sudden occlusion of a major coronary artery in the anaesthetized open-chest dog. Lastly, the effects of restoration of arterial flow on ischaemic viable cells and ischaemic irreversibly injured cells will be presented. Most of the observations summarized here have been presented in detail elsewhere.[3 4 5]

Acute Myocardial Ischaemic Injury

The early changes in tissue structure or metabolism resulting from the sudden onset of ischaemia can be studied only in the experimental animal and cannot be done unless samples known to be ischaemic are available for analysis. The posterior papillary muscle (PP) infarct preparation we described in 1957 is a satisfactory, readily identifiable source of small quantities of tissue known to be severely ischaemic[6] and is the preparation we have used in most of our experiments.

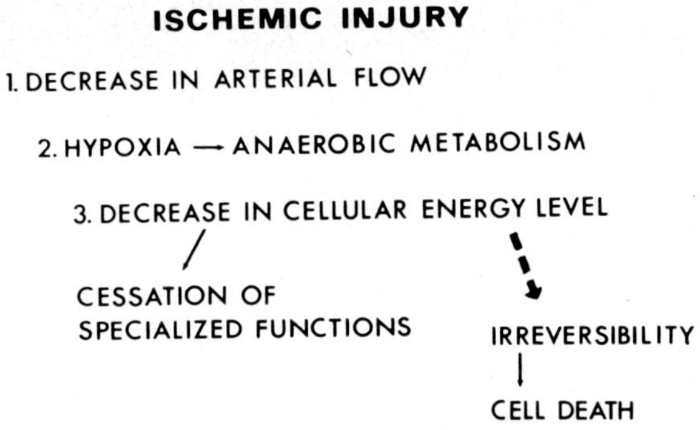

Fig. 5, 1. Diagram of sequential changes in myocardium resulting from sudden occlusion of a coronary artery. Reprinted with permission from Reference 2.

Biological features of ischaemia. Before considering the alterations in myocardial ultrastructure occurring as a consequence of ischaemia, it is important to recognize that sudden occlusion of a major branch of a coronary artery in the dog does not result in uniform reduction in blood flow to all parts of the tissue supplied by this vessel. For example, occlusion of the circumflex branch of the left coronary artery near its origin results in a large posterolateral area of ischaemia which becomes visible a few seconds later as cyanotic, acontractile myocardium. However, cell death usually is restricted to the subendocardial region including the PP and parts of the midmyocardial region (Fig. 5, 2). The superficial epicardium and much of the midportion of the myocardium, although obviously ischaemic, according to the presence of cyanosis and failure of contraction, does not usually die (Fig. 5, 3). We assume that cell death does not occur because collateral arterial flow is adequate to maintain the cells' viability, even though it is inadequate to support function. Gregg and co-workers[7 8] have shown, by inducing slow occlusion of the circumflex artery, that it is possible to stimulate enough growth of collateral vessels to prevent cell death even in the subendocardial region. If one accepts the likely premise[9] that myo-

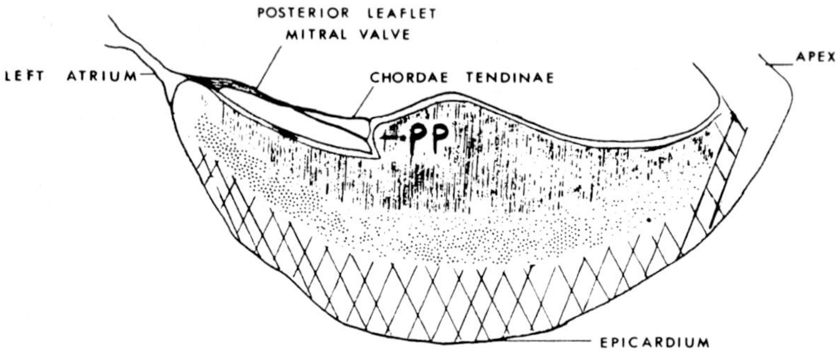

FIG. 5, 2. Diagram of the posterior wall of the dog left ventricle sectioned parallel to the long axis of the posterior papillary muscle (PP) and including a part of the apex and the posterior leaflet of the mitral valve. The shaded portion of the posterior wall is supplied by the circumflex branch of the left coronary artery. Immediately after occlusion of this vessel within 1·0 cm of its origin, ischaemia is most marked in the subendocardial and mid-myocardial region, as evidenced by the fact that necrosis occurs in these inner zones. The endocardium, however, always is spared. The lightly cross-hatched subepicardial myocardium is believed to be less ischaemic than the other zones. Cells in this region are injured reversibly, as are cells in the lightly cross-hatched area at the juncture of the region supplied by the anterior descending and circumflex branches of the left coronary artery. Since no cells die in this lightly cross-hatched zone, and it is similar structurally, chemically, and metabolically to the inner zones,[3 27 28] cell death is related best to differences in blood flow. Reprinted with permission from Reference 9.

cardial cells in the endocardium are not intrinsically more susceptible to injury than those in the epicardium, these observations mean that study of tissue removed from subepicardial myocardium will reveal the changes of mild ischaemia in the sense that it is not sufficiently severe to cause cell death, while cells removed from the subendocardial myocardium will show similar changes acutely but later will become irreversibly injured and will demonstrate progressively increasing signs of damage including coagulation necrosis and, finally, phagocytosis.

We have not studied this phenomenon of differential degrees of ischaemia in detail. However, experiments with intravenous methylene blue do illustrate clearly that ischaemia is present throughout the entire wall of the ventricle, even though cell death is generally localized to the inner layers of the ventricle (Fig. 5, 2). Methylene blue is a deep blue oxidation-reduction dye which diffuses into the myocardium and turns it blue. If a part of the tissue then is made

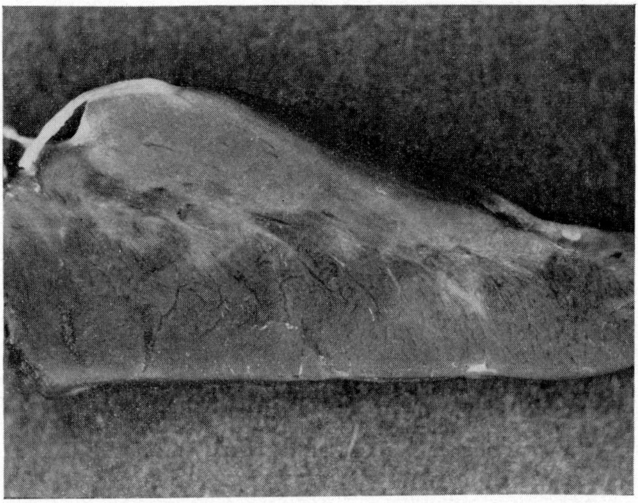

FIG. 5, 3. Midline longitudinal section through the PP after 60 minutes of ischaemia induced by permanent occlusion of the circumflex branch of the left coronary artery. This dog exhibited a large area of cyanosis which included most of the posterior surface of the heart and about 0·5 cm of the anterior surface of the apex of the left ventricle. Note the pale grey irreversibly injured tissue. This section was fixed for 60 seconds in formalin prior to photography. (Mag. 3/4 ×.)

ischaemic by arterial occlusion, it promptly loses its blue colour as the hydrogen ions produced by metabolism accumulate in the absence of oxygen and reduces the methylene blue to its colourless reduced form.[10] In such animals, the ischaemic focus, including the PP, is sharply delimited from non-ischaemic tissue and includes the entire wall of the left ventricle even though cell death eventually becomes manifest only in the inner layers of the affected myocardium.

The recent studies of Becker, Fortuin and Pitt[11] also support the idea that the entire canine myocardial wall supplied by a vessel is not equally ischaemic after sudden occlusion. They have made instantaneous estimates of the magnitude of flow in different parts of dog myocardium by injecting radioactive plastic microspheres of 15μ diameter labelled with isotopes of different energy into the left heart of the dog before and after occlusion. Their studies were made after periods of ischaemia of less than one minute and demonstrate that occlusion of the circumflex artery results in a much greater proportionate decrease in flow in the subendocardial than in the subepicardial myocardium. Since coronary arterial flow occurs primarily during diastole,[12-14] elevations in left ventricular and diastolic pressure or cardiac rate occurring as a consequence of ischaemia might be the reason why subendocardial flow is reduced to a greater extent than subepicardial flow. These factors remain to be investigated in detail but do not alter the fact that the subendocardial myocardium represents a suitable site to study the effects of severe ischaemia.

Permanent ischaemia. No gross changes are seen in the PP for the first 20 to 30 minutes after occlusion of the circumflex artery. By 40 minutes, the PP of some dogs is slightly more pale, and at 60 minutes the irreversibly injured tissues is readily identifiable as a uniformly pale grey focus (Fig. 5, 3). At this time, however, the tissue appears normal to routine techniques of light microscopy. The PP becomes paler and more yellowish as the period of ischaemia is prolonged. All of the final events characteristic of dead cells occur within this area; its electrolytes are identical to those in the extracellular fluid, nuclei disappear, intracellular enzymes disappear or become inactive, etc.[6 9]

Transient ischaemia. An episode of transient ischaemia of 1 to 18 minutes' duration produces no detectable change in tissue structure, even if the arterial flow is restored to the area of ischaemia. On the other hand, obstruction of the artery for 40 minutes, which is the period of permanent ischaemia noted above at which a significant colour change without oedema first becomes manifest, results in striking gross changes in the PP and subendocardial myocardium. Within minutes of the onset of arterial reflow, the irreversibly injured tissue swells markedly, develops contraction bands, unusual mitochondrial changes and other chemical findings which have been reported in detail elsewhere.[4 15 16] Suffice it to state that exposure of irreversibly injured cells to reflow of arterial blood produces a condition in which cell death is occurring in the presence of arterial flow and that electrolyte changes, etc., occur quickly and differ to some extent from those noted in an area of permanent ischaemia. Also, it should be noted[16] that a few cells of the PP of some animals are irreversibly injured after as little as 20 minutes of ischaemia.

Effects of Acute Ischaemia on Cellular Structure

Control. Myocardial tissue removed from well-oxygenated left ventricle shows cells which are moderately contracted and covered with a sarcolemmal membrane which is indented at the Z bands and is covered with a thin fuzzy basement membrane (Fig. 5, 4). The myofibrils show A and Z bands. The nuclear chromatin is evenly distributed, although the nuclear membrane often is indented. The cytoplasm usually contains an abundance of small

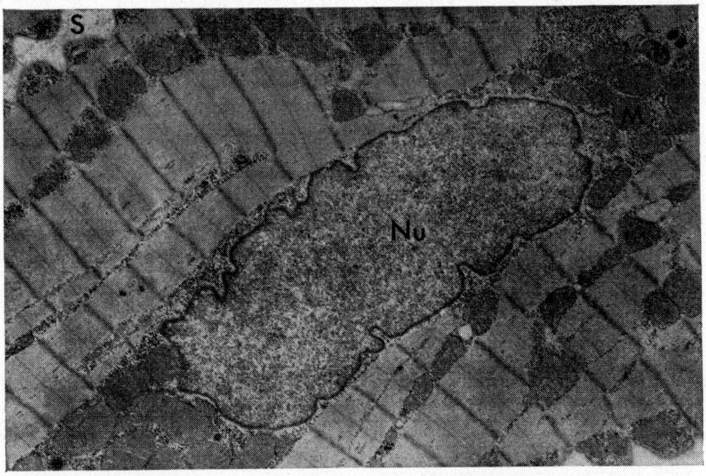

Fig. 5, 4. Section of part of a non-ischaemic left ventricular cell from a dog in which the circumflex branch of the left coronary artery had been occluded for 40 minutes. The sarcolemma (S) is scalloped. Myofibrils are contracted. Mitochondria (M) are abundant and show moderately dense matrices and numerous cristae. The granular material in the sarcoplasm is glycogen. Note the characteristic even distribution of nuclear (Nu) chromatin. Osmium fixation. (Mag. 9, 100 ×.)

granules of glycogen. Present between the myofibrils are mitochondria, usually about one mitochondrion per sarcomere. These mitochondria have a clear outer membrane and the inner membrane is tightly packed with cristae. The matrix is dense and matrix granules are very small and often not detectable. The sarcoplasmic reticulum is closely applied to the surface of the myofibrils and is best seen in oblique sections. The T tubule system is present at the Z lines and is identified by its structural resemblance to the sarcolemma.

Acute permanent ischaemia; reversible phase. Cells of the PP muscle after 5 minutes of ischaemia show little difference from control, non-ischaemic myocardium of the same animal with the exception of the fact that the myofibrils usually are relaxed. After 10 minutes of ischaemia, glycogen supplies often appear to be depleted and mitochondria to be slighlty swollen or to have a less dense matrix. Moreover, the nuclear chromatin distribution in some cells begins to differ from control, non-ischaemic cells of the same animal in that nuclei of many cells show mild margination. These changes are more marked after 15 minutes of ischaemia; the severely ischaemic viable cell, however, never shows amorphous mitochondrial matrix densities or marked margination of nuclear chromatin. Also, the sarcolemma, T tubules and sarcoplasmic reticulum appear similar to control throughout the first 15 minutes of ischaemia. Not all cells studied in different parts of the PP exhibit detectable changes in nuclear, myofibrillar and mitochondrial morphology. This presumably is a function of sampling and/or the severity of the injury (Fig. 5, 5).

Acute permanent ischaemia; irreversible phase. Irreversibly injured cells of the PP are recognizable with the naked eye at 60 minutes, a fact which allows precise sampling of damaged tissue (Fig. 5, 3). Accordingly, the findings in this tissue will be described first (Fig. 5, 6). The affected cells are markedly relaxed. The myofibrils show prominent I bands, and N, M and H bands are seen as well. Glycogen is virtually absent from the sarcoplasm and occasional rough endoplasmic reticulum is observed. The mitochondria are all altered. They appear to be swollen, to have markedly decreased matrix density as well as cristae which often appear to be slightly disorganized and, in addition, contain one or more amorphous osmiophilic matrix densities. These matrix densities will be discussed in more detail in a subsequent section. Some broken mitochondria also are noted. The nuclear chromatin shows marked margination. The sarcolemma usually is flattened over the relaxed myocardial cells and still contains a clearly discernible basement membrane. Without stereological study it is im-

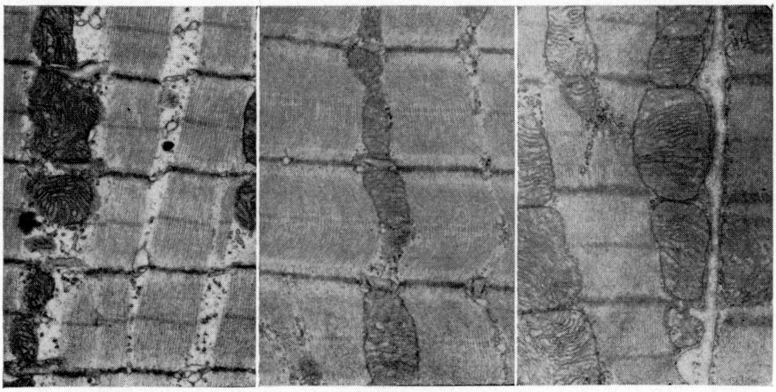

A B C

FIG. 5, 5. Fifteen minutes of ischaemia. Representative sections from three sites from a PP muscle which was grossly normal but was known to have been ischaemic for 15 minutes. Parts of 3 cells are shown. Each, though severely ischaemic, is viable in the sense that restoration of arterial flow would prevent cell death and allow almost instantaneous restoration in function. Site A shows the most severe changes in that glycogen is virtually absent and relaxation is marked. The mitochondria are similar in all 3 sections and are not objectively different from mitochondria in control LV of the same animal. There is a suggestion of swelling with a slight decrease in matrix density. Note that glycogen is present in cell B and quite abundant in cell C. The sarcolemma is intact in section C. Figure 5 in reference 3 is from the same dog and shows slight to mild margination of nuclear chromatin in addition to the changes noted in 5A. Osmium fixation. (Mag. ~16,600 ×.)

possible to state that the affected cells are swollen, but mitochondrial swelling usually is obvious. Capillaries are patent and are lined by intact endothelial cells.

Study of sections of PP between 30 and 45 minutes of ischaemia show variable findings. Some cells show the changes characteristic of ischaemic but viable cells (reversibly injured); others show changes similar to but less marked than those found in dying cells injured by 60 minutes of ischaemia (Fig. 5, 7). This qualitative variation in the type of changes noted was expected since transient ischaemia studies with prolonged periods of reflow[15] had shown that the number of irreversibly injured cells in the PP increases with time after the phase of reversible injury. About 50 per cent of dogs surviving a 20 minute transient occlusion show cell death in isolated cells or tiny groups of cells in the PP,[17] while about half the cells are dead at 40 minutes and almost all the cells are dead after 50 to 60 minutes of transient ischaemia.[15 18]

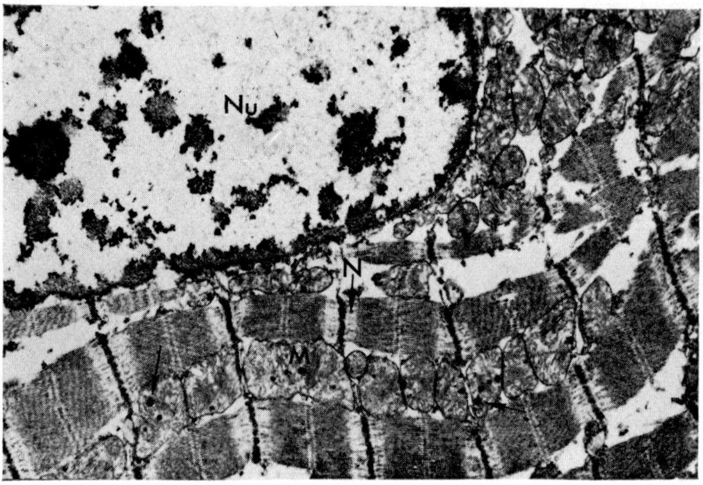

FIG. 5, 6. Sixty minutes of ischaemia. This section was taken from the pale PP tissue of the dog illustrated in Figure 5, 3 and illustrates the characteristic features of irreversible injury. The chromatin of the nucleus (Nu) shows marked margination. The mitochondria are enlarged and contain amorphous matrix densities (arrows). Figure 5, 11 is a high-power view of a mitochondrion from this tissue and shows the swelling, matrix densities and altered arrangement of cristae characteristic of damaged mitochondria. Glycogen is virtually absent from most cells irreversibly injured by 60 min of ischaemia, but the change is exaggerated in this section because of the method of fixation. The myofibrils are relaxed and show N bands in each I band region. Osmium fixation with uranyl acetate in block. (Mag. 13,300 ×.)

Small mitochondrial matrix densities first were noted in some affected myocardial cells at 40 minutes, while decreased matrix density and mitochondrial swelling were clearly observed in some cells of the PP after only 30 minutes of ischaemia. The preceding considerations about the diminishing incidence of cell death as the period of ischaemia is shortened precludes establishment of the earliest time at which the amorphous matrix densities first appear.

The various changes observed at 60 minutes become more marked with prolonged periods of ischaemia (Fig. 5, 8). The amorphous mitochondrial densities are larger and more abundant, 2 to 3 per mitochondrial profile. Also, the outer membrane of the mitochondrion often appears ruptured and the sarcolemma often shows discontinuities in its unit membrane structure.

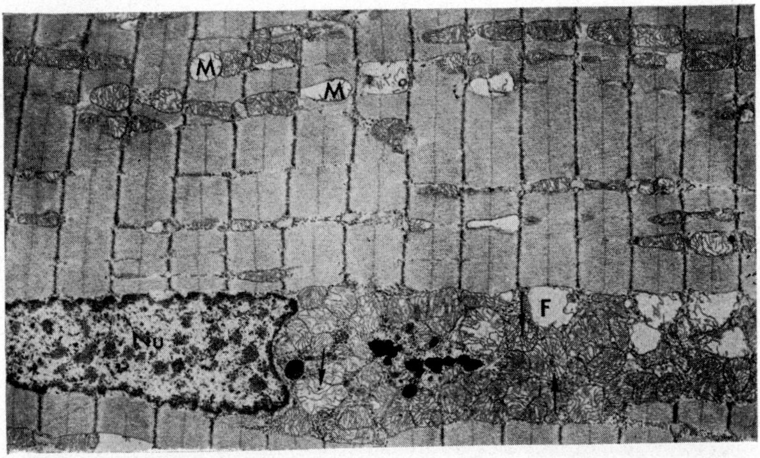

FIG. 5, 7. Forty minutes of ischaemia. Portion of a myocardial cell early in the phase of irreversible injury. Margination of the chromatin of the nucleus (Nu) is prominent as is relaxation of myofibrils and mitochondrial swelling (M) and fragmentation (F). A few small matrix densities are present (arrows). Glycogen granules are present, especially in the sarcoplasm adjacent to the nucleus. Osmium fixation. (Mag. 7,800 ×.)

Sections of ischaemic subepicardial myocardium, i.e. the lightly cross-hatched zone in Figure 5, 2, have not been studied in detail. The morphological and chemical changes in this zone of living ischaemic cells need investigation. The changes in ultrastructure observed during the reversible and irreversible phase are summarized in Table 5, 1.

Autolysis. Many of the chemical and structural changes found in an area of permanent ischaemia are mimicked *in vitro* by incubation of control myocardial tissue at 37°C in a sealed, moist environment.[5] The morphologic changes in this tissue follow a similar time

Table 5, 1. *Ultrastructure changes in acute ischaemia**

Reversible phase	Early irreversible phase
1. Myofibrils—relaxed	1. Same, often stretched
2. Sarcolemma—flattened	2. Stretched; shows defects after 60 minutes
3. Glycogen Early—no change Late—often decreased	3. Glycogen—low to absent
4. Nucleus Early—no change Late—slight margination	4. Nucleus—marked margination
5. Mitochondria Early—no change Late—swelling?	5. Mitochondria Swelling Fragility increased Amorphous matrix densities present

* References 3, 4, 5 and 21 contain the detailed studies which are the basis of this summary table.

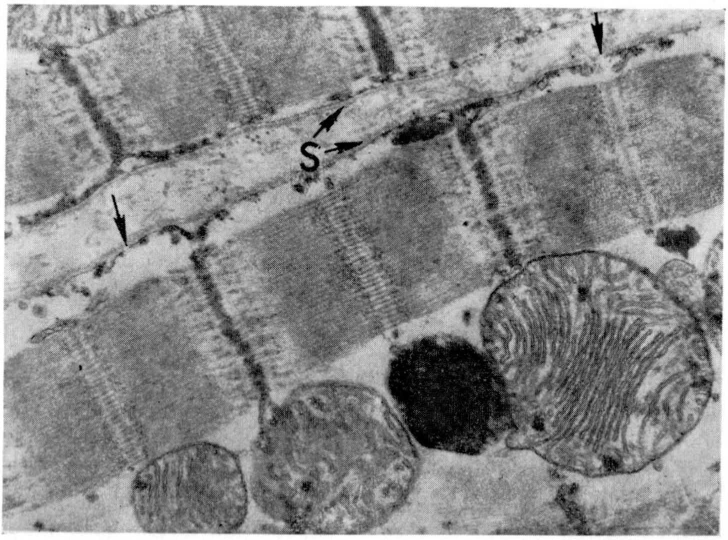

FIG. 5, 8. Four hours of ischaemia. Note extreme relaxation of myofibrils and defects in the plasma membrane of the sarcolemma (arrows). The mitochondria are swollen and contain matrix densities. The dense circular profile between the mitochondria is lipofuchsin. Osmium fixation. (Mag. ~18,900 ×.)

course to that found in permanent ischaemia (Fig. 5, 9) and include the appearance of similar mitochondrial and nuclear changes as well as the virtual disappearance of glycogen.[5] There are two principal differences between autolysis *in vitro* and permanent ischaemia *in vivo*. First is the fact that a variable amount of oxygenation is provided *in vivo* by collateral flow in contrast to the no-flow situation *in vitro*. The second difference involves the effect of the continuous massage of the damaged cells *in vivo* by the contracting non-ischaemic left ventricle. Whether trauma in particular and perhaps partial oxygenation accelerate ischaemic cell death in heart compared to other well-differentiated tissues such as the kidney[19] remain to be established.

Relaxation of the myofibrils is one morphologic change distinctive of permanent ischaemia *in vivo* which is uncommon in autolysis, presumably because stretching of the acontractile myocardium during systole does not occur *in vitro*.

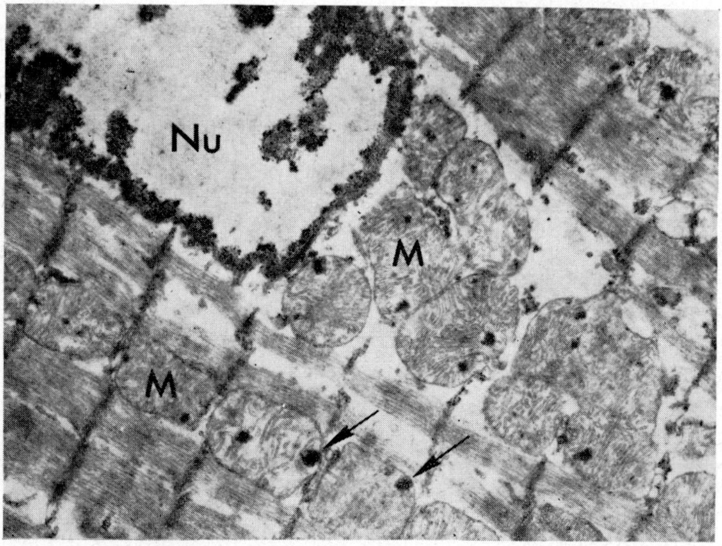

FIG. 5, 9. Two-hour autolysis. Portion of a myocardial cell showing peripheral aggregation of chromatin in the nucleus (Nu) and numerous amorphous matrix densities (arrows) in the mitochondria (M). Picture taken by Dr P. B. Herdson and is of the same field illustrated in Figure 4 of Reference 4. Osmium fixation. (Mag. 12,322 ×.)

Temporary ischaemia. It is important to note that myocardial cells killed by an episode of ischaemia of 40 minutes' duration and allowed varying intervals of arterial reflow develop striking changes in morphology which are different from those noted in equivalent periods of permanent ischaemia. The cells show very marked swelling, prominent contraction bands and swollen mitochondria which have not one but two kinds of intramitochondrial density. The first is the amorphous matrix density induced by 40 minutes of permanent ischaemia, while the other is a granular density of non-crystalline calcium phosphate and unknown components located in the region of the cristae.

Mitochondrial changes. The mitochondrial changes found in irreversibly injured myocardial cells require separate commentary not only because they appear to be one of the earliest structural features pathognomonic of irreversible injury in ischaemia but because adequate function of these organelles is important to the viability and adequate function of the myocardium.

The diagram in Figure 5, 10 illustrates the sequence of mitochondrial changes as a function of time. The mitochondria swell slightly and later develop amorphous densities in the matrix (Fig. 5, 11); these densities are first known to be present after 40 minutes of permanent ischaemia. As ischaemia persists, the number and size of these amorphous matrix densities increase, but they appear to stabilize in size and number after 2 to 3 hours of ischaemia.[5 20] We have not studied this preparation in detail for longer periods of time but have observed amorphous densities in myocardial infarcts several days old. The outer membrane of the mitochondria often is disrupted in tissue sections after as short a period of ischaemia as 40 minutes, but intact mitochondria with an outer membrane can still be isolated from PP after 60 minutes of ischaemic injury.[18, 21]

The amorphous matrix densities also appear in autolysis but are first noted at 60 minutes instead of 40 minutes and often are not abundant until after 90 minutes of ischaemia.[5] Preliminary histochemical results[22] have shown these amorphous densities to contain a high proportion of lipid. They also contain some calcium ions[23] but in insufficient quantities to leave an ash.[24] These findings are summarized in Table 5, 2.

The mitochondria of cells irreversibly injured by ischaemia and reperfused with arterial blood actively accumulate larger quantities

Table 5, 2. *Amorphous intramitochondrial matrix densities*

1. *Composition*
   (a) lipid
   (b) Ca^{++}
   (c) protein?
   (d) other?

2. *Formation**
   (a) irreversible ischaemic injury
   (b) *in vitro* autolysis < mitochondria / tissue
   (c) irreversible toxic injury

* Amorphous matrix densities are found in irreversible ischaemic injury in heart, Figures 5, 7 and 5, 12, or kidney,[19] in autolysis of myocardium, Figure 5, 10, liver or kidney[19] or of myocardial mitochondria *in vitro*.[22] They also are observed in cells irreversibly injured by toxins such as Hg.[26]

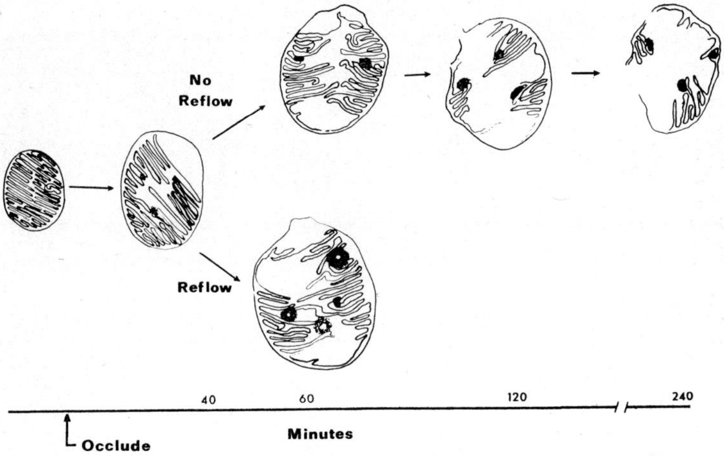

FIG 5, 10. Sequential changes in mitochondrial morphology as a function of ischaemia with and without arterial reflow. With permanent ischaemia (no reflow), the amorphous matrix densities first appear at 40 min. They enlarge and increase in number for the next 3 to 4 hours. Also, the mitochondria swell and often show ruptured outer membranes. If arterial reflow is allowed at 40 min, granular densities of calcium phosphate appear in or on the cristae of the involved mitochondria. Diagram made by Dr A. C. Shen and based on experiments described in References 24 and 25.

of calcium phosphate, presumably in the form of hydroxyapatite. These dense bodies are deposited on or in close proximity to the mitochondrial cristae, can be isolated and leave an ash after micro-incineration (Fig. 5, 10).[25] The accumulation of $CaPO_4$ densities by

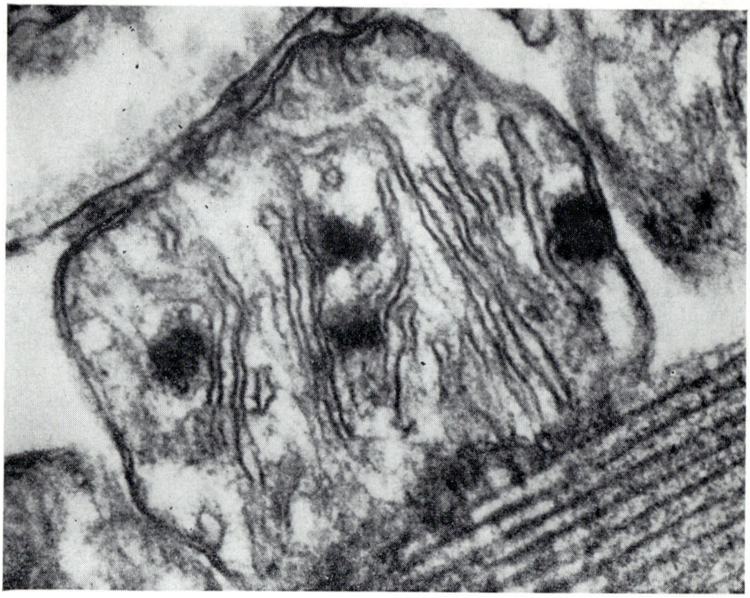

FIG. 5, 11. Sixty minutes of ischaemia. High-power view of a mitochondrion containing 4 amorphous matrix densities. Note that the outer membrane of the mitochondrion appears to be intact and that the cristae are widely separated compared to control mitochondria. Sarcolemma is at the upper left. Osmium fixation with uranyl acetate in block. (Mag. 75,000 ×.)

mitochondria probably is evidence that the cell membrane permeability of the irreversibly injured cell is sufficiently altered to allow calcium ions and perhaps phosphate to enter the cell in large enough quantities to be available for active accumulation by the mitochondria of the damaged cells. Thus, alterations in membrane permeability may be one of the earliest features of irreversible injury in myocardial cells.[20 24]

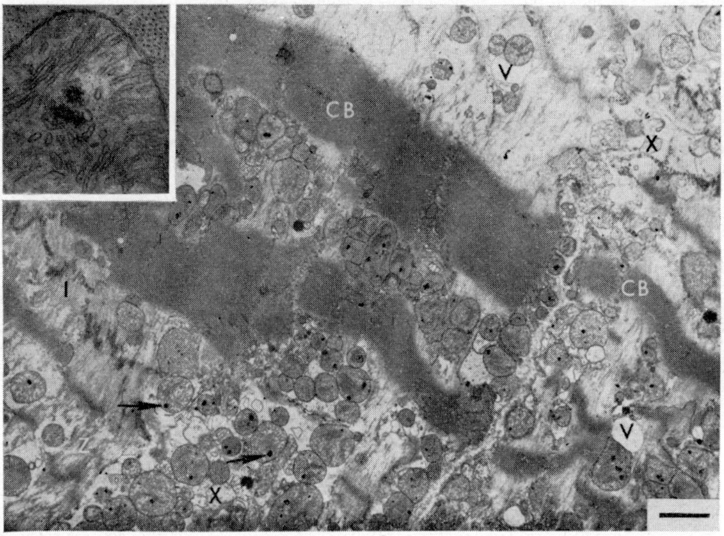

FIG. 5, 12 Posterior papillary muscle after 40 min of temporary ischaemia followed by 20 min of arterial blood flow. Note the disruption of myofibrillar architecture by prominent contraction bands (CB). Adjacent myofibrils are disrupted; remnants of Z lines are visible (Z) as is an intercalated disc (I). Except in the contraction bands, mitochondria appear to be swollen. Almost all mitochondrial profiles contain one or more prominent dense bodies (arrows). Partially disrupted mitochondria are present (X) as are membrane bound vacuoles (V). *Mark*=1 μm (lead acetate, ×9400). *Insert* shows a portion of a typical mitochondrion from the PP of this dog. It contains several clearly discernible densities. They are very electron opaque and exhibit a granular periphery and each exhibits a central clear zone (lead acetate, ×26,000). Reprinted with permission from Reference 24.

SUMMARY

The sequential ultrastructural changes occurring in myocardial cells of the dog heart after exposure to various degrees of ischaemic injury are described. The changes induced by ischaemia include depletion of glycogen and relaxation of myofibrils. Severe ischaemia of 10 to 15 minutes' duration also produces mild alterations in mitochondrial and nuclear morphology. Irreversible ischaemic injury is associated with margination of nuclear chromatin, virtual absence of glycogen, marked relaxation of myofibrils and characteristic mitochondrial abnormalities which include swelling, loss of matrix density and the appearance of amorphous matrix densities. Cells irreversibly injured by ischaemia and then reperfused with arterial blood show striking cellular swelling, severe contraction bands and the appearance of granular mitochondrial densities of $CaPO_4$ in addition to the amorphous matrix densities found in permanent ischaemia.

ACKNOWLEDGMENTS

Over the course of these experiments, P. B. Herdson, M.B., Ch.B., Ph.D.[3 4 5 21 23] and A. C. Shen, M.D., Ph.D.[23 24 25] have contributed much to the evaluation of the changes in ultrastructure associated with ischaemic injury. Hannah Schellin, W. B. Taylor, Barbara Moulton and Saideh Safavi have provided expert technical assistance.

REFERENCES

1 JENNINGS, R. B. (1970). Myocardial ischemia—observations, definitions and speculations. *Journal Molecular and Cellular Cardiology* **1,** 345-348.

2 JENNINGS, R. B. & REIMER, K. A. (1972, in press). In *New perspectives in diagnosis and management of myocardial infarction.* Edited by: E. Corday and H. J. C. Swan. Baltimore Md.: Williams & Wilkins.

3 JENNINGS, R. B., BAUM, J. H. & HERDSON, P. B. (1965). Fine structural changes in myocardial ischemic injury. *Archives of Pathology* **79,** 135-143.

4 HERDSON, P. B., SOMMERS, H. M. & JENNINGS, R. B. (1965). A comparative study of the fine structure of normal and ischaemic dog myocardium with special reference to early changes following temporary occlusion of a coronary artery. *American Journal of Pathology* **46,** 367-386.

5 HERDSON, P. B., KALTENBACH, J. P. & JENNINGS, R. B. (1969). Fine structural and biochemical changes in dog myocardium during autolysis. *American Journal of Pathology* **57,** 539-551.

6 JENNINGS, R. B., WARTMAN, W. B. & ZUDYK, Z. E. (1957). Production of an area of homogenous myocardial infarction in the dog. *AMA Archives Pathology* **63,** 580-585.

7 ELLIOT, E. C., JONES, E. L., BLOOR, C. M., LEON, A. S. & GREGG, D. E. (1968). Day-to-day changes in coronary hemodynamics secondary to constriction of circumflex branch of left coronary artery in conscious dogs. *Circulation Research* **22,** 237-250.

8 KHOURI, E. M., GREGG, D. E. & MCGRANAHAN, G. M. (1971). Regression and reappearance of coronary collaterals. *American Journal of Physiology* **220,** 655-661.

9 JENNINGS, R. B. (1969). Early phase of myocardial ischemic injury and infarction. *American Journal of Cardiology* **24,** 753-756.

10 JENNINGS, R. B., KALTENBACH, J. P., SOMMERS, H. M., BAHR, G. F. & WARTMAN, W. B. (1963). In *The Etiology of Myocardial Infarction* (Henry Ford Hospital International Symposium) p. 189. Edited by: T. M. James and J. W. Keyes. Boston: Little Brown & Co.

11 BECKER, L. C., FORTUIN, N. J. & PITT, B. (1971). Effect of ischemia and antianginal drugs on the distribution of radioactive microspheres in the canine left ventricle. *Circulation Research* **28,** 263-269.

12 GILLESPIE, W. J. & LOVE, W. D. (1967). Gradients in the regional rates of myocardial rubidium-86 clearance in tranquilized dogs. *Circulation Research* **20,** 606-615.
13 MOIR, T. W. & DEBRA, D. W. (1967). Effect of left ventricle hypertension, ischemia and vasoactive drugs on the myocardial distribution of coronary flow. *Circulation Research* **21,** 65-74.
14 KIRK, E. S. & HONIG, C. R. (1964). An experimental and theoretical analysis of myocardial tissue pressure. *American Journal of Physiology* **207,** 361-367.
15 JENNINGS, R. B., SOMMERS, H. M., SMYTH, F. A., FLACK, H. A. & LINN, H. (1960). Myocardial necrosis induced by temporary occlusion of a coronary artery in the dog. *AMA Archives of Pathology* **70,** 68-78.
16 JENNINGS, R. B., SOMMERS, H. M., KALTENBACH, J. P. & WEST, J. J. (1964). Electrolyte alterations in acute myocardial ischemic injury. *Circulation Research* **14,** 260-269.
17 SOMMERS, H. M. & JENNINGS, R. B. (1972). Ventricular fibrillation and myocardial necrosis after transient ischemia. *Archives of Internal Medicine* **129,** 780-789.
18 JENNINGS, R. B., SOMMERS, H. M., HERDSON, P. B. & KALTENBACH, J. P. (1969). Cardiopathies and factors influencing myocardial degeneration. *Annals of the New York Academy of Science* **156,** 61-78.
19 REIMER, K. A., GANOTE, C. E. & JENNINGS, R. B. (1972). Alterations in renal cortex following ischemic injury. *Laboratory Investigation* **26,** 347-363.
20 JENNINGS, R. B. & SHEN, A. C. (1972). In *Myocardiology, Volume I* p. 639. Recent advances in studies of cell structure and metabolism. Edited: E Bajucz & C.. Rona. Baltimore, London, Tokyo: University Park Press.
21 JENNINGS, R. B., HERDSON, P. B. & SOMMERS, H. M. (1969). Structural and functional abnormalities in mitochondria isolated from ischemic dog myocardium. *Laboratory Investigation* **20,** 548-557.
22 GANOTE, C. E., JENNINGS, R. B., & SHEN, A. Unpublished results.
23 JENNINGS, R. B., MOORE, C. B., SHEN, A. C. & HERDSON, P. B. (1970). Electrolytes of damaged myocardial mitochondria. *Proceedings of the Society of Experimental Biology and Medicine* **135,** 515-522.
24 SHEN, A. C. & JENNINGS, R. B. (1972). Myocardial calcium and magnesium in acute ischaemic injury. *American Journal of Pathology* **67,** 417-440.
25 SHEN, A. C. & JENNINGS, R. B. (1967). Kinetics of calcium accumulation in acute myocardial ischaemic injury. *American Journal of Pathology* **67,** 441-452.
26 GRITZKA, T. L. & TROMP, B. F. (1952). Renal tubular lesions caused by mercuric chloride. Electron microscopic observations: degeneration of the pars recta. *American Journal of Pathology* **52,** 1225-1277.
27 JENNINGS, R. B., KALTENBACH, J. P. & SMETHERS, G. W. (1957). Enzymatic changes in acute myocardial ischemic injury; glutamic oxaloacetic transaminase, lactic dehydrogenases and succinic dehydrogenase. *AMA Archives of Pathology* **64,** 10-16.
28 JENNINGS, R. B., SOMMERS, H. M., KALTENBACH, J. P. & WEST, J. J. (1964). Electrolyte alterations in acute myocardial ischemic injury. *Circulation Research* **14,** 260-269.

DISCUSSION

Parratt. Within 5 minutes of sampling blood from a coronary vein draining an ischaemic region, the P_{CO_2} goes up by 20 mm and the pH and oxygen content fall. These changes reach a peak after 30 min and then tend to recover over the next 4 hours. Blood sampled after 4 hours is essentially the same as that sampled before ligation. Can you relate these metabolic changes to what is happening in the cells? Presumably at this time there is a mixture of completely dead cells and dying cells with cells that are for some reason extracting more oxygen than normal, otherwise it is difficult to explain the fact that oxygen extraction by the ischaemic region is ' normal '. Could you perhaps comment on the relationship between these metabolic changes and the ultrastructural changes you have described?

Jennings. The basic question here involves many points which are not known. In order to determine with precision the relationship between what one is measuring in effluent blood with cellular changes occurring in the area of injury, one must know the character of the area of injury, the state of the vascular bed, and the sources of blood draining into the vein. Since I am certain that the metabolic state of the cells in the area is continuously changing, at least for the first day after occlusion, and since I suspect that flow is changing as well as a function of time, I don't think you can relate the observed changes in venous blood constituents to anything but the general effects of ischaemia. Recently published data[11] makes it clear to me that during the acute phase most of the venous blood must be coming from the collateral flow going to the subepicardial myocardium. It should reveal, therefore, changes which are the consequence of mild ischaemia. Venous blood from a local vein in the ischaemic area should show more marked changes than one would observe in the coronary sinus, because of the great dilution of ischaemic blood in the coronary sinus by blood draining non-ischaemic areas.

Since the area of ischaemia is a dynamic focus of continuously changing character (see ref. 9 for a more detailed discussion), I would expect the venous blood drawn several hours after occlusion to show different changes than would be observed acutely. After all, a proportion of the cells in the area of ischaemia have died. In Figure 5, 3, the densely shaded subendocardial area should be largely ametabolic at 1 hour and certainly at 4 hours. Also, I have well-founded suspicions that arterial flow through the densely shaded focus probably ceases at some future time. I have never investigated the flow in detail but would point out that it heals from the outside in rather than throughout as one would expect it to if it still received uniform arterial flow.

Lassers. My question is about the microscopic appearances of lipids accumulated in the myocardium during ischaemia. First, do you ever see this accumulation in those areas which have been completely deprived of their blood supply? Secondly, if you do see lipids, or if you only see them in areas which are relatively ischaemic, rather than totally ischaemic, how long does it take before they begin to be visible microscopically?

Jennings. First, we have never seen much histologically detectable lipid in the posterior papillary muscle area of injury. The neutral fat which appears in most cells that are injured by ischaemia or other processes, i.e. so-called fatty change, is lipid which is delivered to the cell as FFA and then is synthesized to neutral fat. Thus, cells in an area of total ischaemia, i.e. with no blood flow, or cells which are very severely injured will not accumulate lipid. Secondly, cells will accumulate lipid if they are receiving some exogenous flow for a significant period of time, that is a long enough period of time to have taken in some lipid and turned it to neutral fat. At this time one can detect it histologically. We haven't studied this phenomena in this particular area of infarction but in collaboration with Wartman and Yozoyana (*Archives of Pathology,* **62,** 318-323, (1957)) have studied it a long time ago in another infarct. This is a small infarct produced by ligation of the descending branch of the left coronary immediately above a branch which goes towards the apex. Neutral fat first appeared in the cells which were reversibly injured after 3 to 5 hours of occlusion. Lipid did not appear in necrotic cells. This is not necessarily a very sensitive means of detecting lipid but it represents a discrete way of identifying which cells contain this material. Moreover, cells which are severely hypoxic cannot metabolize FFA because of the absence of oxygen, so I assume that potential FFA toxicity would only be a problem in cells which are mildly ischaemic.

Carlson. Dr Jennings, do I understand you correctly when you say that you don't see lipid stores in the normal dog myocardium?

Jennings. Very little in the normal dog heart myocardium.

Carlson. I am surprised because our electron microscopists in Stockholm said they could demonstrate visible lipid droplets in the heart of normal fasting dogs. Chemical methods show there is an appreciable amount of triglyceride present.

Jennings. I have measured it only by histochemical means. I am not saying that there is no triglyceride present for we have seen droplets of lipid in myocardial cells in control as well as in ischaemic tissue, but these are not a prominent feature of healthy mongrel dogs in Chicago. The controls for the 1957 paper referred to earlier also showed very little neutral fat. I should point out that chemical analyses of the myocardium for triglyceride should only be made after removal of epicardial and fibrous tissues which may contain neutral fat.

Carlson. What is the nutritional condition of your dogs?

Jennings. They are healthy mongrel dogs.

Carlson. Are they fasted or fed?

Jennings. They are fasted overnight to prevent regurgitation during anaesthesia. All operations are performed in the morning.

Oliver. This apparent difference of opinion is largely a question of methods of analysis. Dr Jennings bases his views on the results of electron microscopic and staining methods, while we and others have shown by biochemical analyses that there is an appreciable amount of triglyceride in the heart. In normal dogs, there is more in the right ventricle compared with the left: with ischaemia, left ventricular triglyceride increases significantly.

Carlson. *Electron* microscopic pictures prepared by our pathologists at the Karolinska show that the normal dog heart always contains intra-cellular lipid droplets close to the mitochondria.

Jennings. I think the time intervals are very important. What time intervals are you talking about?

Carlson. These were not ischaemic studies but normal dog hearts taken out during pentobarbital anaesthesia after various time intervals.

Opie. Regarding Dr Parratt's comments, Dr Thomas and I presented some data on the local venous changes in the ischaemic dog heart (*American Journal of Cardiology,* **25:**562, 1970; *Lancet* **1:**1187, 1969). Marked metabolic changes, for example lactate discharge, were found in local venous blood for about 20 to 30 minutes and then passed. This raised the question of which part of the tissue was being drained by local venous blood apparently coming from the ischaemic tissue. The addition of coronary flow values was needed. It seems that Dr Parratt can answer this question from his flow studies with xenon.

Parratt. I can't really answer that question. If you measure flow in the infarct within 30 minutes of ligation it is down to about 10 to 20 per cent of normal, and it stays at this level over a 4 hour period during which there are marked differences in the coronary venous blood gases. There is, however, very little change in xenon clearance over this same period.

Jennings. It is very important to recognize that there is a difference between subendocardial and epicardial arterial flow. Again I refer to the work of Becker and colleagues,[11] subendocardial flow occurs during diastole so that one would expect decreased subendocardial flow in any dog with a slight increase in end-diastolic pressure in the left ventricle or any dog with an increased heart rate. I think it would be very difficult by xenon washout to say anything about true difference in regional flow through the wall of the heart, since endocardial xenon is compared to epicardial xenon. All that you would probably obtain is net flow, but net flow doesn't mean much anyway.

Kurien. Wartman (in *Etiology of Myocardial Infarction,* ed. T. M. James and J. W. Keyes. Churchill, London, p. 115, 1963) showed that there is accumulation of neutral fat in the ischaemic area from 1 to 6 hours after coronary artery occlusion. When he restained this area, he showed there was calcium sequestration in the areas in which there was fat deposition. Do you think calcium sequestration occurs in the mitochondria along with deposition of lipid?

Jennings. You will remember the appearance of irreversibly injured cells from an area of permanent ischaemia in the posterior papillary (PP) preparation (see Fig. 5, 2). In Figure 5, 4 the cells are different. One sees disruption in the cellular architecture, enormous swelling, very marked contraction bands containing as many as 10 compressed sarcomeres. Mitochondria are swollen except where they are caught in the contraction bands. Present within the mitochondria are two kinds of density, the kind you are already familiar with and a new kind which is present in or adjacent to the cristae and is composed of calcium: these are entirely different from those which one sees in an area of permanent ischaemia. They represent active calcium accumulation by the involved mitochondria.

The source of the calcium is the arterial flow which is reperfusing the area. Shen and I[25] have shown this clearly by labelling the plasma with a tracer dose of radioactive calcium. This technique reveals uptake of calcium into the irreversibily injured tissue over a period of about 10 minutes. The amount of calcium present increases by about 10 times over the control. The calcium and phosphorus of mitochondria isolated from the tissue also is markedly increased. There is little calcium increase in the PP infarct but probably there is some in a zone 2 or 3 cells wide along the edge of the area of cell death. This zone also shows contraction bands and presumably represents a zone of cell death associated with enough blood flow to provide calcium to induce these increased morphologic changes. The above changes allow me to preach again the philosophy that an acute area of ischaemia is a very dynamic focus which is continuously changing in composition. Some cells in the boundary zone are more ischaemic than the superficial myocardium. An episode of paroxysmal ventricular tachycardia or some other phenomenon which decreases coronary blood flow should induce enough ischaemia to kill more cells in this area of injury. An infarct is not stable until scarred and there is well oxygenated myocardium supported by adequate collateral flow on the superficial surface. To come back to the fat, it occurs in cells which have some exogenous flow, enough flow to keep them alive and deliver FFA to allow accumulation of neutral fat.

Randle. Orth and Morgan (*Journal of Cellular Biology* 1962, **15,** 509-523) reported on triglyceride droplets in electron-micrographs of anoxic muscle. These were in rat hearts perfused with saline, so that there was no question of this triglyceride being synthesized from exogenous fatty acid. We have found that rat heart contains triglyceride by chemical analysis and there are good reasons for thinking it is in muscle fibres and not in any sequestered adipose tissue. Under aerobic conditions, triglyceride cannot be visualized in the normal heart with fat stains. Triglyceride droplets can be seen in the diabetic heart under aerobic conditions where there is about twice or three times as much triglyceride. I think Orth and Morgan concluded that the fat droplets had coalesced under anaerobic conditions to a size where they were visible. In the diabetic heart, where fat droplets can be seen under aerobic conditions, the fat droplets tended to collect around mitochondria.

Herbaczynska-Cedro. Have you studied by histochemical methods which myocardial enzymes might have changed in the early period of myocardial ischaemia?

Jennings. We have not studied the PP infarct with anything but routine histochemical techniques. Depletion of glycogen occurs in the PP infarct as soon as you see the gross colour change associated with irreversibility. We have demonstrated loss of enzyme activity as a function of time.[15] Glutamic oxaloacetic transaminase decreased significantly between 60 min and 120 min after occlusion; LDH activity decreased around 2 hours after occlusion. These decreases were all relative to activity measured in control non-ischaemic myocardium of the same animal. Succinic dehydrogenase activity does not change for 4 to 5 hours; this is exactly what one would expect with an enzyme which is really insoluble and a part of the mitochondrial cristae structure. Some mitochondria do not disappear quickly and one would not expect to detect early changes in the activity of this enzyme.

Wallace. Is there such a thing as chronic ischaemia? You have a very precise way of defining what a reversibly anoxic cell looks like, can that characteristic persist for a long period of time?

Jennings. I think that a very critical and important question. I don't know exactly how to answer it. Ischaemia, by definition, means that there has been a reduction in the arterial flow. Since we don't have a precise technique of measuring changes in arterial flow, except instantaneously with plastic radioactive microspheres, we are restricted to some other definition of whether ischaemia is present or not. So far as I'm concerned that other definition is that ischaemia is present when flow is reduced to the point where one can detect a shift in cellular metabolism from the aerobic to the anaerobic form.

Myocardial cells which survive in the PP infarct in dogs (Fig. 5, 3) must go on for a period of time using some oxygen from collateral flow but presumably they receive an inadequate amount to maintain aerobic metabolism. These cells thus appear to function by a mixture of aerobic and anaerobic metabolism but predominantly by anaerobic metabolism. Since this probably goes on for hours and perhaps days, I think that this represents a kind of 'chronic ischaemia'. It may occur in man as well but I would be very strict in defining its presence by requiring anaerobic metabolism to be identified in the involved zone.[1]

Reduced arterial flow means not only reduced oxygen but decreased clearance of metabolites like lactic acid. This is why I believe Dr Maseri's results in the patient with angina. He showed actual decreased flow in the myocardium in man. Perhaps accumulation of an anaerobic product like lactic acid is the cause of the angina. If chronic ischaemia exists in man, perhaps one should require chronic pain to be present as well.

Riemersma. You described experiments in which you isolated mitochondria from the ischaemic myocardium. Could you isolate from the ischaemic mitochondria enough lipid material to allow you to identify its chemical composition? Can you show that there is increased triglyceride in the mitochondria themselves rather than in the cell as a whole, or were the substances identified as FFA or phospholipid?

Jennings. You can isolate mitochondria from control myocardium and from injured myocardium quite easily in potassium chloride or sucrose, and then can compare the lipid composition of those mitochondria. You have the problem that the mitochondria from the injured tissue are changing in composition relative to the control. An appropriate reference base for comparison must be drawn from dry weight, nitrogen, phospholipid, phosphate or protein. None is ideal unless the measured change is marked.

Riemersma. Did you do this for mitochondria and what did you find?

Jennings. We have not studied neutral fat or triglyceride distribution in mitochondria but have shown that the amorphous matrix densities are soluble in lipid solvents (Shen, Jennings & Ganote, unpublished data).

REPARATIVE PROCESSES FOLLOWING ACUTE CORONARY ARTERY OCCLUSION

S. GUDBJARNASON

THE purpose of this study was to examine the major biochemical alterations observed in cardiac muscle following acute coronary artery ligation in the dog. The reaction of cardiac muscle to acute coronary occlusion may be divided into three phases:

Phase I. This is the early period of ischaemia and reversible biochemical alterations in the ischaemic myocardium (Table 6, 1).

Table 6, 1 *Reversible biochemical changes in ischaemic heart muscle*

1. Diminution in myocardial oxygen tension
   50 per cent decrease in 15 sec
2. Activation of anaerobic glycolysis
   15 sec after coronary occlusion
3. Inhibition of ATP-utilization (energy transfer)
   30 sec
4. Depletion of creatine phosphate (energy reserve)
   30 to 60 sec
5. Diminution in rate of anaerobic glycolysis
   30 to 60 sec
6. Impaired contractile activity
   15 to 30 sec
7. Cessation of contractile activity
   60 to 90 sec

Following diminution in myocardial oxygen tension there is rapid activation of anaerobic glycolysis and myocardial lactate accumulation is observed 15 sec after coronary occlusion or even earlier.[1] The increase in lactate accumulation is followed by an inhibition of ATP-utilization in the presence of unimpaired utilization of creatine phosphate (CP)-stores. Following depletion of CP-stores the rate of lactate-production (accumulation) diminishes again as early as 30 to 60 sec after coronary occlusion (Fig. 6, 1). The rate of energy utilization diminishes rapidly from 0·393 μmole-P/g$\times$beat during the period 15 to 30 sec after coronary occlusion to 0·096 μmole—P/g×beat during the period 15-30 sec after coronary ligation. Contractile activity in the ischaemic area diminishes rapidly and the ischaemic muscle stops contracting about 1 min after coronary ligation, at a relatively high ATP level of 4·5 μmole/g, when only

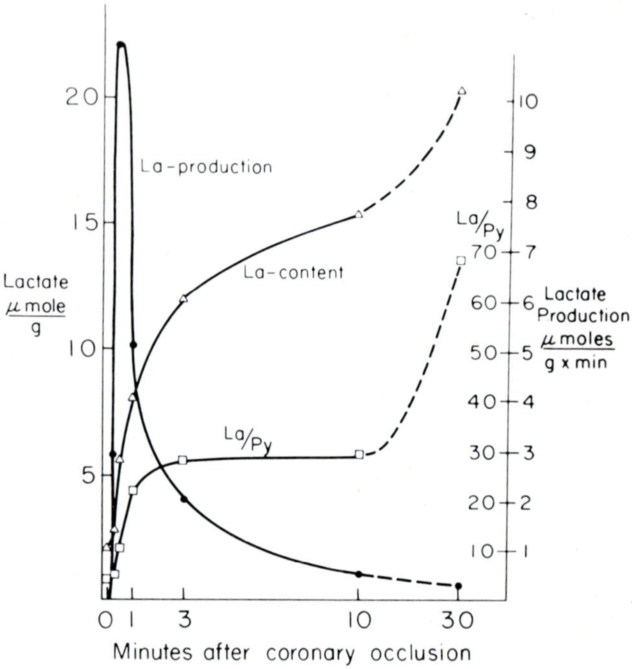

FIG. 6, 1. Changes in the rate of lactate production (μmoles/g x min), lactate content (μmole/g) and lactate-pyruvate ratio (La/Py).

about 20 per cent of the ATP has been utilized. Non-ischaemic cardiac muscle is able to survive and maintain contraction at ATP levels as low as 1·5 to 2·0 μmole/g.[1]

Why does contractile activity stop at relatively high ATP levels in the ischaemic muscle when the non-ischaemic muscle can maintain contractile activity at much lower energy levels? At least two hypothesis have been offered to explain the early cessation of contractile activity in ischaemic cardiac muscle:

1. The increase in intracellular hydrogen ion (H^+) concentration accompanying anaerobic glycolysis depresses the responsiveness of contractile proteins to calcium ions (Ca^{2+}). Katz and Hecht[2] have suggested that H^+ and Ca^{2+} compete for troponin binding sites. The increase in H^+-concentration causes a displacement of the Ca^{2+} bound to troponin reducing the number of troponin molecules bound to Ca^{2+} during systole.[2] The result would be fewer points of release of the inhibition of the actin-myosin interaction, i.e. diminution in Ca^{2+} induced reversal of the tropomyosin-troponin inhibition of the myosin-actin interaction and reduced contractility.

2. The second hypothesis suggests that the increase in intracellular H^+-concentration interferes with intracellular energy-transfer and inhibits the transfer of intramitochondrial energy to the extramitochondrial compartment for utilization in contractile processes.[1]

The loss of contractility is not necessarily permanent and the ischaemic cells regain their contractility if the arterial flow is restored. If the ischaemic period is prolonged beyond 15 to 20 minutes, there is an exponential increase in death of muscle cells with increase in time after cessation of blood flow. More and more dead cells appear with progressive increase in the period of ischaemia and after 45 minutes of ischaemia over 50 per cent of the affected cells have died.

The rapidity of cellular and particularly mitochondrial deterioration appears to depend on the functional state of the ischaemic muscle. Non-functioning ischaemic muscle survives longer than, for example, electrically stimulated ischaemic muscle.

Phase II. Irreversible biochemical changes in infarcted heart muscle during tissue repair.

1. Metabolism

When the ischaemic myocardial cells enter the state of irreversible biochemical alteration, the heart muscle develops myocardial necrosis with subsequent tissue repair and replacement of necrotic muscle by connective tissue[3,4] (Table 6, 2).

The alteration in the energy level of the infarcted myocardium is illustrated by the changes in ATP and CP concentrations of the necrotic tissue. The tissue content of the high energy phosphates decreases by 80 to 90 per cent during the first few minutes of ischaemia. Following death of myocardial cells and commencement of tissue repair, the content of high energy phosphates increases slowly in the infarcted area. The ATP content increases from 1·05 μmole/g 24 hours after infarction, to 2·1 μmole/g on

Table 6, 2. *Irreversible biochemical changes in infarcted heart muscle during tissue repair*

1. *Energy metabolism*		
	a. High energy phosphate levels	
	b. Enzymatic alterations	
	Hexosemonophosphate-shunt enzymes	
	Oxidative enzymes	
	Glycolytic enzymes	
2. *Anabolic (biosynthetic) processes*		
	a. RNA	nucleolar RNA
		messenger RNA
		microsomal RNA
	b. DNA	tissue content
		rate of formation
	c. Protein	nuclear protein
		microsomal protein
		contractile protein
		collagen
3. *Catabolic processes, i.e. removal of necrotic muscle*		
	Lysosomal enzymes	
		Deoxyribonuclease
		Acid phosphatase
		β-Glucuronidase
		γ-Glutamyl-transpeptidase

the tenth day (Fig. 6, 2). The increase in the energy level of the infarcted tissue is accompanied by a marked alteration in metabolism of the necrotic cardiac muscle.

The metabolic activity of infarcted tissue observed 1 to 10 days after infarction represents primarily the activity of invading leucocytes, fibroblasts and other cells involved in removal of dead cells and formation of new connective tissue. The biosynthetic processes and cellular proliferation in the infarcted area requires energy that cannot be provided by aerobic metabolism but must be produced largely in absence of oxygen. The alteration in the enzyme profile of the infarcted tissue illustrates the transition from aerobic to anaerobic metabolism.

Hexosemonophosphate-shunt activity: Following sudden coronary occlusion, the repair process is characterized by a significant increase in hexosemonophosphate shunt (HMP) activity. This increase is illustrated by a continuous increase in the activity of glucose-6-phosphate dehydrogenase (G-6-PDH) and 6-phosphogluconate dehydrogenase (6-PGDH) for at least 10 days following coronary artery occlusion.[8 4 5] Ten days after infarction the activity of

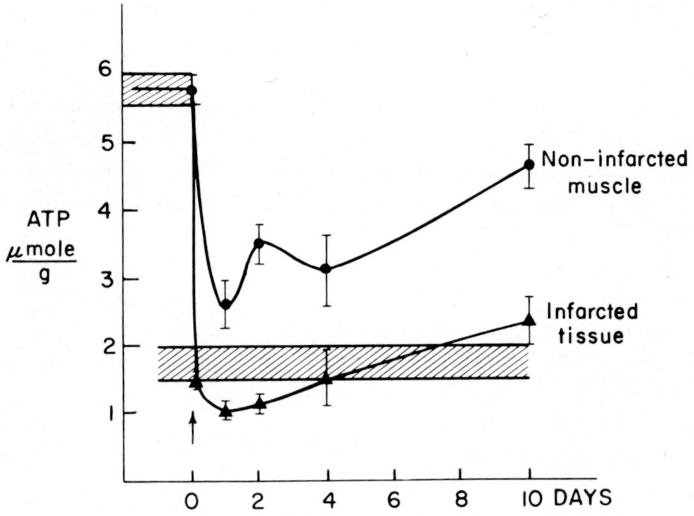

FIG. 6, 2. Changes in tissue content of ATP in infarcted and non-infarcted heart muscle.

G-6-PDH had increased 34-fold in the centre of infarct and 23-fold in the periphery of infarct.[5] The activity of 6-PGDH was similarly elevated in the infarcted tissue.[5] Nine months after coronary occlusion, the activity of G-6-PDH was still significantly higher in the scar tissue of the healed infarct than in normal cardiac muscle.[3] This increase in hexosemonophosphate shunt activity may in part be due to phagocytosis and the earliest appearance of G-6-PDH and 6-PGDH in the periphery rather than in the centre of the infarct provides some biochemical evidence that these enzymes may be carried by leucocytes. However, the persistent elevation of G-6-PDH as late as nine months after the infarction suggests that the elevated hexosemonophosphate shunt activity in the affected area is not due to phagocytosis alone, but may reflect the fibroblastic proliferation in the developing scar tissue.

An important role of the HMP-shunt in cell proliferation and accumulation of specific cell products has been observed in developing organs. Studies on the development of pig heart,[6] sea urchin embryo,[7] and chick brain[8] indictate that the development of an organ and the increased demand for specific substrates for RNA and DNA synthesis and cell proliferation require a high level of HMP-shunt activity. A high level of the HMP-shunt was observed in irreversibly injured necrotic heart muscle when connective scar tissue replace necrotic muscle cells.

The increase in HMP-shunt activity of injured heart muscle is not limited to the infarcted area but also extends, to a smaller degree, to non-infarcted areas of the left ventricle.[4] This increase in non-infarcted muscle probably reflects the development of compensatory cardiac hypertrophy in the surviving muscle. The adjustment of the muscle to the increased workload requires, according to Meerson,[9] an increased activity of the HMP-shunt thus facilitating nucleic acid and protein synthesis. This provides the necessary substrates for development of cardiac hypertrophy. An increase in fibroblastic proliferation in cardiac muscle has also been observed in cardiac hypertrophy.[10] It is therefore not possible to ascribe the increased HMP-shunt activity exclusively to heart muscle cells, since the increase in number of fibroblasts in the hypertrophied heart might also be responsible for the increased HMP-shunt activity.

Glycolytic and oxidative enzymes

In contrast to the marked increase in activity in the HMP-shunt, there was a significant decline in the activity of both oxidative and glycolytic enzymes in infarcted cardiac muscle.[3,4] Mitochondrial enzymes, such as NAD- and NADP-specific isocitrate dehydrogenase, malate dehydrogenase and glutamate oxaloacetate transaminase reached the lowest level in the centre of the infarcted tissue ten days after infarction with 8 to 13 per cent of normal activity. Ten weeks after infarction, there was some recovery of enzyme activities with an increase to 17 to 40 per cent of the control.[3,4]

The activity of glycolytic enzymes was also significantly decreased. Aldolase and lactate dehydrogenase (LDH) activity decreased to 14 and 21 per cent of original activity respectively, whereas the activity of glyceraldehyde phosphate dehydrogenase (GAPDH) was reduced somewhat less to 32 per cent of control ten days after infarction.[3,4]

The periphery and centre of the infarct showed similar enzyme activity 24 hours after infarction, but 10 days and even 10 weeks after infarction the periphery had about 2 to 3 times higher activity than the centre of the infarct.[3 4] The relatively high activity of GAPDH remaining in infarcted tissue indicates that anaerobic sub-

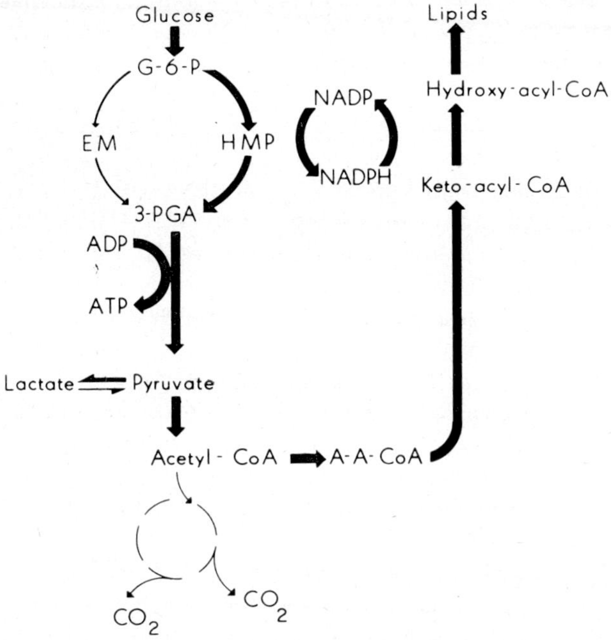

FIG. 6, 3. Metabolism of infarcted heart muscle. The heavy lines indicate metabolic pathways that have increased in activity in the infarcted tissue during tissue repair (hexosemonophosphate-shunt and lipid synthesis). The thin lines indicate diminished activity of the Krebs cycle and a segment of the Embden-Meyerhof pathway.

strate phosphorylation of ADP to ATP can continue at relatively high levels in the ischaemic and infarcted area.

The quantitative decrease in LDH activity of infarcted muscle was also accompanied by qualitative changes in the iso-enzyme pattern.[11]

LDH is a tetrameric molecule made up of four subunits of the two principal molecules, H (heart) and M (muscle) type. The iso-enzymes of LDH represent the combination of these two subunits into five distinct molecular forms: H_4, H_3M, H_2M_2, HM_3 and M_4; classified as isoenzymes, I, II, III, IV and V. The synthesis of the H and M subunits appears to be regulated independently[12] and an example of the independent regulation of H and M genes is provided by alterations in oxygen tension, both *in vivo* and *in vitro*. The changes in the synthesis of LDH subunits with changes in oxygen tension support the proposed physiological role of M and H proteins. The low oxygen tension favours synthesis of M-LDH, the form best suited for anaerobic metabolism. High oxygen tension favours synthesis of the H enzyme, the form which predominates in aerobic tissues.[12]

In normal dog heart muscle LDH displays only three isozymes, with two strong bands representing isoenzyme I (H_4) and II (H_3M), and one weak band representing isoenzyme III (H_2M_2).[4 9] In the infarcted tissue all five isoenzymes can be observed, and in this tissue the relative strengths of bands III, IV (HM_3) and V (M_4) are similar to those of bands I and II.

The diminution in LDH activity of infarcted heart muscle is, in part, due to a release of LDH into the coronary sinus blood and in part due to inactivation of the enzyme or altered enzyme kinetics accompanying the changes in isoenzyme pattern. The release of LDH and other myocardial enzymes into the blood has been utilized to aid in the diagnosis of myocardial infarction.[13] The presence of recent myocardial infarction is characterized by a gross increase in the activity of isoenzyme I (or isoenzyme I and II) in serum, due to necrosis and increased permeability of ischaemic heart muscle.[13] The decrease in isoenzymes I and II in the infarcted, necrotic muscle is paralleled by a relative increase in isoenzymes III, IV and V and probably reflects the replacement of the necrotic muscle by connective tissue. The ischaemic environment of the infarcted tissue, with its low oxygen tension, may thus favour synthesis of M-LDH, the form best suited for anaerobic metabolism[12] and this increase in synthesis of M-LDH is illustrated in the increase in isoenzyme IV (HM_3) and isoenzyme V (M_4) in the infarcted heart muscle.

2. Anabolic processes

The synthesis of new protein and nucleic acids in infarcted heart muscle was studied by examining the incorporation of glycine-2-^{14}C

into protein, DNA and various types of RNA. ^{14}C-glycine was chosen as a tracer because it constitutes a relatively large portion of the collagen (30 per cent) and because it is also incorporated into the purine ring of both RNA and DNA.

The tissue content of nucleic acids in infarcted muscle changed considerably following coronary occlusion. The tissue content of RNA fell immediately after infarction, but then increased two days after infarction. There was a parallel increase in RNA content and incorporation of glycine-C^{14} into protein. This may be related to the increased quantity of microsomes in growing cells.[14] The decrease in RNA content was not accompanied by a similar change in the DNA content. The content of DNA increased on the second day after infarction and increased by 90 per cent above normal after eight days.[14]

The results illustrated a rapid diminution in incorporation of ^{14}C-glycine into protein of infarcted tissue. The incorporation fell immediately after infarction to 70 per cent of control, but increased two days after infarction and reached a maximum of 20 per cent of the control on the fourth day. The rate of protein synthesis diminished slowly after the first week and approached control values six weeks after infarction. The borderline tissue showed an earlier increase in protein synthesis with maximum incorporation two days after infarction. The rate of incorporation in the borderline tissue approached normal levels sooner than in the infarcted tissue.[14]

The studies on the subcellular fractions indicated that the reparative processes begin in the cell nucleus within 24 hours after coronary occlusion. The nuclear ribosomal fraction showed the earliest increase in incorporation of glycine-C^{14} into protein followed by that in mitochondria and microsomes.[14] True muscle regeneration does not seem to take place as indicated by the decreased incorporation of the tracer into the contractile protein fraction. The early renewal of cell material was further demonstrated by the incorporation of glycine-C^{14} into the nucleic acids of the infarcted tissue. The earliest increase in incorporation was observed in nucleolar RNA followed by nuclear ribosomal RNA. The accelerated rate of protein synthesis after infarction was also reflected in the increased incorporation into RNA which two days after infarction was increased 4·6 times. Similarly, the incorporation into cytoplasmic microsomal RNA also increased 4·6 times two days after infarction. The observed similarity in increase in metabolic activity reflects this functional relationship in the intensified protein synthesis in the infarcted tissue. The rate of DNA synthesis increased 48 hours after infarction, which coincided with the appearance of mitotic figures and an increase in number of fibroblasts.[14]

These observations illustrate the rapid commencement of fibroblastic proliferation in the ischaemic area. The existing fibroblasts appear to react to the injury and death of muscle cells by increased synthesis of nucleolar RNA and nuclear ribosomal RNA which precedes mitotic activity by 1 to 2 days. Following increased synthesis of nuclear material there is an increase in synthesis of microsomes and mitochondria which is subsequently followed by an increase in DNA synthesis and fibroblastic proliferation. Connective tissue formation and collagen synthesis during tissue repair was examined by determining the changes in hydroxyproline and proline concentrations of necrotic tissue. The hydroxyproline content of normal left ventricular muscle was 4·02 mg/g muscle dry weight. Following myocardial infarction the hydroxyproline content, reflecting the amount of collagen in necrotic muscle, decreased slightly at first but increased on the fourth day and rose in a logarithmic fashion until the tenth day. Ten days after infarction the hydroxyproline concentration was 17·6 mg/g, after 3 weeks the tissue content was 25·6 mg/g and 10 weeks after infarction the scar contained 43·14 mg/g hydroxyproline with a proline/hydroxyproline ratio of 1·58 (Fig. 6, 4). The proline content of infarcted muscle increased at first rapidly, but remained then relatively constant from the fourth to the eighth day. After the eighth day the proline content increased again rapidly for two weeks and then increased more gradually (Fig. 6, 4).

The rapid rise in hydroxyproline content during the first 10 days after infarction illustrates the fibroblastic proliferation during this period and the rapid synthesis of collagen. The subsequent period of slower increase in hydroxyproline content reflects not only collagen formation but also the increase in density of the developing scar tissue.

The discontinuous increase in proline content of infarcted muscle probably reflects the balance between degradation of necrotic muscle and synthesis of new scar tissue (Fig. 6, 5). The proline content failed to increase significantly from the fourth to the eighth day after infarction. This period represents the time of maximum lysosomal activity, as illustrated in the change in activity of soluble or non-particle bound β-glucuronidase and acid phosphatase (Fig. 6, 5). When the activity of these hydrolytic enzymes decreases the proline concentration increases reflecting a greater rate of scar tissue formation compared to tissue degradation.

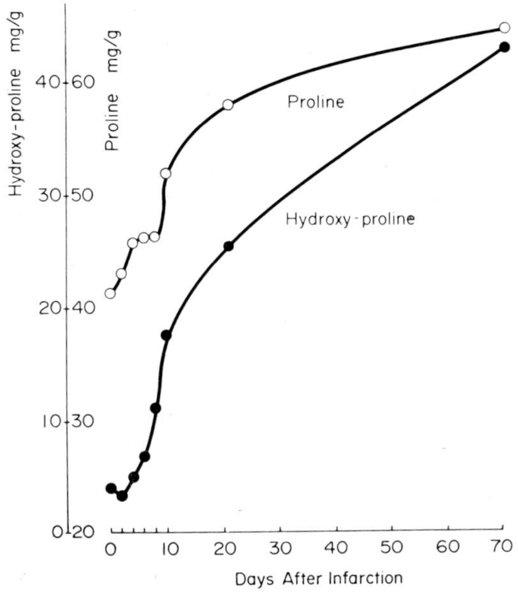

FIG. 6, 4. Changes in proline and hydroxyproline content of infarcted heart muscle.

3. Catabolic processes

The alteration in activity of lysosomal enzymes in the necrotic muscle is a reflection of the rate of catabolic processes i.e. removal of the necrotic tissue. During the early stage of myocardial necrosis, the autolytic phase of cell destruction takes place by release of hydrolytic enzymes from endogenous lysosomes originating in heart muscle cells and local connective tissue cells. This period is characterized by an early increase in free and a decrease in particle-bound enzyme activity.[15] The second stage of tissue degradation, the heterolytic phase, is characterized by an influx of phagocytic cells and a continuous increase in the activity of free lysosomal enzymes which reach a maximum 2 to 6 days after infarction. During the period of highest activities of soluble hydrolytic enzymes the major task of tissue degradation and removal of debris takes place.

The diminution in activity of free lysosomal enzymes 6 to 10 days after infarction is paralleled by an increase in activity of particle-bound enzymes and diminution in catabolic activity.[15]

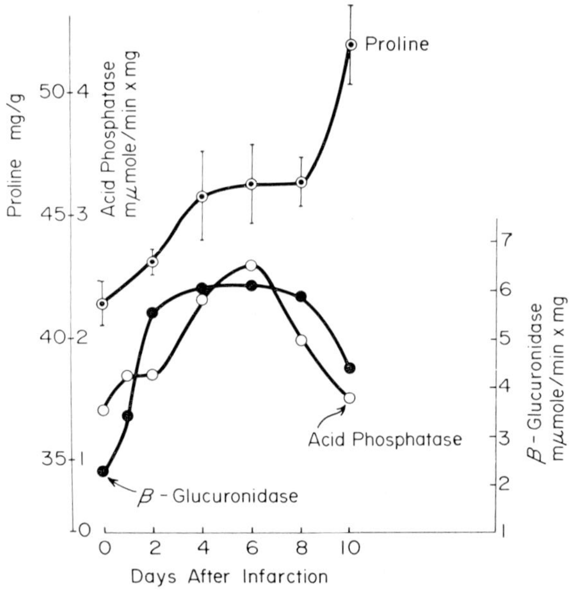

FIG. 6, 5. Changes in proline content and activity of lysosomal enzymes (β-glucuronidase and acid phosphate) in infarcted heart muscle during tissue repair.

The lysosomal enzymes released into the necrotic tissue are transported by lymph and blood vessels into the circulatory system. Significant changes in the serum activity of lysosomal enzymes, such as γ-glutamyl transpeptidase, have been observed in patients with myocardial infarction.[16] In contrast to enzymes, such as LDH and GOT, which indicate acute cellular damage and cell necrosis,[16] changes in serum γ-glutamyl transpeptidase activity may yield information on reparative processes and cellular replacement in the necrotic myocardium.

Phase III. *Reversible biochemical changes in non-infarcted heart muscle following acute coronary artery occlusion*

Biochemical abnormalities in the infarcted heart beyond the ischaemic area are of great importance because the ability of the heart to compensate for the loss of muscle and to survive is largely determined by the metabolic and functional integrity of the non-infarcted muscle (Table 6, 3).

Table 6, 3. *Reversible biochemical changes in non-infarcted heart muscle following acute coronary artery occlusion*

1. Alterations in energy metabolism
   ATP, CP, Lactate, Pyruvate
2. Impairment of myocardial function
   SW, dP/dt
3. Diminution in myocardial catecholamine levels
   Noradrenaline
4. Increase in rate of protein synthesis
   Compensatory hypertrophy

The effects of myocardial infarction upon catecholamine concentration in and energy metabolism of the non-infarcted functioning area of the left ventricle were examined and the findings were related to the functional status of the left ventricle.[17] The results illustrate a significant diminution in ATP and CP content of non-infarcted muscle following myocardial infarction. The ATP concentrations fell from 5·73 μmole/g in normal animals to 2·63 μmole/g 24 hours after infarction and increased to 4·65 μmole/g 10 days after infarction[17] (Fig. 6, 2). The CP concentration in non-infarcted muscle fell from 9·18 μmole/g to 4·87 μmole/g 24 hours after infarction, and increased subsequently to 6·51 μmole/g on the tenth day.[17]

This diminution in ATP and CP stores in non-infarcted myocardium during the post-infarction period may be related to the increase in workload and increased energy-utilization per unit of surviving muscle mass, which may not be proportional to the rate of synthesis. A correlation appears to exist between the diminution in ATP content of non-infarcted muscle and the impairment of left ventricular function following myocardial infarction. One day after infarction the stroke work (SW) and the rate of left ventricular pressure rise (dP/dt) were significantly diminished and increased slowly after that.[17]

The alteration in myocardial performance and energy-stores of non-infarcted muscle were followed by a significant diminution of noradrenaline levels. The infarcted heart muscle showed a rapid decline in noradrenaline content from the control level of 0·96 μg

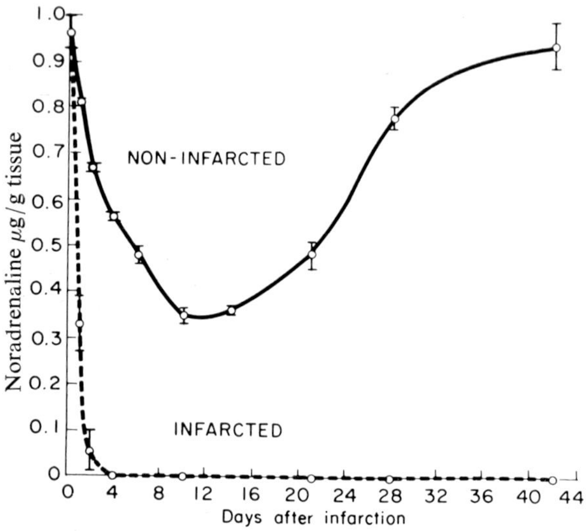

FIG. 6, 6. Changes in tissue content of noradrenaline in infarcted and non-infarcted heart muscle.

to 0·35 μg noradrenaline/g on the 1st day after infarction. On the 2nd day, the infarcted tissue contained 0·06 μg noradrenaline and from the 4th day noradrenaline could not be detected in the infarcted tissue (Fig. 6). The rapid irreversible depletion of noradrenaline stores in infarcted muscle is the result of the death of the ischaemic muscle cells.[17]

In the non-infarcted tissue a continuous decline in noradrenaline content could be observed during the first 10 days following infarction. There was a 67 to 75 per cent decrease in noradrenaline content of left and right ventricles and a 33 per cent decrease in noradrenaline content of both atria.

The changes in myocardial noradrenaline stores could not be

related to an impairment in either transport, binding or enzymatic degradation. Attempts to relate depletion of myocardial noradrenaline stores to changes in myocardial function failed and no correlation was observed between tissue levels and left ventricular function. Both the decline and recovery of left ventricular function after myocardial infarction occurred considerably earlier than the changes in tissue content of noradrenaline.[17]

The results suggest that the increased sympathetic activity following myocardial infarction leads to a gradual diminution of myocardial noradrenaline stores. Upon restoration of normal myocardial function, the activity of the sympathetic nervous system returns to normal, allowing the tissue stores of noradrenaline to return to their original levels six weeks after coronary artery occlusion.

The restoration of normal myocardial function and normal myocardial energy levels depends upon the development of compensatory processes. During the development of compensatory hypertrophy there is an increase in protein synthesis or decrease in the rate of normal myocardial protein degradation or both. The compensatory hypertrophy serves to increase the functioning muscle mass and to compensate for the loss of functioning muscle in the infarcted zone.

Methods to Influence Compensatory and Reparative Processes

Attempts were made to influence the rate of tissue repair and muscle recovery following myocardial infarction. The results indicate that it is possible to accelerate tissue repair in the infarcted area and to enhance compensatory processes in non-infarcted heart muscle by treatment with anabolic hormones (Table 6, 4). A protein-free diet results in delayed healing, impaired development of compensatory hypertrophy and markedly increased mortality rate.[18]

Treatment of animals with experimental myocardial infarction with anabolic hormones, such as insulin (NPH, 1 unit/kg), bovine growth hormone and methandrostenolone (Dianabol) increased the rate of incorporation of glycine-2-^{14}C into protein of infarcted tissue by 90 to 250 per cent.[18] A significant increase in amino acid incorporation into the protein of non-infarcted heart muscle was also observed, especially with growth hormone and anabolic steroids.

Table 6, 4. *Methods to influence compensatory and reparative processes*

Stimulation of repair and compensatory processes.
Anabolic hormones:
Stimulation of protein synthesis in infarcted heart muscle (growth hormone, insulin, anabolic steroids, ascorbic acid).

Increased protein synthesis in non-infarcted heart muscle, compensatory hypertrophy (growth hormone, anabolic steroids).

Increased high energy phosphate levels of non-infarcted muscle, compensatory processes (anabolic steroids).

Inhibition of repair and compensatory processes.
Protein-free diet:
Impaired scar formation and aneurysm.
Impaired development of compensatory hypertrophy and increased mortality.

Treatment with anabolic steroids (Norbolethone, 2 mg/kg per day) appeared to stimulate compensatory processes, both formation of new muscle mass and earlier restoration of normal high energy phosphate levels. In treated animals the ATP levels of non-infarcted muscle returned to normal (5·9 μmole/g) 10 days after infarction, whereas the ATP level of untreated animals was significantly lower (4·65 μmole/g; Fig. 6, 7). Treatment with insulin did not change the ATP level of non-infarcted as well as infarcted muscle.

Treatment with protein-free diet resulted in impaired repair of infarcted tissue, i.e. formation of a thin scar and development of left ventricular aneurysm. This treatment affected the compensatory processes of non-infarcted muscle as well and significantly reduced the ATP level of non-infarcted as well as infarcted muscle.

The ATP level decreased from 4·65 μmole/g in untreated animals to 3·1 μmole/g in non-infarcted heart muscle of animals on a protein-free diet. This decrease in high energy phosphate levels of non-infarcted muscle of animals on the protein-free diet was accompanied by a significant increase in mortality rate, from 10 per cent in control animals to 60 per cent in animals on a protein-free diet.

These results indicate that anabolic agents may increase the rate of reparative processes in infarcted muscle and the rate of compensatory processes in non-infarcted heart muscle, whereas protein deficient diet may have the opposite effect.

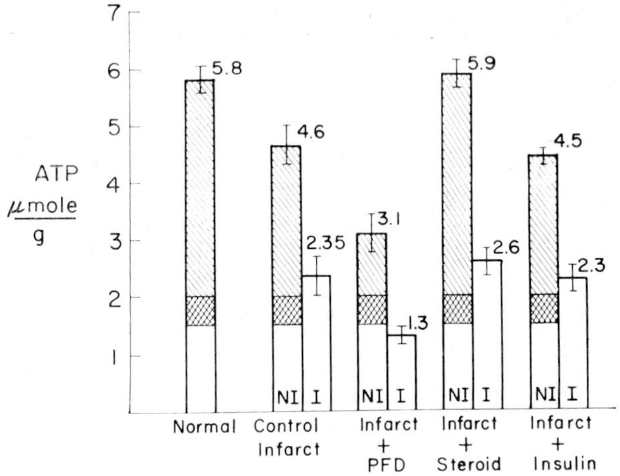

FIG. 6, 7. Effect of anabolic hormones or a protein free diet on tissue content of ATP in infarcted (I) and non-infarcted (NI) heart muscle 10 days after myocardial infarction.
Normal=heart muscle without coronary artery occlusion.
Control infarct=heart muscle with coronary artery occlusion but without treatment.
PFD=animals with myocardial infarction fed a protein free diet.
Steroid=treatment with the anabolic steroid norbolethone 2 mg/kg per day.
Insulin=treatment with NPH Insulin, 0·5 units/kg per day.

ACKNOWLEDGMENTS

This work was supported by the Research Career Development Award from the National Heart and Lung Institute, HE 31271–05, the American Medical Association, Education and Research Foundation and the Michigan Heart Association.

REFERENCES

1 GUDBJARNASON, S., MATHES, P. & RAVEN, K. G. (1970). Functional compartmentation of ATP and creatinine phosphate in heart muscle. *Journal of Molecular and Cellular Cardiology* **1,** 325-339.

2 KATZ, A. M. & HECHT, H. M. (1969). The early 'pump' failure of the ischemic heart. *American Journal of Medicine* **47,** 497-502.

3 GUDBJARNASON, S., BRAASCH, W., COWAN, C. & BING, R. J. (1968). Metabolism of infarcted heart muscle during tissue repair. *American Journal of Cardiology* **22,** 360-369.

4 Gudbjarnason, S., Cowan, C.. Braasch, W. & Bing, R. J. (1967). Changes in enzyme pattern of infarcted heart muscle during tissue repair. *Cardiologia* **51,** 148-159.
5 Gudbjarnason, S., Cowan, C. & Bing, R. J. (1967). Increase in hexosemonophosphate shunt activity during tissue repair. *Life Sciences* **6,** 1093-1097.
6 Jolley, R. L., Chedelin, V. H. & Newburgh, R. W. (1958). Glucose catabolism in fetal and adult heart. *Journal of Biological Chemistry* **233,** 1289-1294.
7 Krahl, M. E. (1956). Oxidative pathways for glucose in eggs of the sea urchin. *Biochimica et Biophysica Acta* **20,** 27-32.
8 Burt, A. M. & Wenger, B. S. (1961). Glucose-6-phosphate dehydrogenase activity in the brain of the developing chick. *Developmental Biology* **3,** 84-95.
9 Meerson, F. Z., Spiritchev, V. B., Pshennokova, M. G. & Djachkova, L. V. (1967). The role of the pentose-phosphate pathway in adjustment of the heart to a high load and the development of myocardial hypertrophy. *Experientia* **23,** 530-532.
10 Meerson, F. Z., Alekhina, G. M., Alexandrov, P. N. & Bazardjan, A. G. (1968). Dynamics of nucleic acid and protein synthesis of the myocardium in compensatory hyperfunction and hypertrophy of the heart. *American Journal of Cardiology* **22,** 337-348.
11 Gudbjarnason, S. & Priver, D. (1968). LDH-isoenzymes in infarcted heart muscle. *Life Sciences* **7,** 623-627.
12 Dawson, D. M., Goodfriend, T. L. & Kaplan, N. O. (1964). Lactic dehydrogenases-functions of the two types rates of synthesis. *Science* **143,** 929-933.
13 Van der Helm, T. J., Zondag, H. A., Hartog, H. A. P. & Van der Kool, M. W. (1962). Lactic dehydrogenase isoenzymes in myocardial infarction. *Clinica Chimica Acta* **7,** 540-544.
14 Gudbjarnson, S., Schrijver, C., Chiba, C., Yamanaka, J. & Bing, R. J. (1964). Protein and nucleic acid synthesis during the reparative processes following myocardial infarction. *Circulation Research* **15,** 320-326.
15 Ravens, K. G. & Gudbjarnason, S. (1969). Changes in the activities of lysosomal enzymes in infarcted canine heart muscle. *Circulation Research* **24,** 851-856.
16 Ravens, K. G., Gudbjarnason, S., Cowan, C. & Bing, R. J. (1969). Gamma-glutamyl-transpeptidase in myocardial infarction. *Circulation* **39,** 693-700.
17 Gudbjarnason, S., Puri, P. S. & Mathes, P. (1971). Biochemical changes in non-infarcted heart muscle following myocardial infarction. *Journal of Molecular and Cellular Cardiology* **2,** 253-276.
18 Gudbjarnason, S., Fenton, J. C., Wolf, P. L. & Bing, R. J. (1966). Stimulation of reparative processes following experimental myocardial infarction. *Archives of Internal Medicine* **118,** 33-40.

Discussion

Oliver. Have you related the shape of the DNA curve to tissue or plasma insulin levels in these animals?

Gudbjarnason. No, we have not attempted to relate the changes in DNA content of the necrotic tissue to the insulin level in these animals.

Oliver. If you prime these animals with insulin, can you advance the peak of DNA concentration?

Gudbjarnason. We measured the RNA and DNA concentration of the necrotic area in animals treated with insulin or bovine growth hormone. Two days after infarction the treated animals showed a greater increase in RNA and DNA in the infarcted muscle as compared to the untreated control animals.

Oliver. Would you go so far as to say that the early administration of insulin is likely to advance repair?

Gudbjarnason. The purpose of these experiments was to attempt to stimulate tissue repair with anabolic agents. Some of the anabolic hormones appear to be effective in stimulating repair. The use of insulin may be difficult because of the danger of hypoglycaemia. We were therefore looking for other anabolic agents with minimal side effects.

Wallace. How do the changes in the catecholamine content observed in the non-infarcted part of the infarcted myocardium compare with changes in the myocardium of sham-operated animals?

Gudbjarnason. The determination of the noradrenaline concentration of cardiac muscle in sham-operated animals was carried out 10 days after operation and no alteration was observed. The study of sham-operated animals was performed at this time, because animals with myocardial infarction showed the maximum decrease in noradrenaline content of non-infarcted muscle 10 days after coronary occlusion.

Maseri. Were you able to correlate the histochemical repair phenomena with any chemically determinable substance that would give us clinicians an idea of when or how the scar formation is proceeding in order to establish when to mobilize patients?

Gudbjarnason. We attempted to do this by determining the activity of γ-glutamyl-transpeptidase (γ-GTP) in serum from patients and animals with myocardial infarction. Alterations in serum activity of this enzyme, and possibly other lysosymal enzymes, might give information regarding the reparative processes in necrotic heart muscle. The activity of γ-GTP increases gradually in the serum after infarction, reaching a maximum 10 to 12 days after infarction, and diminishing subsequently. The increase in serum γ-GTP occurs a few days after a maximum increase in activity of non-particle bound enzyme in the necrotic tissue. The increase in serum activity may be related to a release of this enzyme into the blood and a decrease in rate of hydrolytic, degradative processes in the necrotic tissue may reflect the reparative processes.

Jennings. Have histological studies been carried out to compare the healing process in tissue infarcted by multiple ligation with tissue infarcted by a single occlusion? Collateral flow would be reduced, by definition, to an area with multiple ligations. Also, since all of your changes should be related to the varying kinds of cells present in the samples, it would be important to know the proportions and types of cells in your samples.

The second question concerns your interesting data on the ATP level in the left ventricle 24 hours after occlusion. It seems to me that the ATP level is a function of the rate of utilization of ATP at that time, the rate of degradation or turnover of the ATP pool, the availability of precursors for ATP synthesis, such as adenosine and phosphate, and the stability of your reference base. Is a muscle 24 hours after occlusion the same as that prior to occlusion? Does it have relatively more myofibrillar protein or more mitochondrial protein so that the wet weight or dry weight is different from the control tissue? I would like to hear more about the sham operation: it should be identical to the occlusion procedure. If these changes in ATP are only present in the experimental group and not in the sham-operated controls, then these fascinating results need explanation.

Gudbjarnason. The changes in ATP and creatine phosphate (CP) content of non-infarcted cardiac muscle during the post-infarction period were not observed in sham-operated animals. Sham-operated animals examined 24 hours after operation showed a small but significant fall in CP, but no significant diminution in the ATP content of heart muscle. The alterations in ATP and CP content of non-infarcted muscle were not accompanied by significant changes in water content or hydroxyproline content. The marked reduction in ATP and CP of non-infarcted muscle probably reflects the imbalance between energy utilization and energy production in the surviving, working muscle. Following coronary occlusion the surviving non-infarcted muscle is required to do more work per unit muscle mass and this increase in work load and energy utilization may lead to a diminution in energy supplies if the rate of energy production is insufficient to meet the requirements. This imbalance forces the heart to seek a new state of diminished performance and diminished energy requirement, which can be met by the available muscle. With the development of compensatory hypertrophy and an increase in muscle mass, myocardial performance is gradually restored.

Oliver. This question is rather critical since it raises problems of interpretation. Could you give us more details of the sham-operation?

Gudbjarnason. The sham-operation was carried out in the same way as the operation resulting in coronary occlusion except for the ligation of arteries. The pericardium was opened, the heart was taken out of the pericardium, and then put back in. The anaesthesia was the same and of the same duration, and post-operative treatment was identical.

Shahab. Did you look at the biosynthetic activity of mitochondria during the development of compensatory cardiac hypertrophy?

Gudbjarnason. No.

Randle. I find it difficult to believe that this fall in ATP is due to any sudden increase in turnover. I suppose an obvious experiment is to put a dog which is in poor physical training on a treadmill for a short period of time and see if the same thing happened. Do you have any information on the time scale of *de novo* synthesis of adenine nucleotides in heart muscle? I would imagine there has been some loss as inosine. How quickly does adenosine nucleotide get synthesized *in toto* under conditions where it has been depleted. What fixes its level? Have you measured any inosine levels in the coronary venous blood?

Gudbjarnason. There is a significant drop in total nucleotide levels of the tissue so there appears to be an increase in the irreversible degradation of nucleotides. I do not have any information on *de novo* synthesis of adenine nucleotides in heart muscle. We have not made any measurement of inosine concentrations in coronary sinus blood.

Carlson. Is it possible that formation of cyclic-AMP contributes to the drainage of ATP? Have you measured cyclic-AMP or the activities of either adenylcyclase or phosphodiesterase?

Gudbjarnason. No, we have not measured cyclic-AMP and I doubt whether it could play a role in such a massive loss of ATP.

Barrett. One tends to forget a simple rule of chronic experiments compared with acute studies and that is that animals have to eat to stay alive. I have been led astray in experiments in which I neglected to monitor the food intake in the experimental group. Your figures concerning RNA particularly remind me of experiments in which all the effects of a monoamine oxidase inhibitor—decrease in blood sugar, in growth hormone storage and messenger RNA formation—could be replicated by decreasing the food intake of untreated animals to parallel that of the animals dosed with the drug. Do you know, in this instance, if animals which are sham-operated and animals which have experimental infarction have the same dietary intake and whether this would influence results in long term experiments such as you describe?

Gudbjarnason. We attempted to eliminate specific dietary effects by comparing biochemical changes in infarcted tissue with the same constituents in non-infarcted muscle. This is not a very suitable reference because of the alterations that occur in the non-infarcted muscle. It is likely that an animal with a relatively large myocardial infarct is not going to eat very much during the first 24 hours after coronary occlusion, and I doubt if 24 hours starvation is going to cause a significant decrease in myocardial ATP concentration.

Randle. Forty-eight hours starvation in the rat does not change the adenine nucleotide concentration in the heart at all.

Opie. Nor does 72 hours starvation in the dog.

THE EFFECT OF ACUTE ISCHAEMIA ON CATECHOLAMINES AND CYCLIC AMP LEVELS IN NORMAL AND HYPERTROPHIED MYOCARDIUM

LIANE SHAHAB, ALBERT WOLLENBERGER, ERNST-GEORG KRAUSE and SABINE GENZ

Division of Cellular and Molecular Cardiology, Central Institute of Heart and Circulatory Regulation Research, German Academy of Sciences, Berlin-Buch, German Democratic Republic

THE importance of the catecholamines in regulating metabolism and contractile function in the heart is well recognized. Our special interest in recent years has been directed to determining the role of catecholamines in modifying myocardial energy metabolism following arrest of coronary flow. Evidence was obtained that soon after the onset of myocardial ischaemia endogenous noradrenaline is released from the sympathetic nerve endings of the myocardium. The release of noradrenaline causes a rise in cardiac cyclic-AMP, presumably by activation of adenyl cyclase, which in turn activates phosphorylase *b* kinase and glycogen phosphorylase. As a result glycogenolysis and glycolysis are strongly accelerated.[1 2 3]

It is possible that pathological conditions of the heart which induce a depletion of the myocardial noradrenaline stores would influence the regulation of these processes. In cardiac hypertrophy induced by pathological conditions that place the heart under a permanent strain, the noradrenaline stores of the myocardium become depleted.[4 5 6 7] This depletion has been attributed to increased cardiac sympathetic nerve activity (however see Spilker and Hayden[8]), the positive inotropic influence of which is thought to assist the heart in meeting the increased mechanical demands.[9] In this paper we present preliminary results on catecholamine mobilization and cyclic-AMP levels in the pathologically hypertrophied rat heart during acute myocardial ischaemia.

Resumé of results on hypoxia- and ischaemia-induced noradrenaline release from myocardium of non-hypertrophied hearts

In these experiments our attention was focused on the processes set in motion immediately after the onset of hypoxia or ischaemia.

Isolated Langendorff rat and rabbit heart preparations, aerobically perfused. were exposed to anoxic conditions either by arrest of perfusion or a switch to perfusion with oxygen-free Tyrode-solution. Considerable amounts of noradrenaline were found in the cardiac effluent. The increase in the amine concentration in the perfusate was noted 5 to 10 seconds after the onset of anoxia. Concomitant with the rapid output of noradrenaline (see Fig. 7, 1) into the perfusion

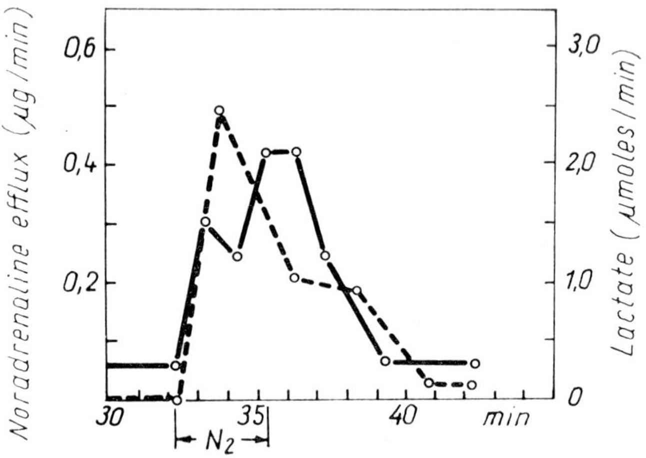

FIG. 7, 1. Release of noradrenaline (solid line) and lactate (broken line) from an isolated perfused rabbit heart following anoxia by switch to anaerobic perfusion.

fluid there was a sharp rise in the lactic acid concentration of the perfusate. Guinea pig hearts did not release noradrenaline after short-lasting periods of anoxia. Pretreatment of experimental animals with reserpine or tyramine, which deplete neuro-transmitter stores, reduced the amount of noradrenaline released by anoxia to a value proportional to the residual quantity of the catecholamine. Similar results were obtained in experiments on dogs *in vivo* in which local myocardial ischaemia was produced by dissecting free the left anterior descending coronary artery for temporary occlusion with a clamp. In one group of animals this vessel was infiltrated with a local anaesthetic (novocaine) in order to prevent stimulation of that branch of the sympathetic nerve localized along the clamped artery. A catheter was introduced into the adjacent interventricular

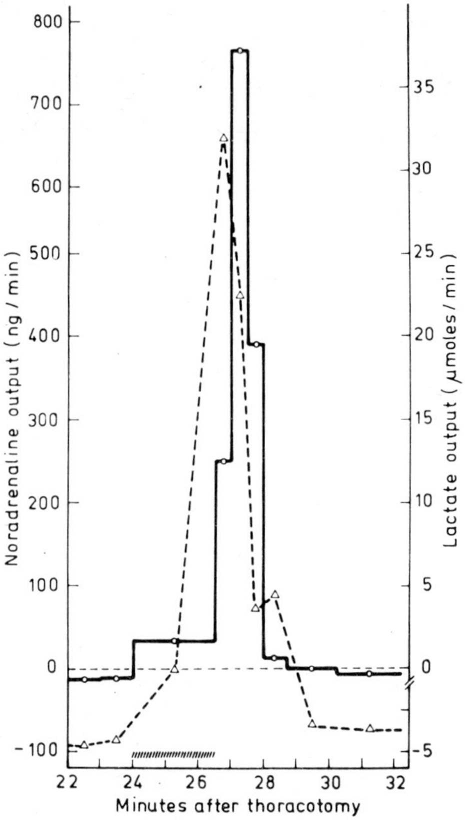

FIG. 7, 2. Net output of noradrenaline and lactate from a portion of a dog's heart. The oblique bars on the abscissa denote the period of occlusion of the left anterior descending coronary artery. Noradrenaline output is represented by the solid line, lactate by the broken line. (From Wollenberger *et al.*[3])

branch of the great cardiac vein for quantitative collection of blood. Simultaneously blood was taken from the left carotid artery. Following clamping of the coronary artery (see Fig. 7, 2) noradrenaline was given off into the catheterized coronary vein. Concomitant with the discharge of noradrenaline, lactate was released into the collected venous blood. The amount of noradrenaline released from myocardium after temporary clamping of the coronary artery was not affected by infiltration of the artery with novocaine. During the time of occlusion of the coronary artery there was still blood flowing through the catheterized vein at about one third of the pre-occlusion rate.

These experiments indicate: 1. Hypoxia causes release of endogenous noradrenaline from the ischaemic myocardium; 2. Hypoxia-induced noradrenaline release is accompanied by release of lactic acid. It is conceivable that accumulation of this and other acid metabolites causes an increase in hydrogen ion concentration which could induce the liberation of neurotransmitter; 3. The amount and rapidity of release differs among various mammalian species; 4. The released noradrenaline is largely responsible for the activation of phosphorylase and initiation of glycogenolysis; 5. The observed noradrenaline release is a direct effect of hypoxia rather than the result of increased sympathetic nerve activity, because it was seen also in isolated heart preparations, where the cardiac nerves were cut.

It was now of interest to investigate how hypertrophied hearts would react in this respect to abrupt ischaemia.

METHODS

Male rats of Wistar strain, 2 months old, were used (see Table 7, 1). Cardiac hypertrophy was induced by constriction of abdominal aorta according to Kogan,[10] renal hypertension, or by an extended programme of enforced swimming. For production of hypertension one kidney was encapsulated and the other kidney was removed after 2 weeks.[11] The animals were killed 4 weeks after the latter operation, at which time their systolic arterial pressure had risen to a mean value of 188 mmHg as compared to 113 mmHg in the controls. The swimming programme was based on the schedule of Crews and Aldinger,[12] using a bath with water circulating at 34°C and progressing from a half-hour swim to 6 hours of swimming daily, 5 days a week to a total time of 300 hours. On the last day of all experiments, which for the exercising animals fell on the 2nd day after the last swim, the rats were anaesthetized with ether and in one group the thorax and pericardium were opened rapidly under artificial respiration with air. The ascending aorta of these rats was cut, the time of cutting being designated as 0 sec, and

Table 7, 1 *Left ventricular hypertrophy and noradrenaline content in aorta-constricted, hypertensive and physically trained rats. Means ± standard errors*

	n	Duration	Blood pressure mmHg	Body weight g		Left ventricle + septum weight mg	Ratio	Noradrenaline content
					I	II	I/II	
				Before	After			ug/g
Control	8	2 months	—	250 ± 10·0	324 ± 10·3	613 ± 51·3	1·89 ± 0·09	0·680 ± 0·08
Control	8	6 months	—	250 ± 12·0	345 ± 6·5	693 ± 60·0	2·30 ± 0·21	0·690 ± 0·05
Aortic constriction	8	2 months	—	250 ± 11·5	305 ± 38·9	1011 ± 93·0	3·32 ± 0·21	0·226 ± 0·04
Aortic constriction	6	6 months	—	250 ± 12·0	348 ± 27·4	1523 ± 74·0	4·17 ± 0·33	0·048 ± 0·01
Control	10	4 weeks	113 ± 3·5	150 ± 12·0	302 ± 8·7	518 ± 18·1	1·71 ± 0·03	0·703 ± 0·08
Renal hypertension	8	4 weeks	188 ± 7·7	150 ± 12·0	214 ± 13·6	694 ± 25·5	3·31 ± 0·18	0·318 ± 0·08
Control	6	3 months	—	150 ± 10·0	265 ± 5·7	552 ± 10·8	2·09 ± 0·10	0·720 ± 0·09
Swimming	8	3 months	—	150 ± 10·0	216 ± 6·5	614 ± 23·4	2·82 ± 0·17	0·522 ± 0·09

the ventricles or parts of them were almost instantly frozen *in situ* with a freezing clamp at 0, 20 and/or 60 sec and analysed for cyclic AMP.[13] The hearts of the other group of anaesthetized rats were rapidly excised without artificial respiration for determination of noradrenaline[14] in the weighted left ventricles plus interventricular septa or for immediate perfusion with Tyrode-solution at 34°C by the Langendorff technique. Discharge of noradrenaline into the perfusate before and after a 3-min interruption of perfusion was determined as in previous experiments.[14]

RESULTS

Cardiac hypertrophy. Aortic constriction, renal hypertension and swimming caused significant increase in left ventricular plus septal mass and in the ratio of this mass to that of the body (Table 7, 1).

Noradrenaline content and release. In agreement with the results of other authors [4 5 6 7] heart hypertrophy due to overloading by chronic outflow obstruction was associated with severe depletion of cardiac noradrenaline. As Table 7, 1 shows, noradrenaline was also low in the hypertrophied left ventricles of the hypertensive rats. On aerobic perfusion with Tyrode-solution (Figure 7, 3) these hypertrophied hearts, in contrast to controls, slowly released noradrenaline into the effluent but failed to release additional amounts of the amine after a temporary stop of perfusion, while relatively large amounts were released after this manoeuvre by the hearts of the control animals. The hearts of the physically trained rats had retained about 80 per cent of the normal amount of noradrenaline per g of myocardium, not quite in agreement with the results of Østman and Sjöstrand,[15] who had found no decrease, and those of De Schrijver *et al.*,[16] who had observed a remarkable decrease. The noradrenaline content of heart hypertrophied by different means and left ventricular weight seem to correlate quite well up to the weight of 800 g (Fig. 7, 4). Further increases in cardiac muscle mass were accompanied by a smaller decrease in noradrenaline.

Cyclic AMP. Interruption of coronary flow to non-hypertrophied hearts caused an immediate rise in cyclic-AMP, peak values of which were reached within 20 sec. The elevated nucleotide level was maintained for at least 1 min. The increase in cyclic-AMP, illustrated in Figure 5, was sensitive to beta-adrenergic blocking

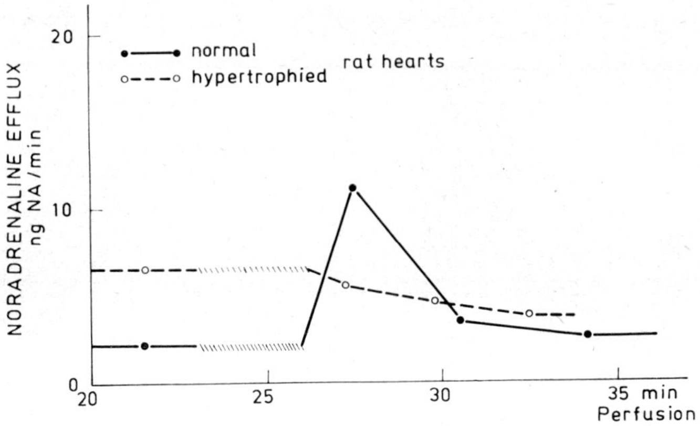

FIG. 7, 3. Noradrenaline release from isolated perfused rat hearts following arrest of perfusion (oblique bars).

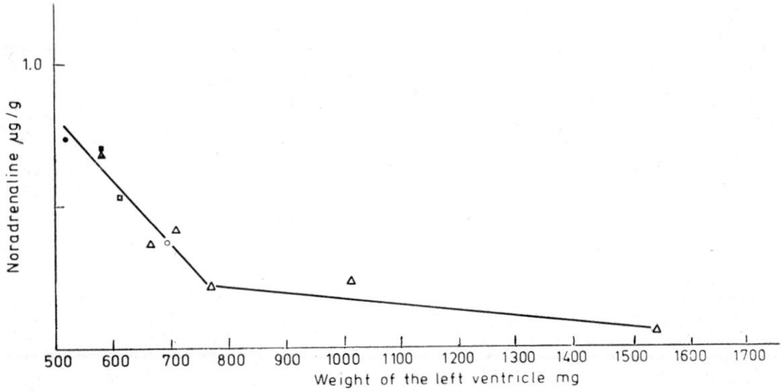

FIG. 7, 4. Noradrenaline content in correlation to left ventricular plus septal weight of hypertrophied rat hearts.

△ Aortic constriction (dark = control).
○ Renal hypertension.
□ Swimming.

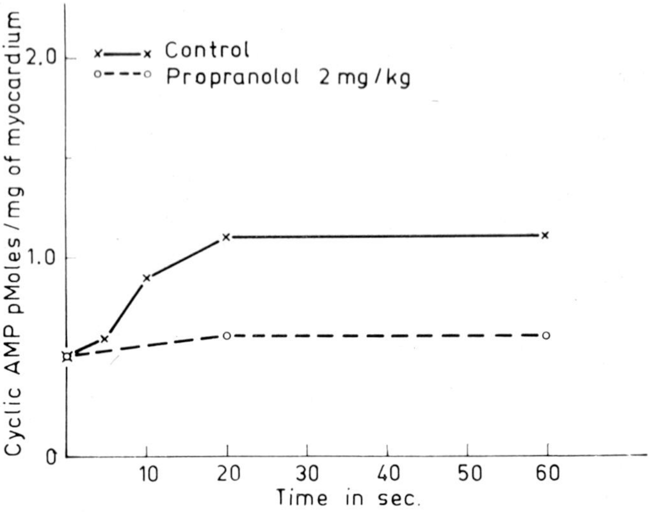

FIG. 7, 5. Cardiac cyclic AMP in the rat heart myocardium following arrest of coronary flow at zero time.

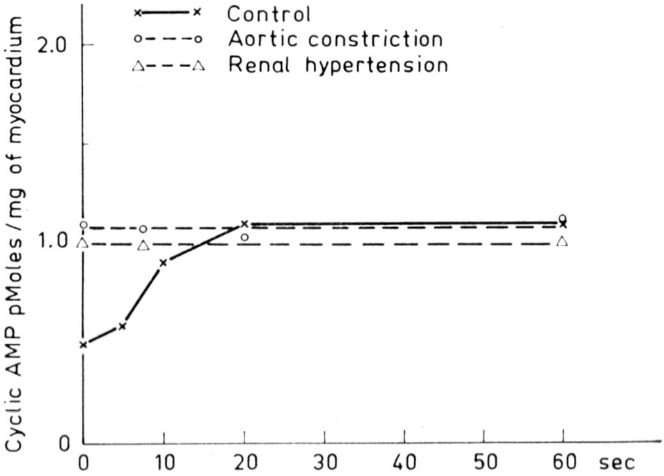

FIG. 7, 6. Formation of cyclic-AMP in normal and hypertrophied rat hearts following arrest of coronary flow.

agents. Rat hearts, hypertrophied either by aortic constriction or renal hypertension showed an elevated level of cyclic-AMP in the non-ischaemic myocardium at zero time. As could be seen from Figure 7, 6 these hearts failed to increase their cyclic-AMP content after sudden ischaemia. This finding corresponds to absence of hypoxia-induced noradrenaline release from hypertrophied hearts, depleted in their catecholamine content.

Discussion

In conformity with the data in the literature we observed a reduction of the noradrenaline content in hypertrophied rat hearts. Furthermore, these hearts failed to mobilize noradrenaline from the depleted stores and did not exhibit the rise in cardiac cyclic-AMP level that is normally seen[13] following the onset of ischaemia. This deviation from the normal response does not imply that the sensitivity of adenylate cyclase in the hypertrophied hearts toward catecholamines was lost or reduced. Henry *et al.*[17] have reported that the hypertrophied and failing guinea pig heart with aortic constriction responds to adrenaline administration with the same rise in cyclic-AMP as does the normal guinea pig heart. How the slow but constant aerobic release from the isolated perfused hypertrophied hearts of the rats with constricted aorta may be related to the depletion of the noradrenaline stores of these hearts, is difficult to say on the basis of the present data. Since the nerve connections to these hearts had been severed, the aerobic release cannot be ascribed to sympathetic nerve activity. This release may reflect an expanded pool of unbound, physiologically active noradrenaline, which by stimulating adenylate cyclase, increases the cyclic-AMP concentration of these hearts.

The difference in the noradrenaline content of markedly hypertrophic (aortic constriction) and moderately hypertrophic (exercised) hearts may reflect a difference in cardiac tissue mass increase or possibly a fundamental difference in the response to pathologically and physiologically induced forms of cardiac hypertrophy. It is worth mentioning in this connection that physically trained rats lose little of their complement of noradrenaline during a bout of strenuous physical exercise.[18]

Experimental analysis of the ischaemia-induced activation of myocardial phosphorylase (conversion of the *b* to *a* form) and of the associated metabolic changes has resolved each of these responses into 2 components, the operation of a humoral (adrenergic) mechanism involving noradrenaline and adenylate cyclase, and a second component that is independent of adrenergic influences and may involve calcium ions.[2 3 19] In the rat the second component preponderates over the first. Nevertheless, in a parallel comparative study of the metabolic response of the normal and hypertrophied rat heart to acute ischaemia, differences in the extent of adrenergically mediated phosphorylase activation and lactate accumulation were found during the first 20 seconds following arrest of blood flow. These differences may partly be explained by the differences in cardiac noradrenaline cyclic-AMP contents in the acutely ischaemic myocardium as influenced by hypertrophy.

The mobilization of endogenous noradrenaline that normally appears to occur in the myocardium immediately or very shortly following the onset of severe myocardial ischaemia helps to support the contractile activity of the muscle and provides it with much-needed energy. On the other hand, the accumulation of free, physiologically active catecholamine in hypoxic cardiac tissue may precipitate arrhythmias.[10 20-24]

Whether the attenuation of these different effects of an ischaemia-induced mobilization of cardiac catecholamines may be of advantage or disadvantage to the hypertrophied ischaemic heart of animals and of human patients, will have to be determined in further studies.

REFERENCES

1 KRAUSE, E. G. & WOLLENBERGER, A. (1967). Uber die Aktivierung der Phosphorylase b-Kinase im Akut ischämischen myokard. *Acta Biologica et Medica Germanica* **19,** 381-393.

2 WOLLENBERGER, A., KRAUSE, E. G. & HEIER, G. (1969). Stimulation of 3′, 5′-cyclic AMP formation in dog myocardium following arrest of blood flow. *Biochemical and Biophysical Research Communications* **36,** 664-670.

3 WOLLENBERGER, A., KRAUSE, E. G. & SHAHAB, L. (1967). In *Coronary Circulation and Energetics on the Myocardium,* p. 200. Edited: G. Marchetti and B. Taccardi. Basel and New York, Karger.

4 CHIDSEY, C. A., KAISER, G. A., SONNENBLICK, E. H., SPANN, J. F. & BRAUNWALD, E. (1964). Cardiac nor-ephinephrine stores in experimental heart failure in the dog. *Journal of Clinical Investigation* **43,** 2386-2393.

5 FISCHER, J. E., HORST, W. D. & KOPIN, I. J. (1965). Nor-epinephrine metabolism in hypertrophied rat heart. *Nature* **207,** 951-953.

6 MEERSON, F. Z., MANUKHIN, B. N., PSHENNIKOVA, M. G. & ROZANOVA, L.S. (1963). On mediator metabolism of the myocardium in compensatory hyperfunction and hypertrophy of the heart. *Patologie Fiziologie Experimentele Terapie* **7,** 32-36.

7 SPANN, J. F. JR., CHIDSEY, C. A., POOL, P. E. & BRAUNWALD, E. (1965). Mechanism of norepinephrine depletion in experimental heart failure produced by aortic constriction in the guinea pig. *Circulation Research* **17,** 312-321.

8 SPILKER, B. A. & HAYDEN, M. L. (1970). Spontaneous sympathetic activity in experimental heart-failure. *Experientia* **26,** 512-514.

9 BRAUNWALD, E. & CHIDSEY, C. A. (1965). The adrenergic nervous system in the control of the normal and failing heart. *Proceedings of the Royal Society of Medicine* **58,** 1063-1066.

10 KOGAN, A. K. (1961). A new simple method of controlled constriction of the renal and other arteries in small laboratory animals in chronic experiment. *Bulletin Eksertie für Biologie und Medicin* **51,** 112-115.

11 PAGE, I. H. (1939). Production of persistent arterial hypertension by cellophane perinephritis. *Journal of the American Medical Association* **113,** 2046-2048.

12 CREWS, L. & ALDINGER, E. E. (1967). Effect of chronic exercise on myocardial function. *American Heart Journal* **74,** 536-542.

13 GILMAN, A. G. (1970). A protein binding assay for adenosine 3′, 5′-cyclic monophosphate. *Proceedings of the National Academy of Science* **67,** 305-312.

14 SHAHAB, L. & WOLLENBERGER, A. (1967). Freisetzung von Noradrenalin aus dem isolierten durch strömten Herzen bei Akuter Anoxie und nach Gabe von Stoffwechsel giften. *Acta Biologica et Medica Germanica* **19,** 939-959.

15 ØSTMAN, I. & SJÖSTRAND, N. O. (1971). Effect of prolonged physical training on the catecholamine levels of the heart and the adrenals of the rat. *Acta Physiologica Scandinavica* **82,** 202-208.

16 DE SCHRIJVER, C., MERTENS-STRYTHAGEN, I., BECSEI, J. & LAMMERANT, J. (1969). Effect of training on heart and skeletal muscle catecholamine concentration in rats. *American Journal of Physiology* **217,** 1589-1592.

17 HENRY, P. F., SOBEL, B. E., KJEKSHUS, J. K., ROBINSON, H. & STULL JR., J. T. (1971). Cyclic AMP in the perfused failing guinea pig heart. *Proceedings of the Society for Experimental Biology and Medicine* **137,** 768-771.

18 SHAHAB, L., WARBANOW, W. & WOLLENBERGER, A. (1972). *Medische Sport* **12,** in press.

19 WOLLENBERGER, A. & KRAUSE, E. G. (1968). Metabolic Control characteristics of the acutely ischemic myocardium. *American Journal of Cardiology* **22,** 349-359.

20 BARRERA, F., ASCANIO, J. H., BOUTWELL, M. P., PAMIS, J. L. & OPPENHEIMER, M. J. (1966). Importance of myocardial catecholamines in myocardial infarction. *American Journal of Medical Science* **252,** 177-183.

21 CEREMUZINSKI, L., STASZEWSKA-BARCZAK, J. & HERBASZYNSKA CEDRO, K. (1969). Cardiac rhythm disturbances and the release of catecholamines after acute coronary occlusion in dogs. *Cardiovascular Research* **3,** 190-197.

22 CLARK, B. B. & CUMMINGS, J. R. (1956). *Annals of the New York Academy of Science* **64,** 543.

23 MALING, H. M. & MORAN, N. C. (1957). Ventricular arrhythmias induced by sympathomimetic amines in unaesthetized dogs following coronary artery occlusion. *Circulation Research* **5,** 409-413.

24 SCHAAL, S. F., WALLACE, A. G. & SEALY, W. C. (1969). Protective influence of cardiac denervation against arrhythmias of myocardial infarction *Cardiovascular Research* **3,** 241-244.

Discussion

Oliver. Does the concentration of ATP fall inversely with the increase in cyclic AMP?

Shahab. In the short time used to produce ischaemia, there was no significant fall in ATP.

Mjøs. What happens to lactate uptake if you deplete myocardial catecholamines by reserpine and then produce ischaemia?

Shahab. Uptake and release of lactate were unaffected by pre-treatment with reserpine.

Oliver. How long have you continued these experiments?

Shahab. We have continued these experiments in the dog heart for 10 minutes, and found cyclic AMP to be elevated.

Oliver. What proportion of the total catecholamines of the myocardium are released in ten minutes?

Shahab. In the isolated rabbit heart, after 3 or 4 minutes interruption of perfusion, one third of the total noradrenaline present in the left ventricle was released.

Fitzgerald. If anoxia caused interruption of the uptake '1' process, this would explain why you have a large increase in the effluent catecholamine since the mechanism of uptake '1' is energy dependent. Secondly, in the hypertrophied heart, a large increase in the uptake '2' mechanism, which is now regarded as being of physiological as well as pharmacological importance, might explain why there is no greater increase during hypoxia.

Shahab. Uptake '1' seems to be unaffected by ischaemia as long as energy from glycolysis is available. It is known that severe hypertrophy of the myocardium is associated with a reduced uptake mechanism. In our experiments with the hypertrophied rat heart, the noradrenaline stores were depleted from 0·7 mg/g to 0·05 mg/g in the left ventricle.

Fitzgerald. Did the group of dogs with aortic constriction show progressive depletion in catecholamine stores? How critical was the stenosis? Have you followed the time-course of the effects of this constriction?

Shahab. We have not followed the fate of animals with aortic constriction for a long time.

Kaijser. You expressed the myocardial catecholamine figures in amounts of amine/unit myocardial weight. Since catecholamines are mainly stored in nerves along the blood vessels, the decreases in catecholamine concentrations in the hypertrophied heart might partly reflect a decrease in vessel density.

Shahab. There is one part of the sympathetic innervation belonging to the vessels and another part located near to the muscle cells. Which part is more or less involved in the reaction to ischaemia is difficult to say. We have not done any histochemical work in order to answer your question.

Kaijser. But do not most of the adrenergic nerves in the ventricles follow the vessels?

Oliver. What contribution to plasma levels do myocardial catecholamines make compared with that from the catecholamines released by sympathetic nerve endings?

Shahab. The earliest time at which we observed an elevated noradrenaline level in the cardiac effluent was about 10 sec after the onset of ischaemia. This was in an isolated heart preparation. The largest part was released following reopening of the circulation.

Taggart. With a heart weight of 500 g and a mean catecholamine content of about 1μg/g fat free weight, an increase in the concentration of plasma catecholamine would last only 15 to 30 minutes.

Shahab. When considering the relatively high values of noradrenaline observed in the dog experiments one must take into account that the mean ischaemic area is only about 40 g.

Wallace. You indicated that noradrenaline stores are reduced in hypertrophied hearts and that these hearts have reduced release of noradrenaline in response to hypoxia. The normal rise of cyclic AMP in response to hypoxia was also reduced in hypertrophy. However, several investigators have suggested that the reason for reduced noradrenaline stores with hypertrophy is increased sympathetic activity. If that were the case, wouldn't we expect elevated levels rather than reduced levels of cyclic AMP? Do you think that other hormonal factors might be at play, for example, growth hormone? How do you explain reduced adenyl cyclase activity in hypertrophy?

Shahab. Maybe hormonal influences are involved in noradrenaline release from hypertrophied hearts, but I have no knowledge which of the hormones could be involved in this phenomenon. Our explanation was that these hearts need support in maintaining function, and this is done by utilizing the endogenous neurotransmitter.

Barrett. Are you using a trihydroxyindole method for catecholamine determination?

Shahab. Yes.

Barrett. You mention that you estimate catecholamine levels in blood from the heart and that you also take blood from a carotid artery as a reference. Since some of your figures show a negative value, has there been a subtraction made between these two levels?

Shahab. The effect either of noradrenaline or of lactate was calculated from the arterio-venous differences corrected by the flow through the ischaemic area.

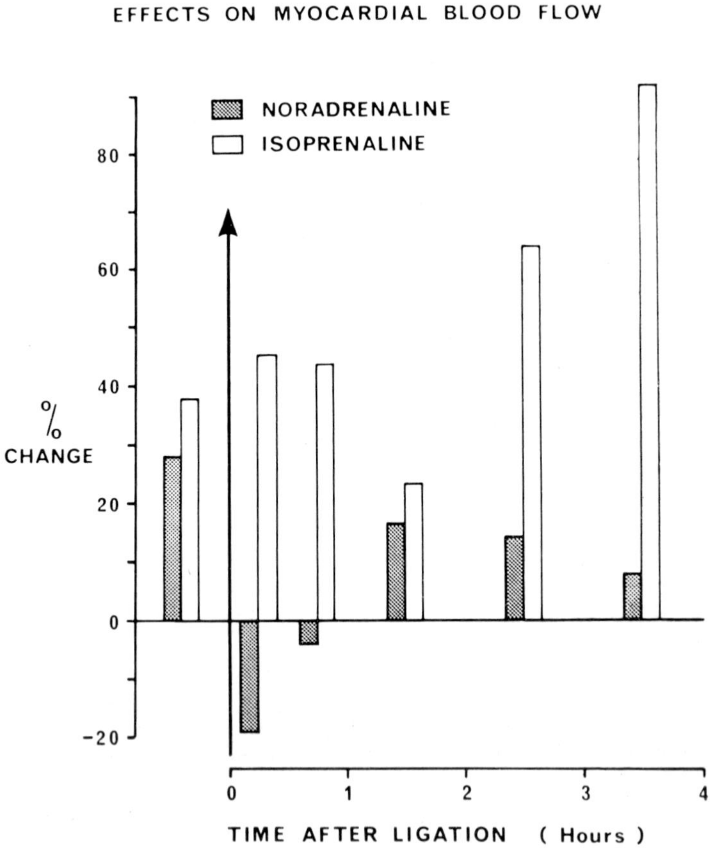

FIG. 7, 7

Barrett. So this represents a subtraction between the two concentrations actually measured?

Shahab. Yes.

Parratt. We have studied the effects of noradrenaline and blood flow in cats by means of heated thermocouples placed in different parts of the myocardium. One thermocouple recorder is in the normal region, one is in the area below the point of ligation of the descending coronary artery and one is at the boundary of the potentially ischaemic region. Blood flow is measured in these three regions. Moore and I have found that with ligation of a coronary artery in the cat, the flow only falls to about 50 per cent of normal, so they have a very good collateral circulation. We were interested in looking at the effect of noradrenaline on flow in the myocardium in the first hour after ligation which, as Dr Shahab has shown, is the time when release of myocardial noradrenaline occurs. Figure 7, 7 shows changes in blood flow in the ischaemic region at different times after ligation during intravenous infusions of noradrenaline (1·0 mg/kg/min) and isoprenaline (0·5 mg/kg/min). With noradrenaline there is a 50 per cent *increase* in flow in the normal myocardium but in the first hour after ligation noradrenaline infusion results in a 20 per cent *decrease* in flow. In other words, there is a complete change in the reactivity of the blood vessels in the ischaemic region from vasodilatation to vasoconstriction.

Wallace. Where do you infuse? How do you know the catecholamines reach the heart in reasonable concentration?

Parratt. They get there, because if you give isoprenaline intravenously there is no difference in the blood flow change after ligation (Fig. 7, 7). You get a 40 per cent increase in flow before ligation and the same increase in the first hour after ligation. Since haemodynamic changes are the same before and after ligation, I think that this noradrenaline reversal is a vascular effect.

Taggart. What about the uptake by the lungs of noradrenaline as compared with isoprenaline?

Parratt. We have looked at myocardial changes (left ventricular dP/dt, heart rate and ventricular volume) at the same time as measuring flow and the myocardial changes induced by noradrenaline after ligation are the same as those before ligation. So I am sure that the drug is getting to the heart and also to the ischaemic region. It looks very much as though there must be a change in the reactivity of the vessels in the ischaemic region.

There is one other thing. The first hour after ligation is the only time when ventricular arrhythmias occur in the cat during noradrenalin infusion. I wonder if there is any relationship between changes in flow in the ischaemic myocardium and the occurrence of ventricular arrhythmias.

Shahab. For how long have you observed this effect? Was it during the hour following ligation or is it more persistent?

Parratt. It is only in the first hour that you get this reversal. After the first hour, there is an increase in flow with noradrenaline.

LOSS OF MYOCARDIAL ENZYMES IN RELATION TO ENHANCED ADRENALINE SECRETION IN AN EARLY STAGE OF EXPERIMENTAL INFARCTION

KRYSTYNA HERBACZYNSKA-CEDRO

THIS study was undertaken to investigate the activity of myocardial enzymes after experimental infarction and their relation to the increased adrenergic response which may follow acute ligation of the coronary artery.

The need for this work was indicated initially by the results of experimental studies on the adrenergic response to myocardial infarction. Within minutes after coronary ligation the release of catecholamines, mainly adrenaline, into the circulation is increased and is maintained in the early post-infarction period.[1] A correlation has been observed between the enhanced adrenaline secretion and the incidence of ventricular arrhythmias[2] and the role of the neuroflex mechanism in the activation of adrenergic response has recently been established.[3]

A further problem considered in this study concerned the possibility that catecholamines produce an injurious effect on the myocardium. The possibility that catecholamines could cause myocardial damage comes mainly from the studies of their deliberate administration or induced release. Their effects on the myocardium can be summarized in terms of functional overload, biochemical changes[4 5 6 7] and morphological consequences.[8 9 10 11] Biochemical effects of circulating catecholamines, however, are difficult to distinguish from those induced by an excessive function alone. A deleterious effect may appear when a limited supply of substrate and of oxygen is associated with an increased requirement for energy. Morphologically, hearts exposed to increasing amounts of catecholamines and their derivatives exhibit eosinophilia, swelling and, ultimately, massive necrosis.[8 9 12 13 14] Early consequences of catecholamine excess, such as intracellular lipid accumulation, mitochondrial changes and abnormalities in enzymatic activity were shown by electronmicroscopic and histoenzymatic studies before any lesions detectable by classical histological methods appeared.[8 12 15]

Since catecholamines may be released following experimental infarction and since their effect may be deleterious it was the purpose of the present study to examine these factors in relation to each other. Clinical findings of an increased blood catecholamine level and of an increased catecholamine excretion in patients with recent infarction[16 17 18] indicate the relevance of this study to the effects of sympathoadrenal response accompanying clinical infarction.

METHODS

Thirty mongrel dogs of either sex, weighing from 6·5 to 13 kg were used in the study. Anaesthesia was induced with hexobarbitone sodium 40 mg/kg i.v. and then maintained with chloralose 100 mg/kg i.v. Positive-pressure ventilation was maintained with a Starling pump. The blood pressure was recorded from the carotid artery and the electrocardiogram from standard leads with an Elema Schönander Mingograf 42B. The chest was opened in the midline by sternal section. Coronary occlusion was induced by ligation of the anterior descending branch of the left coronary artery, two-thirds of its length from the coronary ostium.

Blood catecholamine estimation

Changes in the concentration of adrenaline and noradrenaline in the circulating blood were continuously determined by the use of blood-bathed organ technique.[19] The carotid artery was cannulated after administration of heparin 1000 units/kg i.v. and the arterial blood was used to superfuse two isolated organs—chick rectum and rat stomach strip; the blood then returned to the animal via a cannula in the jugular vein.

The principle of this bioassay is based on differential sensitivity of two isolated organs to the relaxing effects of adrenaline and noradrenaline. The rat stomach strip relaxes to both catecholamines[20] whereas the chick rectum relaxes only to adrenaline.[21] The amount of amine released into the circulation is determined by comparing its effect on isolated organs with that of a known dose of amine infused intravenously. Simultaneous use of these two organs, therefore, allows the proportion of adrenaline and noradrenaline in a mixture to be quantitatively estimated.[22]

Morphological and histoenzymatic methods

The morphological and histoenzymatic examination involved extensive sampling of both anterior and posterior left ventricular walls from animals with coronary occlusion. In dogs in which no coronary ligation was performed the sections were taken only from the anterior wall of the heart. The pieces of the myocardium were immediately placed in buffered 10 per cent formal saline, in Carnoy's fluid and in a dry ice-acetone mixture and were then subjected to staining reactions. Routine staining with hematoxylin and eosin was performed on 4μ paraffin sections prepared from Carnoy's fluid-fixed tissue blocks.

Histochemical techniques[23 24] applied to formalin-fixed sections cut on the freezing microtome at 12 to 15μ included the detection of:

1. nonspecific esterases using α-naphthol acetate as a substrate. Gomori;[25]

2. alkaline phosphatase using β-glycerophosphate as a substrate, adapted from Gomori;[26]

3. adenosine triphosphatase; Wachstein and Meisel;[27]

4. for the demonstration of succinate dehydrogenase (succinate-tetrazolium reductase—STR) and lactate-tetrazolium reductase (LTR) cryostat sections of about 7μ were used. Succinate dehydrogenase was demonstrated by the method of Nachlas *et al.* (1957) which employs nitro-BT as an electron acceptor.[28] Lactate-tetrazolium reductase was demonstrated by the method of Nachlas *et al.* (1958) in which nitro-BT is also used as an electron acceptor.[29] In the literature this technique is commonly referred to as a method for the demonstration of lactate dehydrogenase.

Design of the study

Of 30 animals used, 23 were subjected to coronary ligation. The level of circulating catecholamines was estimated for 2 hours following coronary occlusion and the hearts were then taken for morphological and histoenzymatic study. Hearts were also taken from seven open-chest dogs in which no coronary ligation was performed. Five of them were given continuous adrenaline infusion at a rate of 1 to 4 μg/min for 2 hours. In the remaining two dogs the endogenous blood catecholamine level was continuously measured for two hours prior to histoenzymatic study.

Results

Estimation of blood catecholamine level

Continuous monitoring of catecholamine concentration in the circulating blood showed that in 14 out of 23 dogs coronary occlusion was followed by an increased release of amines into the circulation. Adrenaline was released in the majority of animals; its increased secretion occurred within two to 35 min of coronary ligation in 11 out of 14 dogs (Fig. 8, 1). Increase in blood noradrenaline level was

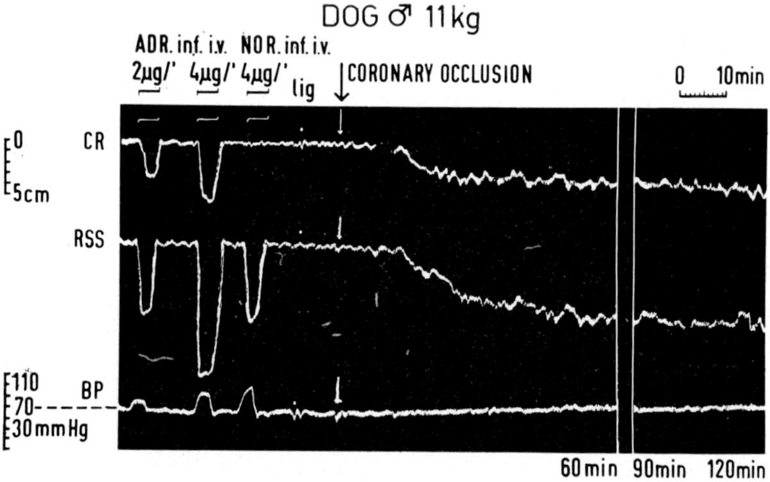

FIG. 8, 1. A chick rectum (CR-top record) and a rat stomach strip (RSS-middle record) were superfused with carotid arterial blood. The lower record is blood pressure. An initial calibration shows differential sensitivity of assay organs to adrenaline and noradrenaline. The ligature was inserted under the carotid artery (lig.) and 10 min later the artery was occluded. This was followed by gradually increasing relaxation of both assay organs indicating an increasing release of adrenaline into the blood. Increasing secretion of adrenaline started within about 15 min after coronary occlusion and at its maximum was equivalent to 2 μg/min.

detected in 2 dogs only, in another animal both amines were released together. The maximal amounts released varied with each animal, the range being 1 to 8 μg/min for adrenaline, 3 to 4 μg/min for noradrenaline. These values, calculated per kilogram of body weight, did not exceed 1·2 μg/min for adrenaline and 0·36 μg/min for noradrenaline.

The results of this part of the study confirmed earlier observations[1 2] that:

1. an increased release of adrenaline into the circulation rather than that of noradrenaline occurs after acute coronary occlusion;

2. an increased output of catecholamines begins within minutes of coronary ligation and increases over the next half hour;

3. the pattern of release is not uniform but shows a gradual increase followed by steady release, or repetitive outbursts of amine into the circulation;

4. the adrenal medulla is the main source of adrenaline released into the circulation as adrenalectomy effectively abolished its enhanced secretion;

5. ventricular arrhythmias are associated with an elevated catecholamine release. Disturbances of rhythm occurred in 9 out of 14 catecholamine-secreting animals. In dogs with no detectable release and with similar electrocardiographic evidence of ischaemia, cardiac arrhythmias occurred in only 3 out of 9 animals.

As the amine released was primarily adrenaline, our further results refer to this amine. It was for this reason that adrenaline was chosen to be administered to animals which were not subjected to coronary ligation. The dose infused corresponded to the amounts released spontaneously.

Results of morphological and histoenzymatic examination

Routine haematoxylin and eosin staining was performed to exclude pre-existing myocardial abnormalities rather than to identify lesions due to coronary occlusion as a low incidence of evident histological changes in the early period of myocardial ischaemia has been commonly found. This technique revealed occasional local vascular congestion, slight acidophilia and a loss of cross-striation of myocardial fibres. These were present in a few preparations in the ischaemic region and in some were unrelated to the area of involvement as shown by other techniques. No significant changes were observed in the sections from the posterior wall of the left ventricle in dogs with coronary occlusion. In those without coronary ligation the histological pattern of the myocardium did not show any evident abnormalities.

Staining reactions for esterases, alkaline phosphatase and adenosine triphosphatase showed no evident differences between tissues from control, adrenaline-infused or coronary-ligated animals. Sections of myocardium were strongly positive for esterases, the activity of alkaline phosphatase, confined to the endothelium of capillaries and adventitia of moderate size arteries was well preserved; the staining reaction for adenosine triphosphatase showed high activity in all the sections studied.

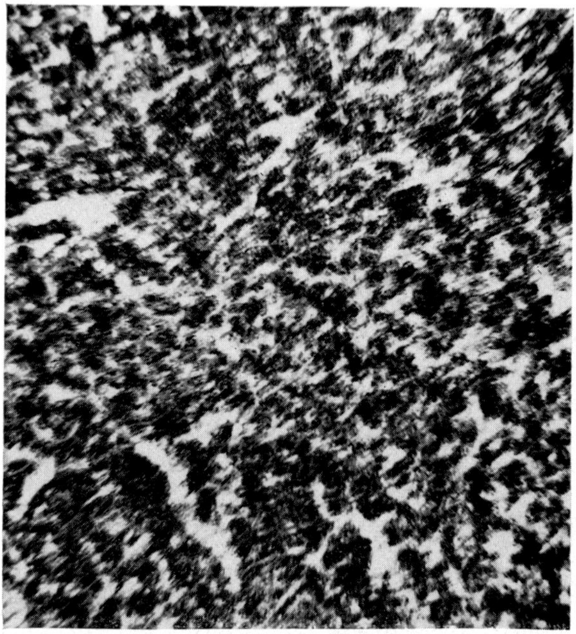

FIG. 8, 2. Succinate-tetrazolium reductase (STR) staining reaction in a control animal. Grade of staining intensity + + +. This pattern of staining was found in uninfarcted part of the left ventricle in dogs without detectable increase in blood catecholamine level after cororonary ligation (×100).

In contrast to these findings, staining reactions for the demonstration of succinate dehydrogenase and lactate-tetrazolium reductase showed evident differences between the samples examined. To summarize the results of this staining reaction a grading system corresponding to the degree of staining reduction and to the size of the area involved was established. Normal (+ + +) intensity of the histoenzymatic reaction was recognized when the sections showed a positive and uniform distribution of formazan granules. Grade I (++) represented a slight focal diminution of staining interspersed with normally reacting fibres. Grade II (+) indicated a marked decrease in staining intensity in the multiple areas of the myocardium. Grade III (0) showed a generalized reduction of histoenzymatic reaction with diffuse areas in which the staining was absent.

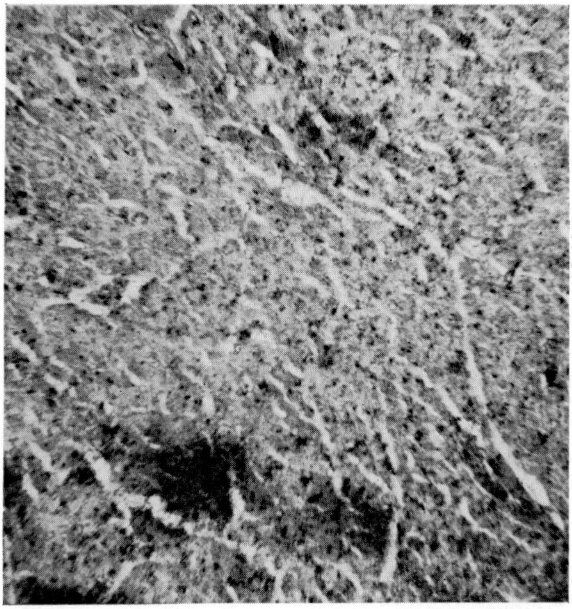

FIG. 8, 3. Infarcted area of the myocardium. Diffuse reduction of STR staining reaction (grade 0) in a dog with increased adrenaline secretion maintained for two hours after coronary ligation. Reaction for the demonstration of LTR showed this pattern of staining in majority of adrenaline-secreting animals (×100).

Strongly positive and uniformly distributed staining intensity, considered as normal in our grading system, was found in heart samples from the control dogs. The changes in the pattern of staining detected in the remaining animals are summarized in Table 8, 1. Although staining intensity has to be considered only as a qualitative basis for the evaluation of the results, the differences in

Table 8, 1. *Changes in staining reactions for lactate-tetrazolium reductase (LTR) and succinate-tetrazolium reductase (STR) in left ventricular myocardium in relation to catecholamine (CA) release after coronary occlusion (cor. occl.)*

NUMBER OF EXPERIMENTS	EXPERIMENTAL GROUP		ENZYMES	HISTOENZYMIC CHANGES (number of animals) Grade of activity Normal +++	I° ++	II° +	III° o
9	COR OCCL WITHOUT CA RELEASE	infarcted area	LTR	2	6	1	
			STR	6	3		
		posterior wall	LTR	8	1		
			STR	9			
12	COR OCCL WITH ADRENALINE RELEASE	infarcted area	LTR		1	3	8
			STR		3	8	1
		posterior wall	LTR		3	9	
			STR		11	1	
5	ADRENALINE INFUSION WITHOUT COR OCCL	anterior wall	LTR		2	3	
			STR		3	2	

histoenzymatic pattern between animals were clearly evident and it appeared that the intensity of histoenzymatic changes shows a correlation with the incidence of the humoral response detected in the first part of the study. Usually animals which demonstrated an increase in blood adrenaline concentration after coronary occlusion also demonstrated a decrease in the histoenzymatic activity of myocardial samples. Direction of changes in both histoenzymatic reactions was parallel; the tendency to decrease, however, was more evident for lactate tetrazolium-reductase than for STR.

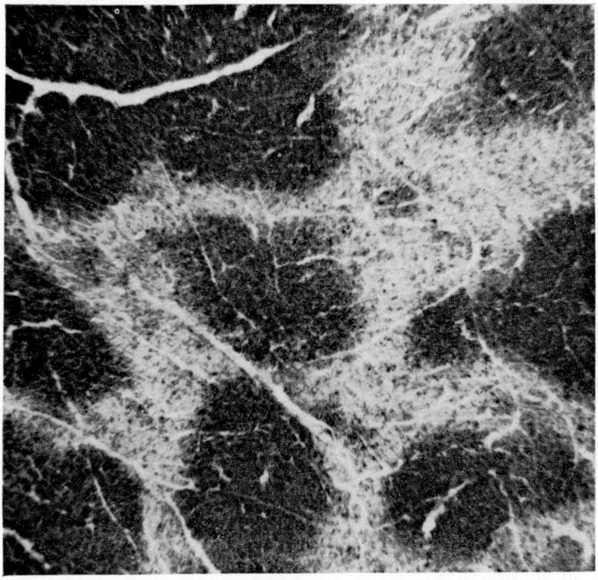

FIG. 8, 4. Decreased intensity of STR reaction (grade +) observed in majority of preparations from ischaemic area in adrenaline secreting animals. Similar decrease in histoenzymatic reaction was found in uninfarcted part of the left ventricle in a dog with maintained adrenaline secretion (×100).

In the animals without detectable increase in blood catecholamine level after coronary ligation, the sections from the posterior wall of the heart showed unchanged STR staining intensity (Fig. 8, 2). This was also found in the infarcted area in the majority of these animals. In three dogs only a slight decrease in STR reaction in ischaemic myocardium could be detected and was manifested by a focal diminution of staining intensity recognized as grade I (+ +) in our classification system.

In dogs in which blood adrenaline level after coronary ligation was increased, the sections from the infarcted area showed a considerable loss of staining intensity (Fig. 8, 3). In most of the preparations histoenzymatic reaction for STR showed a marked decrease of staining recognized as grade II (+) (Fig. 8, 4); this was even more pronounced in lactate-tetrazolium reductase reaction

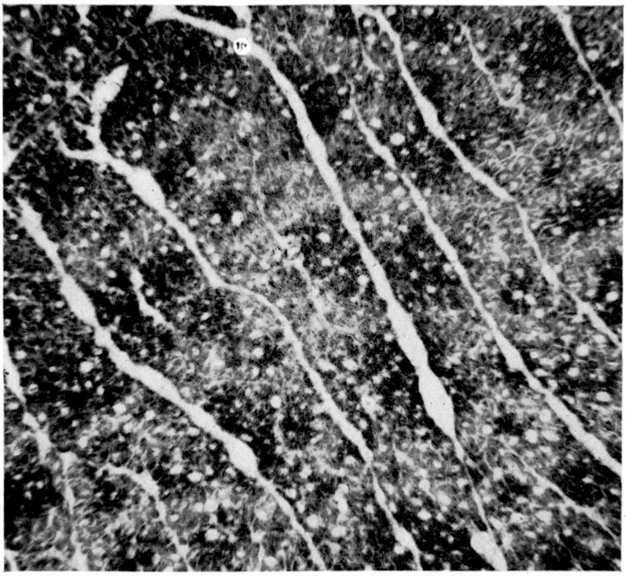

FIG. 8, 5. Diminution of staining for STR (grade + +) in intact region of the myocardium in adrenaline secreting dogs. Similar changes of staining intensity were induced by adrenaline infusion ($\times 100$).

which showed a complete absense of staining in the majority of hearts. Multiple areas of decreased histoenzymatic activity and a variable intensity of staining were found in the sections from the posterior, uninfarcted myocardial wall in adrenaline-secreting animals and this appeared to be a constant finding in this experimental group (Figs. 8, 4 and 8, 5).

Adrenaline infusion at a rate of 1 to 4 μg/min, the mean total dose 25 $\pm$ 1·5 μg/kg, given to dogs without coronary ligation, induced detectable changes in the pattern of staining such as an unequal formazan distribution and a slight focal diminution of staining intensity.

Discussion

The results of the study have shown that in the hearts exposed to adrenaline the histochemical reactions for lactate and succinate dehydrogenase systems were more affected than in those from animals without detectable humoral response, the entire myocardium being involved. The unchanged activity of the other enzymes studied was an expected finding since their decrease is considered to occur late after the onset of ischaemia.[30 31] The lack of difference in these staining reactions between controlled and infarcted hearts provided validity of our histochemical procedure and confirmed the results of others using similar techniques.

The demonstration of dehydrogenase systems by the methods used in the study depends on the reduction of a tetrazolium salt to insoluble formazan which is generally assumed to be deposited within the cells at the site of enzymatic activity. Tetrazolium salts, however, are not reduced by the specific dehydrogenases but rather by an intermediate flavoprotein.[32 33] The problem as to what extent staining intensity reflects the activity of primary dehydrogenase or the activity of the whole system has not been satisfactorily resolved.[34 35 36] Thus, for methodological reasons staining intensity should be interpreted as reflecting the activities of an enzymatic system rather than of a single dehydrogenase.

The time relationship between the onset of acute ischaemia and the first changes in staining reaction for the demonstration of lactate dehydrogenase system detected in our study parallels the results of others who used this technique to identify early myocardial lesions.[30 37] A detectable decrease in staining for succinate dehydrogenase occurred earlier in our study than in other studies. The average time for the decrease in succinate dehydrogenase activity in the ischaemic myocardium has been reported to be more than four hours,[30 32 37 38 39] and this is in agreement with the direct assay of succinate dehydrogenase in the homogenate of infarcted muscle.[40] But without regard to the time of onset of decreased staining in our study it seemed meaningful that the degree of histoenzymatic changes was correlated with an increase in the blood adrenaline level which followed acute ligation of the coronary artery.

The explanation for the decreased histoenzymatic reaction might be a decrease in the enzyme protein itself, following an altered permeability of the membrane. This is the probable explanation for the appearance of lactic dehydrogenase in serum[41] and also for the decrease of lactic dehydrogenase concentration in tissue which has been reported to occur in infarcted heart muscle at times corresponding to those of our study.[40] Extensive myocardial damage and increased serum levels of myocardial enzymes can be produced by the administration of catecholamines to the animals with intact hearts.[8 15 42] Thus, catecholamines cause a depletion of enzyme from the ischaemic myocardium which results in a decreased staining reaction.

Leakage of enzyme from the cells may not, however, be the only basis for the observed decrease in staining reaction. Biochemical data[40] makes it seem unlikely that the decrease in the reaction for succinate dehydrogenase is caused by loss of enzyme from the cells. An alternative explanation for the decreased staining reaction may be the loss of enzyme activity rather than of enzyme protein. Decreased enzymatic activity in the ischaemic myocardium, as shown by histochemical techniques, reflects metabolic and structural disorganization at different levels induced by acute ischaemia. The tendency for greater decrease in histoenzymatic reaction in animals with increased secretion of adrenaline suggests that catecholamines may contribute to the development of these alterations. The possibility that catecholamines potentiate structural lesions is reasonable, as these can be induced by catecholamine administration to intact hearts. A potentiated decrease in histoenzymatic activity in ischaemic heart muscle in animals with increased secretion of adrenaline may also be a function of the synergistic metabolic effects of anoxia and catecholamines on the myocardium. Although histochemical technique does not provide precise information regarding the biochemical changes that occur, a consideration of factors which might cause a decrease in enzymatic activity includes, among other possible factors, the changes in coenzyme and cofactor concentration and the changes in the conditions which control the rate of enzymatic activity, such as ATP/AMP ratio or intracellular electrolyte levels. Thus, decreased enzymatic activity in ischaemic myocardium and its evident tendency to decrease more in animals with increased secretion of adrenaline might be explained on the basis of known metabolic events induced both by anoxia and by catecholamines in the myocardium.[7 43 44 45 46 47] It is known that both anoxia and catecholamines cause an acceleration of substrate utilization and an increased demand for the synthesis of high-energy phosphates. This could subsequently lead to the changes in the ratio of these substances which is known to control or to influence the rate of enzymatic activity. Both anoxia and catecholamines cause similar ionic redistribution and corresponding shifts in the concentration of substrates and products of the anaerobic pathway. Another factor which might be induced by anoxia and/or catecholamines is a loss of metabolites involved in the electron transport system between cytoplasm and mitochondria.[48] In view of these links between anoxia and catecholamines in their action within the tissue, the increase of adrenaline in the conditions when oxygen supply is limited may potentiate histochemical indices of ischaemia. This seems to account for the correlation between decreased staining intensity, ischaemia and an elevated blood adrenaline level and may explain intensified loss of histoenzymatic activity in animals with maintained adrenaline secretion.

A striking decrease in staining intensity in the non-infarcted portion of the heart was not an expected finding in view of biochemical data on its increased metabolic efficiency due to increased function.[49] Decreased intensity of histoenzymatic reaction in the non-infarcted area occurred in animals with increased secretion of adrenaline. The development of these lesions in the myocardium whose functional and metabolic load was further increased by catecholamines may reflect the state of metabolic imbalance when the capability to maintain the energy supply becomes critical. Although catecholamines may induce the increase in blood flow, substrate and oxygen availability, this beneficial response may be offset by their effect in increasing function and their metabolic action. This is reflected in our study by the decreased histoenzymatic reaction in the non-infarcted area of the hearts, which being already seriously affected, were confronted with an increased work load.

All these effects were caused by the spontaneous release of much lower amounts of catecholamines than any doses deliberately applied. This fact should be considered with regard to the possible relevance of these findings to the pathology of human infarction. Caution is needed, however, before attempting to interpret the results of this experimental study in terms of human physiopathology, but the data available so far make this approach worth considering. It may be suggested that the results of this study are relevant to clinical observations in the following ways:

1. Myocardial damage potentiated by catecholamines may partially account for the observations that the most severe rhythm disturbances, haemodynamic and metabolic complications accompanying acute infarction are usually correlated with an excessive sympathetic overactivity, as measured by blood and urine concentrations of catecholamine.[16 17 18 50 51]

2. If the heart is exposed to maximal endogenous catecholamine drive, not only the potentiation of changes in the infarcted area may occur, but also the supportive effect of sympathoadrenal discharge on residual non-infarcted myocardium may be overcome by a risk of total ischaemia. This might be added to other possible causes for the development of cardiogenic shock.

3. If histological examination fails to provide an adequate explanation for the fatal outcome of myocardial infarction, catecholamine-induced histoenzymatic changes may do so.

The author is greatly indebted to Dr M Kałczak for his help in histochemical part of this work and to Professor H. Feinberg for valuable discussions and his help in preparing the manuscript.

REFERENCES

1 Staszawska-Barczak, J., Ceremuzynski, L. (1968). The continuous estimational catecholamine release in the early stages of myocardial infarction in the dog. *Clinical Science* **34,** 531-539.

2 Ceremuzynski, L., Straszewska-Barczak, J. & Herbaczynska-Cedro, K. (1969). Cardiac rhythm disturbances and the release of catecholamines after acute coronary occlusion in dogs. *Cardiovascular Research* **3,** 190-197.

3 Staszewaka-Barczak, J. (1971). The reflect stimulation of catecholamine secretion during the acute stage of myocardial infarction in the dog. *Journal of Clinical Science* **41,** 419-439.

4 Sarnoff, S. J., Gilmore, J. P., Weisfeldt, M. L., Daggett, W. M. & Mansfield, P. B. (1965). Influence of norepinephrine on myocardial oxygen consumption under controlled hemodynamic conditions. *American Journal of Cardiology* **16,** 217-226.

5 Klocke, F. J., Kaiser, G. A., Ross, J. Jr., & Braunwald, E. (1965). Mechanism of increase of myocardial oxygen uptake produced by catecholamines. *American Journal of Physiology* **290,** 913-918.

6 Ellis, S. (1956). The metabolic effects of epinephrine and related animals. *Pharmacological Review* **8,** 485-565.

7 Williamson, J. R. (1966). Metabolic effects of epinephrine in the perfused rat heart II Control steps of glucose and glycogen metabolism. *Molecular Pharmacology* **2,** 206-220.

8 Schenk, E. A. & Moss, T. J. (1966). Cardiovascular effects of sustained norepinephrine infusions. II morphology. *Circulation Research* **18,** 605-615.

9 Maling, H. M. & Highman, B. (1958). Exaggerated ventricular arrhythmias and myocardial fatty changes after large doses of norepinephrine and epinephrine in unanesthetized dogs. *American Journal of Physiology* **194,** 590-596.

10 Hunt, D. & Gore, I. (1972). Myocardial lesions following experimental intracranial hemorrhage: prevention with propranolol. *American Heart Journal* **83,** 232-236.

11 Raab, W., Stark, E., MacMillan, W. H. & Gigee, W. R. (1961). Sympathogenic origin and antiadrenergic prevention of stress-induced myocardial lesions. *American Journal of Cardiology* **8,** 203-211.

12 Ferrans, V. J., Hibbs, R. G., Black, W. C. & Weilbaecher, D. G. (1964). Iso proterenol-induced myocardial necrose. A histochemical and electron microscopic study. *American Heart Journal* **68,** 71-90.

13 Rosenblum, I., Whol, A., Stein, A. A. (1965). Studies in cardiac necrosis. I. Production of cardiac lesions with sympathomimetic amines. *Toxicology and Applied Pharmacology* **7,** 1-8.

14 Roma, G., Chappel, C. L., Balasz, T. & Gaudry, R. (1969). An infarct-like myocardial lesion and other toxic manifestations produced by isoproterenol in the rat. *Archives of Pathology* **67,** 443-455.

15 Schenk, E. A., Galbreath, R. & Moss, A. J. (1966). Cardiovascular effects of sustained norepinephrine infusion III lactic dehydrogenase isoenzyme release. *Circulation Research* **18,** 616-619.

16 Valori, C., Thomas, M. & Shillingford, J. (1967). Free noradrenaline and adrenaline excretion in relation to clinical syndromes following myocardial infarction. *American Journal of Cardiology,* **20,** 605-617.

17 Jewitt, D. E., Mercer, C. J., Reid, D., Valori, C., Thomas, M. & Shillingford, J. (1969). Free noradrenaline and adrenaline excretion in relation to the development of cardiac arrhythmias and heart failure in patients with acute myocardial infarction. *Lancet* **1,** 635-641.

18 Prakash, R., Parmley, W. W., Horvat, M. & Swan, H. J. C. (1972). Serum cortisol, plasma free fatty acids, and urinary catecholamines as indicators of complications in acute myocardial infarction. *Circulation* **45,** 736-745.

19 Vane, J. R. (1969). The release and fate of vaso-active hormones in the circulation. *British Journal of Pharmacology* **35,** 209-242.

20 Vane, J. R. (1957). A sensitive method for the assay of 5-hydroxytryptamine. *British Journal of Pharmacology* **12,** 344-349.

21 Mann, M. & Wesr, G. B. (1950). Nature of hepatic and splenic sympathin. *British Journal of Pharmacology* **5,** 173-177.

22 Armitage, A. K. & Vane, J. R. (1964). A sensitive method for the assay of catecholamines. *British Journal of Pharmacology* **22,** 204-210.

23 Pearce, A. G. E. (1960). In *Histochemistry Theoretical and Applied.* London: J. & A. Churchill, Ltd.

24 Krygier, A. & Godlewski, K. (1963). In *Histochemical Methods.* Edited: Pol. Histochem. Cytochem. Soc., Warsaw (in Polish).

25 Gomori, G. (1952). The histochemistry of Esterases. *International Review of Cytology* **1,** 323-335.

26 Fredericsson, B. (1956). Distribution of alkaline phosphatase in rat lung. *Acta Anatomica* **26,** 246-256.

27 Wachstein, M., Meisel, E. (1957). Histochemistry of hepatic phosphatases of a physiologic pH; with special reference to demonstration of bile canaliculi. *American Journal of Clinical Pathology* **27,** 13-23.
28 Nachlas, M. M., Tsou, K. C., de Souza, E., Cheng, C. S. & Seligman, A. M. (1957). Cytochemical demonstration of succinic dehydrogenase by the use of a new p-nitrophenyl substituted ditetrazole. *Journal of Histochemistry* **5,** 420-436.
29 Nachlas, M. M., Walker, D. G. & Seligman, A. M. (1958). A histochemical method for the demonstration of diphosphopyridine nucleotide diaphorase. *Journal of Biophysical and Biochemical Cytology* **4,** 29-38.
30 Fine, G., Morales, A. R. & Scerpella, J. R. (1966). Experimental myocardial infarction. *Archives of Pathology* **82,** 4-8.
31 Kent, S. P. & Diseker, M. (1955). Early myocardial ischemia; study of histochemical changes in dogs. *Laboratorial Investigations* **4,** 399-405.
32 Nachlas, M. M. & Shnitka, T. K. (1963). Macroscopic identification of early myocardial infarcts by alterations in dehydrogenase activity. *American Journal of Pathology* **42,** 379-405.
33 Kun, E. (1951). Mechanism of enzymatic reduction of triphenyl tetrazolium chloride. *Proceedings of the Society for Experimental Biology and Medicine* **78,** 195-197.
34 Farber, E., Sternberg, W. H. & Dunlap, C. E. (1956). Histochemical localization of specific oxidative enzymes. *Journal of Histochemistry* **4,** 254-265.
35 Nachlas, M. M., Walker, D. G. & Seligman, A. M. (1958). A historical method of the demonstration of diphosphopyridine nucleotide diaphorase. *Journal of Biophysical and Biochemical Cytology* **4,** 29-38.
36 McCabe, M., Maple, A. J. & Jones, G. R. N. (1945). Variations in dehydrogenase and neotetrazoleum reductase (diaphorase) activities in various buffers studied in frozen sections. *Journal of Histochemistry and Cytochemistry* **13,** 541-546.
37 Morales, A. R. & Fine, G. (1966). Early human myocardial infarction. *Archives of Pathology* **82,** 9-14.
38 Kaufman, N., Gavan, T. L. & Hill, R. W. (1959). Experimental myocardial infarction in the rat. *Archives of Pathology* **67,** 482-488.
39 Shnitka, T. K. & Nachlas, M. M. (1963). Histochemical alterations in ischaemic heart muscle and early myocardial infarction. *American Journal of Pathology* **42,** 507-521.
40 Jennings, R. B., Kaltenbach, J. P. & Smetters, G. W. (1957). Enzymatic changes in acute myocardial ischemic injury; glutamic oxaloacetic transaminase, lactic dehydrogenase and succinic dehydrogenase. *AMA Archives of Pathology* **64,** 10-16.
41 Wroblewski. F. & LaDue, J. S. (1955). Lactic dehydrogenase activity in blood. *Proceedings of the Society for Experimental Biology and Medicine* **90,** 210-213.
42 Highman, B., Maling, H. M. & Thompson, E. C. (1959). Serum transaminase and alkaline phosphatase levels after large doses of norepinephrine and epinephrine in dogs. *American Journal of Physiology* **196,** 436-440.
43 Bing, R. J. (1965). Cardiac metabolism. *Physiological Reviews* **45,** 171-213.
44 Scheuer, J. (1967). Myocardial metabolism in cardiac hypoxia. *American Journal of Cardiology* **19,** 385-392.
45 Williamson, J. R. (1966). Glycolytic control mechanisms II. *Journal of Biological Chemistry* **241,** 5026-5036.
46 Wollenberger, A. & Krause, E. G. (1968). Metabolic control characteristics of the acute ischemic myocardium. *American Journal of Cardiology* **22,** 349-359.

47 WOLLENBERGER, A., KRAUSE, E. G. & HEIER, G. (1969). Stimulation of 3', 5'-cyclic AMP formation in dog myocardium following arrest of blood flow. *Biochemical and Biophysical Research Communications* **36,** 664-670.
48 BOXER, G. E. & DEVLIN, T. M. (1961). Pathways of intracellular hydrogen transport. *Science* **134,** 1495-1501.
49 BRAASH, W., GUDBJARNASON, S., PURI, P. S., RAVENS, K. G. & BING, R. J. (1968). Early changes in energy metabolism in the myocardium following acute coronary artery occlusion in anaesthetized dogs. *Circulation Research* **23,** 429-438.
50 OLIVER, M. F., KURIEN, A. & GREENWOOD, T. W. (1968). Relation between serum-free-fatty-acids and arrhythmias and death after acute myocardial infarction. *Lancet* **I,** 710-714.
51 MCDONALD, L., BAKER, C., BRAY, C., MCDONALD, A. & RESTIEAUX, N. (1961). Plasma-catecholamines after cardiac infarction. *Lancet* **II,** 1021-1023.

DISCUSSION

Opie. What is the advantage of using histochemistry? Is it not much easier to quantitate exactly if tissue enzymes are measured biochemically?

Herbaczynska-Cedro. As I have said, a number of objections can be raised against the grading system which we used, but for this particular experimental design it seemed to us much more applicable than biochemical methods. Histochemical methods, although less quantitative, are generally closer to the biological system than assays of homogenates. These methods also allow the position and extent of the infarction to be established and this would not be possible using techniques which require tissue homogenization.

Noble. With histochemical techniques, you are measuring the activity of the hydrogen transport chain in the tissue and not the amount of enzyme present.

Herbaczynska-Cedro. Staining intensity in our techniques reflects an activity of the enzymatic systems linked with aerobic and anaerobic metabolic pathways and thus gives a general insight into the metabolic state of the myocardium, but certainly doesn't provide information as to the amount of any specific enzyme. Before more precise histochemical methods for the absolutely quantitative determination of enzymes in the tissues are available the use of this technique is a way of getting more general information on the biological state.

Thomas. I wonder whether it is really fair to speak of these changes as indices of ischaemia? Clearly you demonstrate that they occur in regions with presumed normal blood flow, maybe even greater than normal blood flow. Assuming that the coronary vasculature in this area responds to catecholamine-induced oxygen demand, it is not difficult to believe that the biochemical changes are peculiar to catecholamines and not ischaemia.

Herbaczynska-Cedro. In view of the metabolic links between anoxia and catecholamines, it seems reasonable to consider their effects in ischaemic tissue as synergistic and thus to consider the effect of catecholamines as potentiating ischaemia.

Kaijser. Dr Levi and I studied the effects of prolonged stress on sixty army volunteers. Under conditions intended to mimic those of combat, the subjects excreted increased amounts of catecholamines and 10 per cent of them showed depressed or negative T waves; these remained abnormal for a further two to three days.

Oliver. Is there any difference in serum enzyme levels if you give a beta blocker before ligating the coronary artery?

Herbaczynska-Cedro. There are numerous studies on the protective effect of beta blockers on the development of morphological lesions in the myocardium, but I don't know whether there is any data on the effect of beta blocker pretreatment on serum enzymes in myocardial infarction.

Burges. I wonder what would happen if these dogs were pretreated with nicotinic acid? Is there any chance that these changes are due to the large elevation in serum free fatty acid levels accompanying these rises in adrenaline secretion? Dr Mjøs' experiments show quite clearly that the rises in free fatty acid levels induced by infusions of catecholamines intravenously cause an increase in myocardial oxygen consumption and this surely could be relevant to a system involving electron transport changes.

Mjøs. From experiments on the effect of intravenous isoprenaline on myocardial performance and oxygen consumption in the normal dog heart, it is clear that one can increase the mechanical activity of the heart to the same extent before and after the administration of nicotinic acid. However, this is accompanied by a smaller increase in myocardial oxygen consumption in dogs pretreated with nicotinic acid. So perhaps one consequence of the adrenergic activation within the heart during coronary artery occlusion is increased oxygen demand by free fatty acids within the myocardium.

Taggart. I was unaware that adrenaline raises plasma free fatty acids in man. Dr Carruthers and I have extensive experience of simultaneous plasma catecholamine and free fatty acid measurements and it is very clear that it is noradrenaline not adrenaline that elevates plasma free fatty acids.

Burges. In dogs it may be different.

Kurien. Dr Herbaczynska-Cedro's study is the only one in which adrenaline levels are higher than noradrenaline levels. In human beings it has been shown that the adrenaline level rises only when there are complications like heart failure or shock. Do you think these dogs were in shock or in failure before you started the experiment? Secondly, I think it has been well established that in young people who die of cerebral haemorrhage you can show areas of focal myocytolysis in the myocardium in association with changes in the electrocardiogram at a time when there is no overt evidence of myocardial ischaemia.

Herbaczynska-Cedro. The development of myocardial lesions following cerebral haemorrhage has been reported in man and prevention against the development of these lesions by β-blockade occurs in animals. In our experimental model, increased catecholamine secretion follows acute coronary ligation in about 70 per cent of animals whereas in the remaining 30 per cent there is no response at all. It is difficult to say why one group of animals responds and the other doesn't. The suggestion that the sympathoadrenal response in humans depends on the basal state of sympathoadrenal system may be also applicable in dogs. Adrenaline was secreted in the majority of animals, and noradrenaline was released in excess in a minority. It is also difficult to say why noradrenaline and not adrenaline was released in any particular experiment and vice versa. Increased catecholamine secretion which occurs in the early post-ligation period was not due to the fall in the blood pressure and was not due to baroreceptor activation. It began within minutes following coronary ligation and was maintained for a few hours usually without change in systemic blood pressure. It has been shown in studies of Hodge *et al.* that in dogs very strong baroreceptor activation due to carotid occlusion induces relatively small changes in the peripheral catecholamine levels, and also the lowering of blood pressure by haemorrhage often fails to induce detectable changes in circulating amines. The mechanism of increased sympathoadrenal discharge in our experiments was studied in detail by Staszewska-Barczak[3], who found that it was induced reflexly by stimulation of cardiac receptors at the site and at the boundary of infarction.

EFFECTS OF ISCHAEMIA ON THE ACTION POTENTIAL

A. G. WALLACE

THE electrophysiological consequences of ischaemia are manifest on the electrocardiogram as characteristic alterations of initial (Q waves) and terminal portions of the QRS complex, elevation of the ST segment and inversion of the T wave. During the acute phase of ischaemia, but also following infarction for many months there is an increased propensity to a variety of disturbances of cardiac rhythm, particularly the ventricular extrasystole. The purpose of these remarks will be to review certain aspects of our knowledge about the electrophysiological basis of ischaemic changes and other data which may be relevant to the genesis of arrhythmias during infarction.

In order to build this story I would like to begin with the human heart and human electrocardiogram and to try and work backwards towards the single cell. This is important, because at least in my view the data which are available in experimental preparations and in studies of the single cell need to be viewed in the context of what is known about infarction in man. In the lower portion of Figure 9, 1 the precordial leads of a patient with a previous anterior myocardial infarction are shown. The patient also had angina pectoris and underwent aortocoronary saphenous vein bypass grafting which permitted this study. The electrocardiogram shows large Q waves in leads $V_{1\text{-}4}$ characteristic of an old anterior infarction. In the upper portion of the figure four epicardial unipolar recordings are shown from sites A, B, C and D which are indicated on the diagrammatic picture of the heart. Notice that recording [A] is taken from the trabecular zone of the right ventricle adjacent to the anterior descending branch of the coronary artery. Tracings B, C and D are taken from the anterior and lateral portions of the left ventricle at its apical portion and over the zone of old infarction. Unipolar tracing [A] reveals an initial R wave which reflects endocardial to epicardial activation. The sharp deflection which occurs 22 msec after the onset of the QRS complex represents local epicardial activation at site [A]. This wave form, that is an RS complex, is what one expects to record over normal epicardial regions of the heart. Data from a large number of normal hearts have defined the normal range of epicardial activation at each region of the right and left ventricle. Tracings

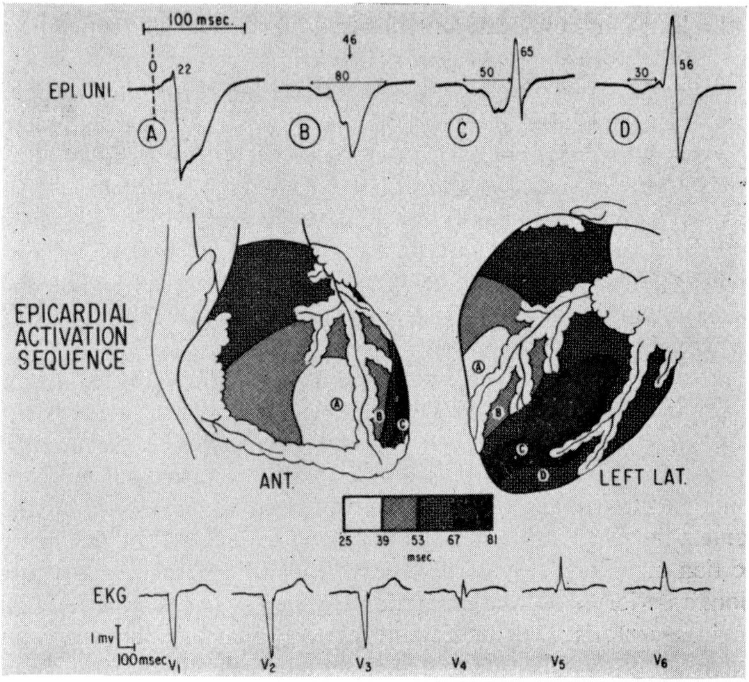

FIG. 9, 1

B, C and D are taken over the zone of infarction. You will note that rather than having an initial R wave these recordings demonstrate an initial Q. This is abnormal in this region of the heart. In addition, the rapid component of the deflection which represents local activation on the epicardial surface occurred 46 to 65 msec after the onset of the QRS complex. These local activation times, particularly that noted in Panel C, are delayed with respect to what would be expected at these locations in a normal ventricle. Activation times at approximately 50 points over the epicardial surface were used to construct the map of the sequence of epicardial excitation shown in the middle of the slide. The region overlying the infarct in the anterior apical portion of the left ventricle is the last area to depolarize and is depolarized during the terminal portions of the QRS complex.[1 2] From these direct studies of the human heart one can conclude that the Q wave which is observed on the body surface after myocardial infarction is accompanied

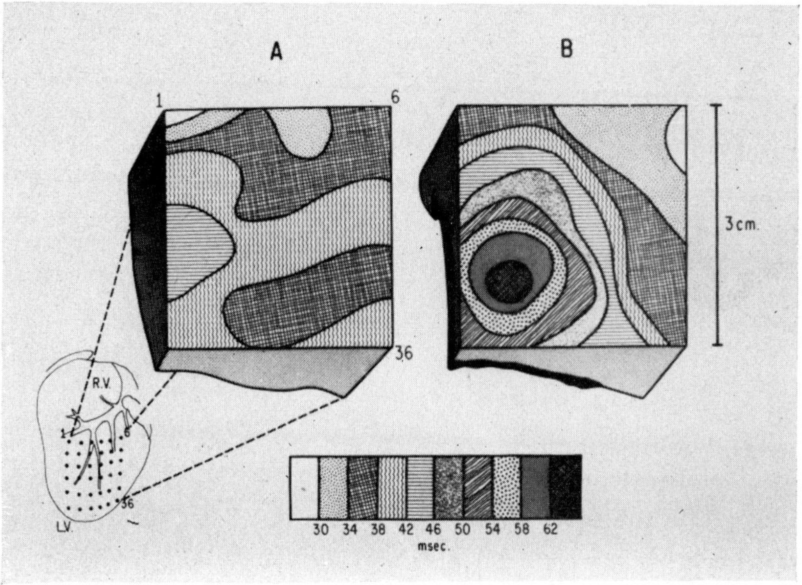

FIG. 9, 2

by Q waves recorded from unipolar epicardial leads over the zone of infarction. These Q waves result from an absence of early endocardial to epicardial forces in the region of the infarct and because electrical forces generated in other regions of the heart, and oppositely directed to those beneath the electrode, predominate. These data confirm the window theory of the Q wave. Despite the presence of Q waves, however, almost all patients with infarction except for those with gross ventricular aneurysms show local activity on the epicardial surface over the infarct and this activity is delayed. Thus, the concept of a peri-infarction conduction delay or block is evident in almost all human hearts after infarction.

Figure 9, 2 illustrates an epicardial map from a block of the anterior region of the right and left ventricle before and after myocardial infarction in the dog. Before infarction epicardial breakthrough occurs early in the QRS complex and is nearly simultaneous at multiple sites. Two weeks after occlusion of the anterior descending coronary artery and resulting infarction epicardial activation is delayed. Furthermore, the sequence of spread over this region now forms a series of converging concentric wavefronts with

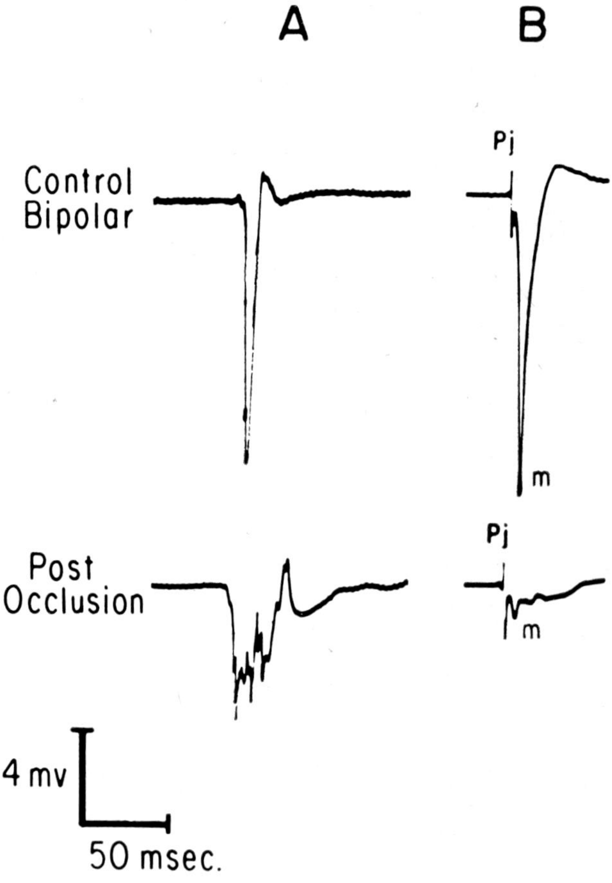

FIG. 9, 3

the last area to be depolarized being at the centre of the infarct and during the terminal portions of the QRS complex.

One can obtain a great deal of insight from epicardial maps over the region of an infarct. However, much of what is actually going on depends on recordings from intramural leads. Figure 9, 3 shows recordings from two electrodes before and after coronary occlusion in the dog. In the upper control tracings the first record is a bipolar electrogram obtained from the epicardial surface of the ventricle and tracing B is a bipolar recording obtained from the endocardial surface from the same plunge electrode. The complexes are single spikes and that the endocardial electrode shows a Purkinje spike with a large amplitude muscle deflection following it. In the lower panel approximately one hour after coronary ligation recordings are illustrated from the same site. In Panel B the Purkinje spike is still present without delay; however the endocardial muscle potential is almost absent. In Panel A there is a broad Q wave and contained within this are multiple fragmented splintered activation waves of low amplitude. Thus, in the intramural portions of an infarction there is loss of amplitude of signals and the delayed splintered complex suggests slow activation.

After infarction, the intramural delay which occurs leads to splintered complexes, but in addition one may observe marked delay and within the ischaemic zone periodic delays of the Wenckebach type. Like Wenckebach periodicity in the AV node, these delays within the wall of the ventricle also can be shown to be rate related. From these observations, one can conclude that there is not only delay of epicardial activation following infarction, but furthermore, within the ischaemic zone there is marked delay, rate dependent conduction and sometimes Wenckebach periodicity. Thus, the infarction zone demonstrates behaviour analogous to the AV node, and behaviour consistent with the requirements for re-entrant beating

Figure 9, 4 shows the early effects of ischaemia on the action potential of Purkinje fibres on the left and ventricular muscle on the right. At least at this level of examination the effects appear to be similar. The normal myocardial action potential is characterized by a resting membrane potential of approximately −90 mv; the upstroke of the action potential is rapid with a prominent overshoot and in Purkinje fibres action potential duration is normally

250-300 msec. Ischaemia produces time dependent changes in the characteristics of the action potential. In both Purkinje fibres and ventricular muscle the first effect of ischaemia is a decrease in the duration of the action potential due to more rapid repolarization. Subsequently there is a loss of resting membrane potential and a corresponding decrease in the rate of rise of the action potential and the overshoot. When Purkinje or muscle fibres are made totally ischaemic they progress from normal through the stages described to a state of considerable loss of membrane potential and finally total inexcitability in about 40 minutes.

EFFECTS OF ISCHAEMIA

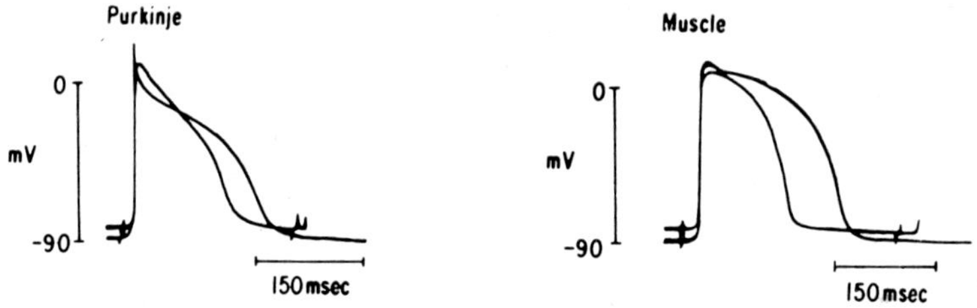

FIG. 9, 4

Figure 9, 5 is taken from a paper published by Scher and his colleagues[3] and demonstrates the relationship between the changes in the action potential and the surface electrocardiogram. The unique features of their study were first the simultaneous recording of action potentials from normal and ischaemic muscle and second the recording of surface electrocardiograms with DC rather than AC amplifiers. Thus, the electrocardiograms noted below are recordings of potential on anterior chest with respect to ground rather than an indifferent lead. With these amplifiers they could analyse whether changes of the ST segment represented true elevation of the ST segment or were a consequence of depression of the T-Q segment. In the control state action potential duration in the two zones was comparable and both the ST and TQ segments were at ground potential. Approximately 5 minutes after coronary ligation action potentials in the ischaemic zone became shortened. There was thus a voltage gradient between the normal and ischaemic zones of muscle because of the early repolarization in the ischaemic zone. This voltage gradient during repolarization was reflected as an elevation of the ST segment on the surface electrocardiogram because unipolar records obtained over this region represented a source for electrical current during repolarization. In the last panel which was recorded later during the course of ischaemia when some cells had lost resting potential there was in addition to the systolic voltage difference between

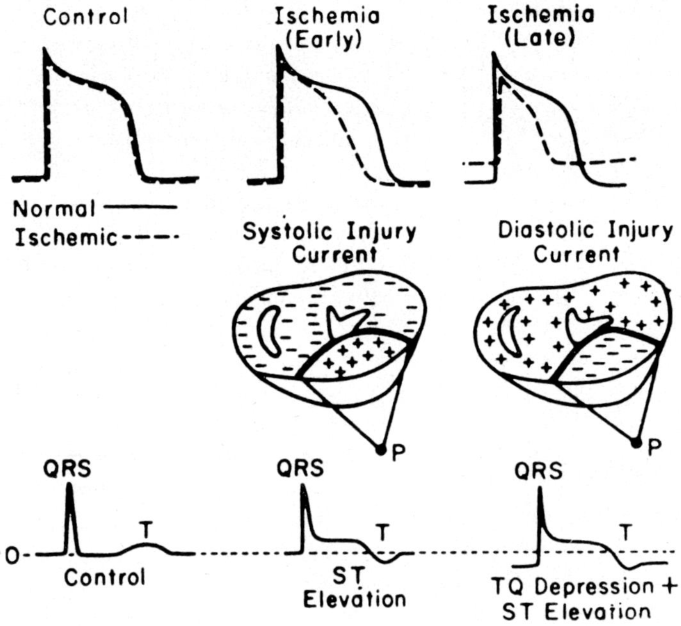

FIG. 9, 5

normal and ischaemic cells a diastolic difference. In this situation the ischaemic zone represented a sink for current and was thus reflected as a deviation negative to ground during the TQ interval on the surface electrocardiogram. From these studies one can conclude that the actual ST segment displacement during the acute phase of myocardial injury is the result of true ST segment elevation in part and also depression of the TQ interval. The Q wave on the other hand as indicated previously is the result of an intramural conduction disturbance or an actual loss of cells in the ischaemic zone.

In an effort to better understand the potential role of re-entry as a basis for ectopic beats arising from depressed tissues, Dr Cranefield and his colleagues have recently presented some very provocative experiments.[4] Isolated Purkinje fibres have been exposed to a high concentration of extracellular potassium by placing them in an agar block which contains excess potassium. One effect of the high potassium is to partially depolarize the fibres resulting in a conduction disturbance.

This of course is not ischaemia but the effects of high potassium do seem to simulate the effects of ischaemia and to the extent that this simulation is accurate one can draw certain conclusions about the nature of arrhythmias which might occur under such conditions. Thus, the basic design of these experiments was to create a small localized area of depression in the Purkinje fibre and to examine propagation along the fibre. In this strand of Purkinje fibres local depression induced by high extracellular K^+ produced a local conduction disturbance. The conduction disturbance was rate related and demonstrated Wenckebach type periodicity. The conduction disturbance was such that spontaneous extra systoles occurred after every seventh beat.

There are many potential mechanisms for arrhythmias in the human heart during ischaemia. Each of these deserves exploration. Evidence from both human and the experimental animal which indicates that a prominent feature of myocardial infarction is a conduction disturbance in the zone of the infarct.

This conduction disturbance has been recorded and can be shown to demonstrate rate dependence, unidirectional block and Wenckebach periodicity each of which are characteristic of circuits which will support re-entry. The apparent changes of the ST segment and the development of the Q wave on the electrocardiogram can be explained on the basis of our present knowledge of the consequences of infarction. Ischaemia produces a decrease in action potential duration, a loss of resting membrane potential and a decrease in the upstroke velocity of surviving cells. These abnormalities possibly together with the interruption of low resistance intracellular connections can account for the conduction disturbance produced by infarction. To the extent that Cranefield's experiments using high potassium to simulate ischaemia are an accurate simulation of the ischaemic process studies have been performed in Purkinje fibres which also demonstrate slow conduction, unidirectional block and re-entry. Thus, it seems possible to account for the phenomenon of ventricular irritability following infarction on a re-entry basis. The data I have presented do not exclude other possibilities but the re-entry hypothesis is an attractive one because it could be used not only to explain the phenomenon of arrhythmias during the acute phase of infarction—but also the persistence of a susceptibility to ventricular ectopic beats long after the acute phase.

ACKNOWLEDGMENT

I wish to express my appreciation to Dr John Boineau who contributed Figures 9, 1 to 9, 3 for this manuscript and did most of the research which forms the basis of this report.

REFERENCES

1 DANIEL, T. M. (1971). Comparison of human ventricular activation with a canine model in chronic myocardial infarction. *Circulation* **44,** 74-89.

2 DURRER, D., FORMIJNE, P., DAM, R. T., VAN LIER, A. A., BULLER, J. & MEIJLER, F. L. (1961). The electrocardiogram in normal and some abnormal conditions, in revived human fetal heart and in acute and chronic coronary occlusion. *American Heart Journal* **61,** 303-316.

3 SAMSON, W. E. & SCHER, A. M. (1960). Mechanism of ST segment alteration during acute myocardial injury. *Circulation Research* **8,** 780-787.

4 WIT, A. L., CRANEFIELD, P. F. & HOFFMAN, B. F. (1972). Slow conduction and re-entry in the ventricular conducting system. *Circulation Research* **30,** 11-22.

DISCUSSION

Opie. What was the concentration of potassium in the hyperkalaemic experiments? How easy is it to measure the epicardial delay in conduction?

Wallace. Your first question relates to Dr Cranefield's experiments[3] which he has done with agar containing potassium in a variety of concentrations. I think that most of the experiments were carried out at a potassium concentration of approximately 10 mM. The second question relates to the recording techniques used for epicardial mapping. Dr Durrer should comment on this because he developed the techniques. We use a recording system which contains two electrodes which are a millimetre apart. We record bipolar signals from the combination of the two and we record unipolar signals from each of the single components of the electrode. Data are accepted for analysis only if this is a sharp deflection of less than 3 or 4 msec duration in the bipolar trace. The instrumentation is a series of high fidelity amplifiers with good frequency response. All data are recorded on tape and then played back on a photographic recorder.

Durrer. Our methods were published in the *American Heart Journal* in 1964 (**68,** 765 to 776).

Reuter. You can see exactly the same effect on the duration of action potential in an isolated perfused organ if you eliminate the oxygen supply from the perfusion fluid. Usually you see first a change in the duration of the action potential and afterwards a loss of the resting potential. However there has been an interesting report by Dr McLeod, who showed that despite the persistence of hypoxia if he added glucose to the solution particularly if he added insulin, he could lengthen the action potential again quite appreciably. Have you any information on this from your own experiments?

Wallace. I don't have any information on raising the blood sugar or the combination with insulin in this preparation. One of the things which I am not clear about is the extent to which the effects of ischaemia are really hypoxia dependant. I have never been certain that oxygen is the critical substrate in determining the phenomena that we see when one reduces blood flow.

Durrer. The concentration of potassium of the interstitial fluid of the ischaemic region is increased. It can be demonstrated that injection of potassium into a branch of a coronary artery may cause similar changes in excitation as occur during ischaemia of this region.

Reuter. If there is an increase in potassium concentration I would not expect spontaneous depolarization to occur in the region of ischaemia because the potassium conductance increases if external potassium concentration is increased and this abolishes spontaneous activity. However if you depolarize the cells by passing a current then you can see regularly spontaneous depolarization occurring even in cells which do not normally have pacemaker potential such as ventricular or atrial cells. I wonder whether you saw during the period of ischaemia, spontaneous depolarization occurring in the region of the ischaemia.

Wallace. Dr Cranefield did not comment on this in his paper. Dr Sherlag from Miami has done some recent studies in which he has resected portions of ischaemic endo-myocardium and studied it using micro-electrodes. He has found spontaneous automaticity in endocardial fibres.

Reuter. If you depolarize into the range where the potassium conductance decreases, spontaneous activity is favoured. Hence, my question as to whether there was an increase in the potassium concentration.

Wallace. I think that most clinical cardiologists would still have considerable difference of opinion as to how frequent the extra-systolic phenomenon that we see in acute infarction meets criteria for being an automatic rhythm. But if you look at all the extra-systoles that occur in people with acute myocardial infarction most of these are of the coupled variety. One certainly sees other rhythms that appear to represent automatic rhythms in acute infarction.

Durrer. It is very difficult to unravel the causative mechanism of VPB in the intact exposed dog heart with acute myocardial infarction. The location of the return pathway is like looking for a needle in a haystack.

Han. Non-paroxysmal ventricular tachycardia or accelerated idioventricular rhythm that we see in some patients with myocardial infarction may be due to enhanced automaticity. It has been shown that Purkinje fibres increase the automaticity, that is, the slope of slow diastolic depolarization is increased under the influence of steady depolarizing current. The ischaemic myocardial tissue may supply such steady depolarizing current to the adjacent Purkinje fibres to increase these automaticity.

Durrer. There are arguments that a paroxysmal ventricular tachycardia in the human heart may be caused by a circus movement in the ventricles. We can stop a paroxysmal ventricular tachycardia in these instances by inducing 1 or sometimes 2 ventricular premature beats at the right time and at the right location.

Vellani. I refer to the experiments of Cranefield in which delayed conduction is well shown. Would you comment on the behaviour of these Purkinje fibres which appear to be excitable surprisingly early during repolarization and the action potentials propagate even though the upstroke begins at less than half the resting membrane potential?

Wallace. It is possible to re-excite a Purkinje fibre when it has repolarized to −50 or −60 mv. This type of re-excitation can be seen by stimulating the cell directly or by propagation from another cell. Let me say that I think there is something here which is pertinent to all of us who are interested in the pharmacology of treating arrhythmias. Most of us are used to putting pharmacological agents on normal myocardial cells, but the pharmacology of diseased tissue may be unique.

Reuter. Pharmacology in this respect is really quite underdeveloped. However there is some information that partially depolarized cells are very sensitive to the application of noradrenaline or adrenaline—particularly adrenaline. You can get much larger potentials with a slow uptake velocity if you apply adrenaline.

Durrer. To ischaemic muscle?

Reuter. Not to ischaemic muscle but to potassium depolarized muscles.

Thomas. Conduction delays over an infarction presumably can cause a shift in mean QRS vector. Do you think that what we call hemiblock these days is in fact a myocardial block and not a fascicular block?

Wallace. Many instances of axis deviation may be the consequence of an intramural conduction disturbance without requiring interruption of the proximal portions of the left bundle branch.

Durrer. I cannot explicitly answer 'yes' or 'no' to Dr Thomas' question, but I think you can have marked axis deviation following a myocardial infarction associated with the abnormal and slow intramural conduction without there being involvement of the fascicles.

VENTRICULAR VULNERABILITY IN MYOCARDIAL ISCHAEMIA

J. HAN

Supported by Grants HE-12498 and HE-14177 from the National Institutes of Health.

VENTRICULAR vulnerability to fibrillation can be demonstrated in experimental animals by stimulating the ventricle during a brief period in the relative refractory period. Weak electrical stimuli applied during this vulnerable period evoke only early premature beats, but if stimuli were increased in intensity, fibrillation results.[1] Such stimuli applied during diastole never produce fibrillation. In clinical practice, spontaneous ventricular premature beats or artificial pacemaker stimuli occurring around the peak of the T wave may precipitate ventricular fibrillation and this is considered as a demonstration of ventricular vulnerability in man. Mechanisms of ventricular vulnerability are not completely clear, but it is generally agreed that a strong stimulus delivered in the vulnerable period sets up a centre of rapidly repetitive impulses which, in turn, initiate fibrillation in the ventricle.[2] Such rapid impulses appear to arise at a site in the ventricle as a result of sustained re-entrant activity. These rapid impulses will be conducted along markedly irregular wave fronts as they are initiated during the relative refractory period when excitability and conductivity are nonuniformly depressed in the ventricle. The nonuniformity of the ventricle with respect to excitability and conductivity should become progressively increased by the repetitive excitation resulting in the development of multiple sites of re-entry and fractionation of wave fronts into many irregular wavelets, i.e., fibrillation.[3]

It has been shown in experimental animals that ventricular fibrillation threshold is significantly lowered (or ventricular vulnerability is increased) in the ventricle after an area of ischaemia has been created by occlusion of a coronary artery branch.[4 5] The incidence of ventricular fibrillation is also increased in patients with acute myocardial infarct. The degree of nonuniformity with respect to excitability and conductivity should be increased in the ventricle during coronary occlusion as a result of marked depression of these properties in the affected area of myocardium. The ventricles with myocardial ischaemia or infarction should, therefore, be more vulnerable to fibrillation since re-entrant activity and fractionation of wave fronts are more likely to occur in such ventricles. The purpose of this paper is to discuss the mechanisms of re-entry and increased vulnerability of the ventricle associated with experimental myocardial ischaemia or infarction.

Re-entrant Activity

There are two basic types of re-entrant activity operating to generate ectopic impulses, namely ' focal ' re-excitation and ' circus ' re-entry.[6 7] Focal re-excitation is re-entrant activity without establishment of a circus movement loop. If neighbouring myocardial fibres repolarize at sufficiently disparate rates, already repolarized fibres may be re-excited by the flow of current between these and neighbouring fibres that are still depolarized.[3 6 7] When neighbouring fibres repolarize within a few milliseconds of each other, re-excitation can not occur because the difference in potential among them will not exceed the threshold of already repolarized fibres; however, increased temporal dispersion of repolarization would increase the potential difference and initiate re-excitation. It appears that the electrotonic interaction among adjacent fibres effectively prevents a gross disparity in their repolarization rates in the normal myocardial tissue; hence, the phenomenon of re-excitation can not occur. However, in the diseased myocardium, adjacent fibres or fibre groups may repolarize at sufficiently disparate times, and the resulting potential difference may initiate re-excitation. Circus re-entry represents propagation of an impulse in a circular path. A necessary factor for the establishment of a circus movement loop (or a circuit) is an area of refractory tissue which initially fails to respond to an impulse propagating in one direction (unidirectional block). This area may recover its excitability in time to accept re-entry of the same impulse returning in the opposite direction. A re-entry circuit can also be established if propagation of an impulse in one area is slow enough to permit other areas to recover from the initial response and be re-entered by the slowly emerging impulse.[6 7] Such re-entry circuits should be more likely to be created in the tissue with localized areas of depressed excitability and conductivity produced by disease processes.

Figure 10, 1 depicts the time course of changes in diastolic threshold, refractory period and conduction time in the affected area after complete occlusion of the anterior descending artery.[8] Diastolic threshold, refractory period and conduction time slightly decreased initially within three min after the artery was totally occluded. Subsequently, they were increased markedly during the remainder of the occlusion period. It appears that excitability and conductivity are initially increased because of moderate ischaemia in the area, but they are depressed later when the area becomes severely ischaemic. These results suggest that increased ventricular ectopic activity during coronary occlusion might be partly due to focal re-excitation resulting from increased asynchrony of recovery at the boundary between the normal area and the moderately ischaemic area with accelerated repolarization.[6-8] It may also occur as a result of re-entrant circuits established between the normal and severely ischaemic areas of the ventricle. Because of marked depression in excitability and conductivity in the severely ischaemic area, an impulse may be delayed through the depressed area long enough to permit re-entry of the same impulse into the normal area and generate a re-entrant response.[6-8]

The results of an experiment shown in Figure 10, 2 suggests that the re-entry between normal and severe ischaemic areas may indeed be established. In the control in part A, the ventricle was paced by basic stimuli (S_1) applied to the ventricle at a cycle length of 500 msec; and the earliest possible premature response was evoked by delivering a premature stimulus (S_2) at 190 msec following the 10th S_1. In part B, about 4 min after occlusion of the anterior descending artery, the premature response of the same timing was followed by a re-entrant response in the normal area (Va). This was observed when the local electrogram of the ischaemic area (Vb) demonstrated a decrease in amplitude and an increase in duration indicating slow conduction in the area. This suggests that the slow propagation of premature response through the ischaemic area allowed a sufficient time for the normal area to recover from the previous response and accept the re-entrant impulse. The re-entrant response was then propagated to the whole ventricle to produce an extrasystole, as indicated in the lead II electrocardio-

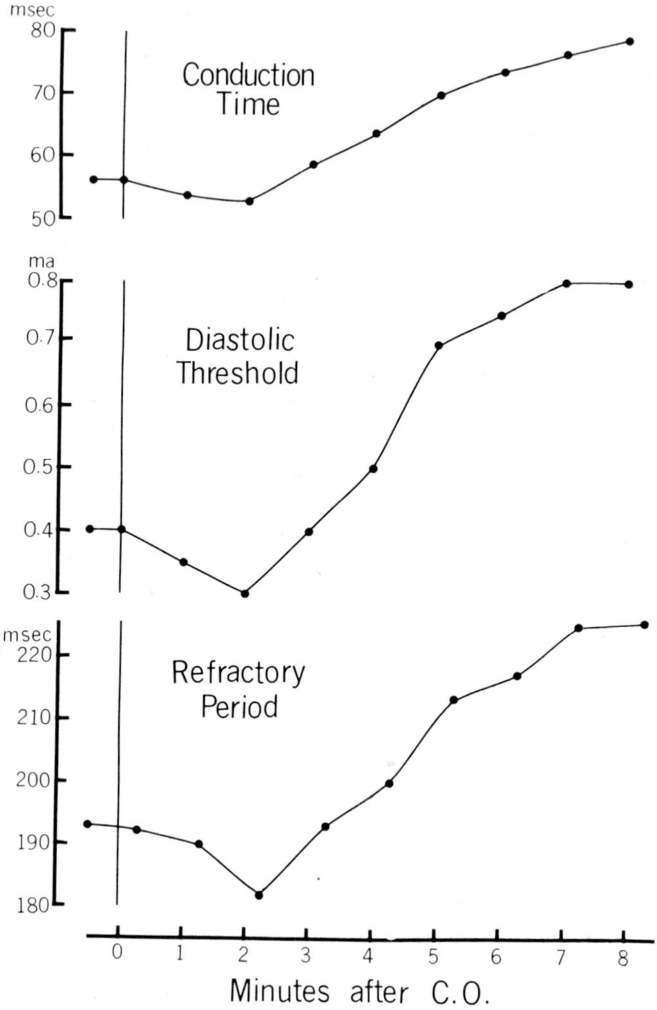

FIG. 10, 1. Changes in diastolic threshold, refractory period and conduction time in the ischaemic area after complete occlusion of the anterior descending artery (C.O.). (From Han[8] by permission of the publisher.)

gram. In part C at 5 min after occlusion of the artery, the premature response propagated to the ischaemic area and returned to the normal area as a re-entrant beat, and this was followed by a number of recurrent responses at the Vb and Va recording sites, suggesting continuation of the re-entry between the ischaemic and normal areas. When the premature response was induced later at

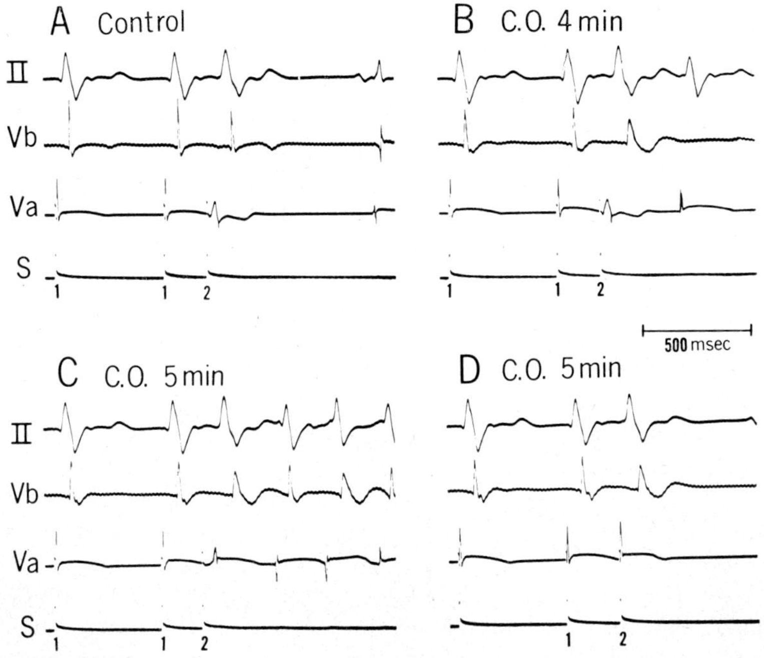

FIG. 10, 2. Re-entrant activity induced by a premature response in the ventricle with an ischaemic area. A, control; and B through C, during coronary occlusion (C.O.). Lead II electrocardiogram was recorded; local electrogram was also recorded at the normal area (Va) and at the area of potential ischaemia (Vb). Stimuli (S) were applied to the normal area at a site close to the Va recording site.

250 msec. following S_1 in part D, it was propagated to the ischaemic site more rapidly (shorter S_2 Vb_2 interval) and was not followed by re-entrant beats. It appears that no re-entry resulted because relatively rapid transmission through the ischaemic area did not allow a sufficient time for the normal area to recover and accept the re-entrant impulse. The results indicate that premature beats, whether generated by enhanced automaticity of Purkinje fibres or

L

re-entry in the ventricular tissues, would be more likely to induce sustained re-entry and tachycardia in the ventricle with myocardial ischaemia.[6-9]

Increased Vulnerability

Ventricular vulnerability to fibrillation can be estimated by determining the fibrillation threshold, i.e., the least intensity of an electrical stimulus applied to the ventricle to induce fibrillation. The fibrillation threshold has been customarily determined by time-consuming repeated scans of the vulnerable period with a single pulse at increasing intensities until fibrillation occurs. However, the fibrillation threshold can be more rapidly determined by applying a train of square pulses occurring at a rate of 100 per second during the vulnerable period.[5] In our experiments, these rapid pulses are applied during an interval between the onset of the basic response and the peak of T wave in the lead II electrocardiogram, within which the vulnerable period would certainly fall (see Fig. 10, 3). The gradual increase in the intensity of these gated pulses results in a progressive decrease in the coupling interval of the first premature beat and a progressive decrease in the number of subsequent repetitive responses preceding the onset of fibrillation.

Figure 10, 3 depicts the results of an experiment in which fibrillation thresholds were determined with the gated pulses in the control state and during coronary occlusion.[5] In the control state in part A, gated stimuli of 21 ma, just short of the fibrillation threshold, evoked two premature responses. When fibrillation was induced by stimuli of 22 ma, it was preceded by the first premature beat coupled to the basic response at 168 msec. In part B at about five min after occlusion of the anterior descending artery, stimuli of 13 ma evoked only one premature beat, but stimuli of 14 ma were successful in inducing fibrillation preceded by the first premature beat with a coupling interval of 180 msec. As shown in the figure, the decreased fibrillation threshold was observed when the local electrogram of the ischaemic area (Vb) demonstrated a decrease in amplitude and an increase in duration indicating depressed conductivity. The results indicate that in the presence of an ischaemic area the ventricle can be fibrillated by premature excitation occurring later in the cycle. Relatively late premature beats can, of course, be induced in the ventricle by test stimuli of a lower intensity, resulting in a lower fibrillation threshold for the ventricle during coronary occlusion.[5 6]

Ventricular vulnerability can be also assessed by increasing the

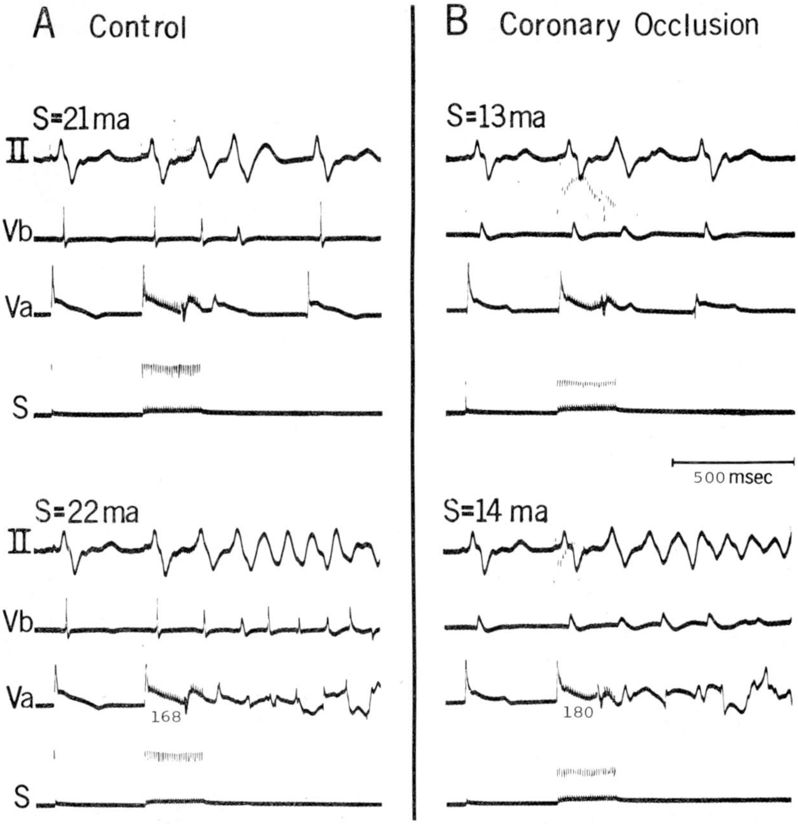

FIG. 10, 3. Fibrillation thresholds determined with the gated stimuli in the control state (A) and during coronary occlusion (B) at an identical site unaffected by ischaemia. Local ventricular electrograms were recorded at a site close to stimulating electrodes in the potentially intact area (Va) and at a site within the area of potential ischaemia (Vb). (From Han[5] by permission of the publisher.)

duration of application of rapid stimuli to increase progressively the number of premature beats until fibrillation occurs.[5] The gated rapid stimuli of twice the diastolic threshold intensity and at a rate of 100 per sec are used in our experiments. As the duration of the gate of rapid stimuli is gradually increased to produce increasing number of premature beats, the cycle length between successive beats decreases progressively and fibrillation is induced when the cycle length is reduced to a critical value. If the ventricle can be fibrillated by premature beats, with relatively long cycle length, i.e.,

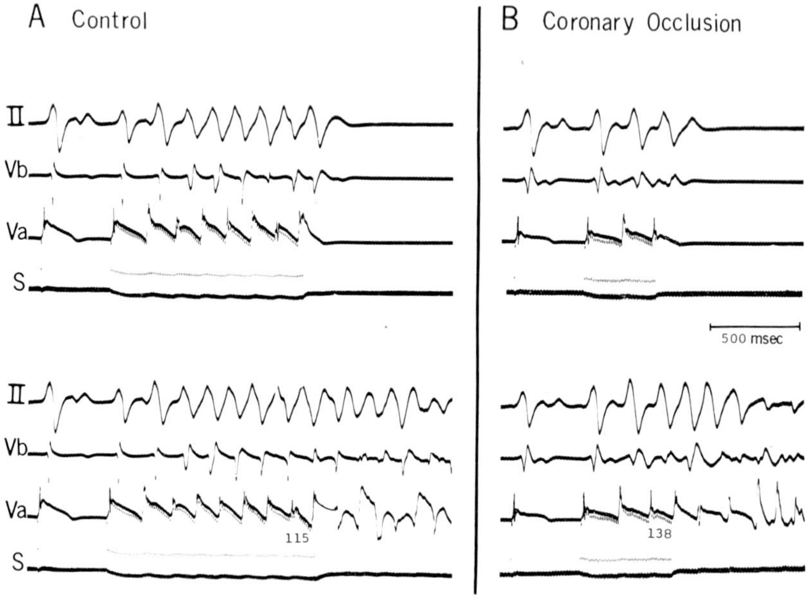

FIG. 10, 4. Numbers of accelerating premature beats required to initiate fibrillation in the control state (A) and during coronary occlusion (B). The gated stimuli were applied to an identical site unaffected by ischaemia. Other conventions as in Figure 10, 3. (From Han[5] by permission of the publisher.)

if the critical cycle length for fibrillation is increased, fibrillation will result from a smaller number of accelerating premature beats, provided that the rate of acceleration is constant. The vulnerability is, therefore, inversely related to the number of accelerating premature beats preceding the onset of fibrillation.[5]

Figure 10, 4 illustrates the results of an experiment in which the number of accelerating premature beats required to induce fibrillation was studied before and during coronary occlusion.[5] In the control state in part A, fibrillation was not induced by seven premature beats, but it resulted when eight premature beats accelerated to reach a critical cycle length of 115 msec. In part B, about six min after occlusion of the anterior descending artery, fibrillation was produced by three premature beats accelerating to a cycle length of 138 msec. As shown in the figure, the observation was made when the electrogram recorded in the ischaemic area (Vb) showed a decrease in amplitude and an increase in duration indicating depressed conductivity. The results indicate that the critical cycle length of premature beats for the initiation of fibrillation was longer in the ventricle with an ischaemic area; the longer critical cycle length was attained by a smaller number of repetitive beats, since the rate of their acceleration remained the same.[5 6]

The irregular excitability and conductivity are the conditions which favour development of re-entrant activity, fractionation of wave fronts of excitation, and total disorganization of impulse propagation, i.e., fibrillation.[5-8] Myocardial ischaemia produces a marked depression of excitability and conduction velocity of the myocardium. The likelihood of re-entrant activity and the resulting fibrillation would be, therefore, increased in the ventricle with an ischaemic area because of the presence of localized areas of depressed excitability and conductivity.[5-10] An early premature impulse is more likely to be delayed through the ischaemic area, and the impulse may then return to the intact area as a re-entrant beat. If such re-entrant activity is sustained, the ventricle will be repetitively activated and eventually thrown into a disorganized state of fibrillation. Because of the increased likelihood of development of re-entrant activity, fibrillation can be more readily induced in the ventricle with an ischaemic area by test stimuli of lower intensities, which evoke premature beats of longer coupling intervals and fewer subsequent premature beats. Such test stimuli would have been ineffective in producing fibrillation in the normal ventricle.[5 6]

Figure 10, 5 illustrates the results of an experiment in which the mode of initiation of fibrillation was studied before and after coronary occlusion.[11] In the control state in A, the ventricle was paced by basic stimuli (S_1) applied to a pacing site (S) near the base of the right ventricle at a cycle length of 400 msec; fibrillation thresholds were determined by repeated scans of the vulnerable period with a single test shock (S_2) at increasing stimulus intensities. The fibrillation threshold was found to be 15 ma at an interval of 160 msec following the basic response. The responses to S_1 and S_2

propagated from the site of stimulation to Va, Vb and Vc recording sites, and subsequent 7 or 8 rapidly repetitive beats preceding the onset of fibrillation were also originated from the site of stimulation as indicated by the repeated sequence of Va–Vb–Vc. In part B

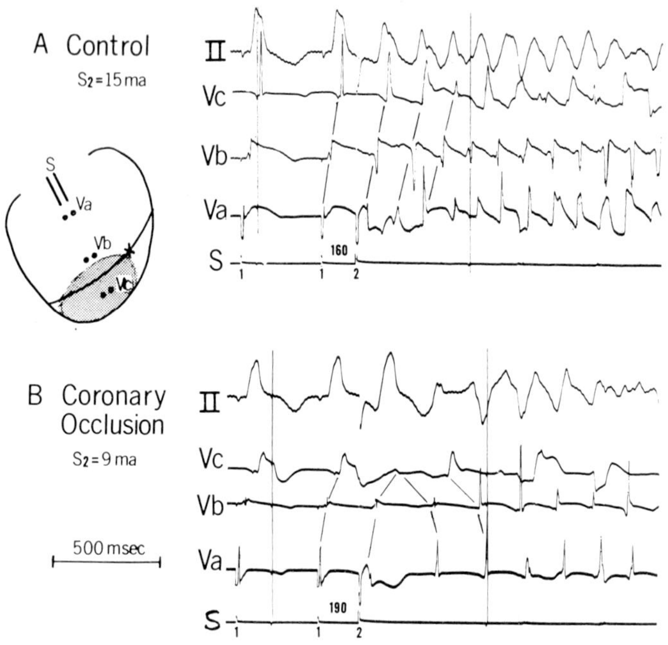

FIG. 10, 5

FIG. 10, 5. Fibrillation thresholds determined with a single pulse applied to the vulnerable period of the ventricle in the control state (A) and during coronary occlusion (B). The diagram in the left shows the arrangement of stimulating and recording electrodes and the area of potential ischaemia (shaded area) on the anterior surface of the ventricles. Basic (S_1) and test (S_2) stimuli were applied to a pacing site (S) near the base of the ventricle. Local ventricular electrograms were recorded at a site close to stimulating electrodes and another site close to the edge of the area of expected ischaemia (labelled Va and Vb). The electrogram was also recorded at a site within the area of potential ischaemia (Vc). (From Han[11] by permission of the publisher.)

after creation of an ischaemic area by occlusion of the anterior descending artery, the fibrillation threshold was found to be 9 ma at 190 msec after the basic response, and 3 or 4 rapid beats preceding the onset of fibrillation were originated near the ischaemic area as indicated by the reversed sequence of responses at the 3 recording sites. The rate of the initial rapid responses was about 440/min (a cycle length of 135 msec) in the control state and it decreased to 340/min (a cycle length of 175 msec) after coronary occlusion. The results again indicate that fibrillation can be induced by the initial premature beat of a longer coupling interval and a smaller number of subsequent repetitive beats in the ventricle during coronary occlusion. The rate of rapid repetitive beats preceding the onset of fibrillation would be slower during coronary occlusion because the length of a re-entrant circuit established between normal and ischaemic areas is expected to be longer than that of focal re-entrant activity set up near the site of stimulation.[11]

SUMMARY

Ventricular fibrillation can be induced by electrical stimuli applied to the ventricle during the vulnerable period. Such stimuli set up a centre of rapidly repetitive impulses which, in turn, precipitate fibrillation in the ventricle. The origin of these rapid impulses appear to be due to sustained re-entrant activity established at a site in the ventricle. These rapid impulses will be conducted along progressively more irregular wave fronts as they are initiated during the relative refractory period when excitability and conductivity are nonuniformly depressed in the ventricle. Fibrillation may then result when the ventricle becomes sufficiently disorganized as a result of the development of multiple sites of the re-entrant activity and independent irregular wavelets. Severe ischaemia produces marked depression of excitability and conductivity in the affected area of myocardium. The presence of ischaemic areas increases the degree of nonuniformity in the ventricle with respect to excitability and conductivity, and this facilitates the development of re-entrant activity and fractionation of wave fronts. Increased vulnerability of the ventricle with ischaemic areas is manifested by a decrease in the fibrillation threshold because fibrillation can be induced in such ventricles by premature beats with longer coupling intervals and fewer subsequent repetitive responses.

REFERENCES

1 WIGGERS, C. J. & WEGRIA, R. (1940). Ventricular fibrillation due to single localized induction and condenser shocks applied during the vulnerable period of ventricular systole. *American Journal of Physiology* **128**, 500-505.

2 Moe, G. K., Harris, A. S. & Wiggers, C. J. (1941). Analysis of the initiation of fibrillation by electrographic studies. *American Journal of Physiology* **134,** 473.
3 Moe, G. K., Abildskov, J. A. & Han, J. (1964). Factors responsible for initiation and maintenance of ventricular fibrillation. In *Sudden cardiac death*; p. 56. Edited by: B. Surawicz and E. D. Pellegrino. New York: Grune and Stratton.
4 Wiggers, C. J., Wegria, R. & Pinera, B. (1940). The effect of myocardial ischaemia on the fibrillation threshold—the mechanism of spontaneous ventricular fibrillation following coronary occlusion. *American Journal of Physiology* **131,** 309-316.
5 Han, J. (1969). Ventricular vulnerability during acute coronary occlusion. *American Journal of Cardiology* **24,** 857-864.
6 Han, J. (1969). Mechanisms of ventricular arrhythmias associated with myocardial infarction. *American Journal of Cardiology* **24,** 800-813.
7 Han, J. (1971). The concepts of re-entrant activity responsible for ectopic rhythms. *American Journal of Cardiology* **28,** 253-262.
8 Han, J. (1972). Ventricular ectopic activity in myocardial infarction. In *Cardiac Arrhythmias,* p. 171. Edited by: J. Han, Springfield and C. C. Thomas.
9 Han, J., Goel, B. G. & Hanson, C. S. (1970). Re-entrant beats induced in the ventricular during coronary occlusion. *American Heart Journal* **80,** 778-784.
10 Lown, B., Klein, M. D., Hershberg, P. I. (1969). Coronary and per-coronary care. *American Journal of Medicine* **46,** 705-724.
11 Han, J. (1972 in press). Ventricular vulnerability to fibrillation. In *The 2nd Hahnemann Symposium on Cardiac Arrhythmias.* Edited by: L. S. Dreifus and W. Likoff. New York: Grune and Stratton.

Discussion

Kurien. In view of the demonstration that there are significant changes in hormonal milieu and the functional and anatomical characteristics of the non-ischaemic myocardium, is it fair to say that the electrophysiological characteristics of the non-ischaemic myocardium do not change?

Han. We have assessed electrophysiological properties such as diastolic threshold, refractory period and conduction rate in the non-ischaemic area during coronary occlusion and found that they were not significantly changed.

Kurien. You demonstrated that if you infuse catecholamine you can reduce the threshold of fibrillation in the non-ischaemic heart.

Han. Yes, sympathetic stimulation may decrease the fibrillation threshold. But the decreased fibrillation threshold during coronary occlusion is mainly due to the presence of ischaemic areas in the ventricle.

Kurien. Then do you need to postulate that the ischaemic area itself is contributing to lowering of threshold?

Han. It was shown in my presentation that the pattern of initiation of fibrillation is different between the control state and after coronary occlusion. Fibrillation was initiated by premature beats with longer coupling intervals and by a smaller number of repetition beats after coronary occlusion. This contributes to lowering the threshold.

Vellani. Would you comment on the relationship between the early beats initiating fibrillation presumably by a re-entry mechanism and the beats seen within 15 min or so after coronary occlusion? Whereas one would expect the position of ectopic beats to be at the end of the T wave i.e. immediately after recovery of excitability, it is surprising how many ectopic beats are distributed throughout diastole and the intervals between the beats reveal periodicity suggesting parasystolic rhythm and, therefore, an automatic basis for their origin. Do you consider that the R-on-T excitation which leads to fibrillation is something different to that which produces ectopic beats in diastole?

Han. Ventricular premature beats that are due to the re-entrant mechanism may be closely coupled to the previous beat, that is the R-on-T phenomenon. Because of their greater prematurity, these beats should be more likely to initiate ventricular tachycardia and fibrillation. The coupling interval of this type of premature beat is usually short and constant because the re-entry is expected to occur as soon as the myocardial tissue recovers from the previous activity. Ventricular premature beats resulting from enhanced automaticity of the His-Purkinje system are expected to occur with late and variable intervals. These may be guidelines for the differentiation between premature beats of re-entry and enhanced automaticity.

Durrer. But you don't think, Dr Han, that these are absolute criteria?

Han. No, I am afraid they are not.

Vellani. An analogue-hybrid computer built in the Department of Medical Physics of the University of Edinburgh has been used to find ventricular ectopic beats in the tape recorded ECG signal and to time these from the preceding beat. The coupling interval histogram (Figure 10, 6) shows the distribution of ectopic complexes which occurred about 10 min after occlusion of the left circumflex coronary artery of a dog by a balloon catheter inserted through the right carotid artery. The ectopic beats are distributed throughout diastole with a preference for late diastole. The intervals between ectopic beats examined by power spectrum analysis revealed the sinus period and in addition the values 0·25 and 0·21 sec which are clearly different from the sinus period. I do not minimize the problems of diagnosing parasystolic rhythm but if ectopic distribution in diastole was random due only to varying conduction times of re-entrant sinus impulses I would not have

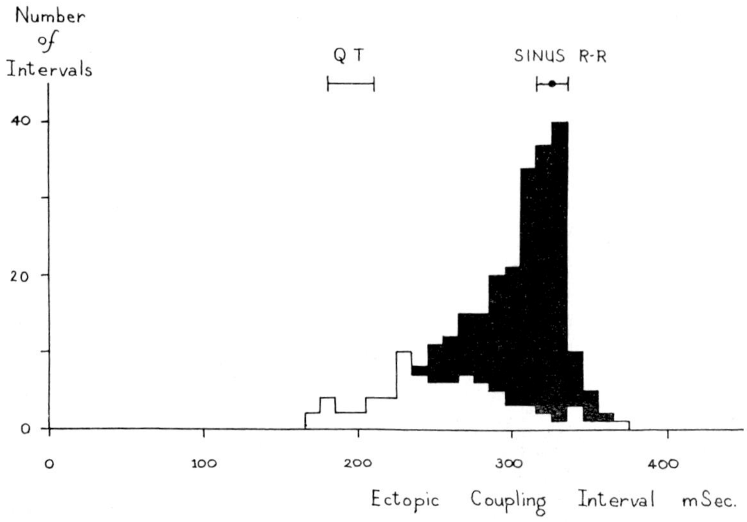

FIG. 10, 6. Shaded area represents coupling intervals of single ventricular ectopic beats. Clear area represents intervals between consecutive 'ectopic' beats.

expected the inter-ectopic intervals to yield a period other than sinus. The sample consists of only 258 intervals; nevertheless. I believe that this example is suggestive of parasystolic rhythm. Finally, the R-on-T phenomenon surely needs explanation for in the normal heart and even in the heart containing ischaemic myocardium a large stimulus is required to achieve this electrocardiographic characteristic. Whatever the mechanism of excitation during the T wave *in vivo,* impulse propagation at this time is not expected.

Han. There are two basic mechanisms for ventricular ectopic activity in myocardial infarction. The re-entry mechanism has been already elaborated in my presentation. Enhanced automaticity of the His-Purkinje fibres, which is the second important mechanism, takes place because of hypoxia, stretch of fibres and catecholamine release in the ischaemic area. Premature beats occurring in diastole with variable coupling intervals may be due to the enhanced automaticity.

Durrer. You could differentiate between these different tissues by recording intracellular potentials from the acutely ischaemic area.

Mjøs. Is it possible to increase the fibrillation threshold by giving glucose or glucose/insulin intravenously?

Han. I am not aware of any studies dealing with glucose.

Jennings. There has been a great deal of discussion about electricity without regard to its source. It requires energy to pump sodium out and allow potassium to accumulate and produce a membrane potential. In an area of ischaemia we have a very variable situation which changes with time. Eventually cells die and the energy level should decrease to the point that no membrane potential is generated. I would like to make two observations about this. First, it is very unusual ever to see histological evidence of Purkinje cell injury in ischaemia with dog heart and I think this is because these cells receive enough oxygen by diffusion from the oxygenated blood in the cavity of the left ventricle to survive intact. Purkinje cells have much glycogen, few myofibrils and presumably a better capacity to function by anaerobic metabolism than left ventricular cells. So my first question is: in the dog how is the Purkinje system involved in the development of arrhythmias and if it is, what is the evidence for its involvement? Second, it seems to me that 40 to 60 min of ischaemia in the dog results in the death of a number of cells. I think that dead cells probably have no membrane potential; consequently arrhythmias at 60 min should originate from the cells that are still ischaemic in mid-myocardial and epicardial regions of the zone of ischaemia. The studies that Dr Han is referring to were done after 15 min of ischaemia. Have you repeated the studies at a later time intervals, and if you have, do you observe differences in susceptibility to arrhythmias?

Han. First, I have no idea whether the His-Purkinje system plays a part in the establishment of re-entry pathways in our experiments. Secondly, the dead tissue will not be involved in arrhythmia formation; the boundary between ischaemia and normal areas probably plays an important role in the genesis of ectopic activity. The boundary is expected to have depressed excitability and conductivity and this will facilitate re-entrant activity.

Taggart. Could anybody enlarge on the observations of Noble who demonstrated an outward stabilizing potassium current in phase 3 of the action potential in Purkinje fibres, this current being small? It is catecholamine sensitive and it has been suggested that it might be one of the mechanisms of producing arrhythmias by catecholamines.

Han. I have no real answer to that question.

Durrer. I would like to ask Dr Wallace if in his experiments on the mini-pig he finds injury in the myocardial Purkinje system?

Wallace. Yes, you may see injury of the Purkinje system in many instances. I don't believe that Dr Jennings would really want to go on record as saying that the action potential is generated metabolically. I believe that the ionic conductance changes which result in the action potential are passive.

Reuter. The Purkinje fibres are electrophysiologically very sensitive to all sorts of alteration in the extracellular condition. They depolarize very easily before you see any morphological changes. It is likely that you can get changes in electrical properties of the membranes of Purkinje fibres and metabolically they are only dependent in that the cation gradients across the membrane have to be maintained. For example, in the case of the squid giant axon it is possible to extrude the axoplasm and perfuse the system with appropriate salt solution and still get propagated action potentials in spite of the fact that you have completely depleted the cell of metabolism and mitochondria. Secondly, Noble in Oxford has determined the pacemaker potential in Purkinje fibres. One should not refer to it as a stabilizing current but rather as a labilizing current when it re-creates the diastolic potential change of the Purkinje fibres. This preparation is very sensitive to noradrenaline and adrenaline activities.

CATION MOVEMENTS DURING EXCITATION OF THE HEART

H. REUTER, L. S GETTES AND B. G. KATZUNG

IN cardiac fibres as in nerve, rapid depolarization is caused by the rapid inward Na current (I_{Na}). The maximum rate of rise $(dV/dt)_{max}$ of the action potential spike is proportional to I_{Na}.[1] In the steady state, I_{Na} decreases i.e. is inactivated along a sigmoid curve as the membrane potential prior to depolarization falls from −90 to −40 mV.[1] When the membrane potential falls to potentials which are less negative than −40 mV, as during a propagated action potential, I_{Na} is completely inactivated. By studying the time course with which the $(dV/dt)_{max}$ of test responses regained the steady state value after a prior conditioning action potential, we were able to assess the kinetics of the reactivation of the Na system following its complete inactivation. By changing the resting membrane potential of the cardiac fibre between −90 and −60 mV, we assessed the effects of changes in membrane potential on these kinetics.

The experimental procedure and the results are illustrated in Figure 11, 1. Mammalian ventricular and Purkinje fibres were stimulated at a basic rate of 1 per 2 seconds. The maximum rate of depolarization was measured by electronically differentiating the upstroke of the action potential. The $(dV/dt)_{max}$ of the action potentials induced at the basic rate (the conditioning action potentials), represent the steady state values at the resting potential level. Test action potentials were induced progressively earlier between two conditioning action potentials. The $(dV/dt)_{max}$ of the test action potentials were plotted as a function of the interval (msec) between the end of the conditioning and the test action potentials. The resting membrane potential was then progressively lowered from control value of −85 to −90 mV, to −60 mV by adding KCl to the Tyrode's solution and the introduction of test action potentials was repeated.

Our results can be summarized as follows:

1. At each of the studied resting membrane potential levels, $(dV/dt)_{max}$ of the test responses decreased exponentially as the interval preceding the test action potential was shortened, even

though the test action potentials continued to arise from a constant membrane potential (Fig. 11, 1).

2. The decrease in $(dV/dt)_{max}$ became greater and persisted for a longer time as the resting membrane potential was made less negative by the addition of KCl to the perfusate (Fig. 11, 2A).

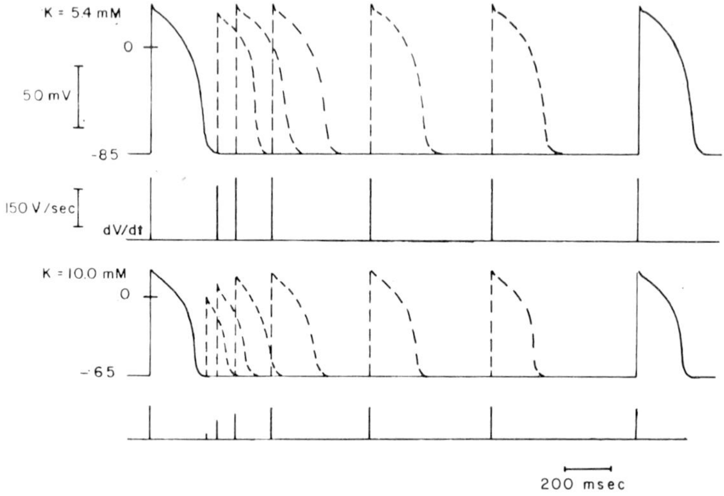

FIG. 11, 1. Ventricular action potentials (guinea pig heart) and maximal upstroke velocities $(dV/dt)_{max}$ (=differentiated traces below each action potential) arising from two different resting potentials (−85 mV upper part; −65 mV lower part). Action potentials during constant driving rates (0·5/sec) are indicated by heavy lines; premature responses elicited of various intervals after the first action potential are drawn as dashed lines. The resting potential was changed from −85 mV to −65 mV by increasing the K concentration in the Tyrode's solution from 5·4 to 10·0 mM.

3. The time constant whereby $(dV/dt)_{max}$ of the test action potentials regained the steady state value increased from less than 20 msec when the resting potential ranged between −90 and −80 mV, to more than 100 msec when the resting potential ranged between −70 and −60 mV (Fig. 11, 2B).

It is known that an increase in external Ca concentration shifts the curve describing the steady state relationship between membrane potential and I_{Na} (the inactivation curve) along the voltage axis in the depolarizing direction.[1] Thus, dV/dt_{max} recorded when the membrane potential is −65 mV in a fibre perfused with 1·8 mM Ca containing solution is similar to dV/dt_{max} when the membrane potential is −60 mV in the same fibre perfused with 7·2 mM Ca containing solution. This shift is believed to be due to an alteration in the negative fixed charge at the surface of the membrane. Figure 11, 2 shows the results of an experiment assessing the effects of a 4-fold increase in external Ca concentration on the steady state

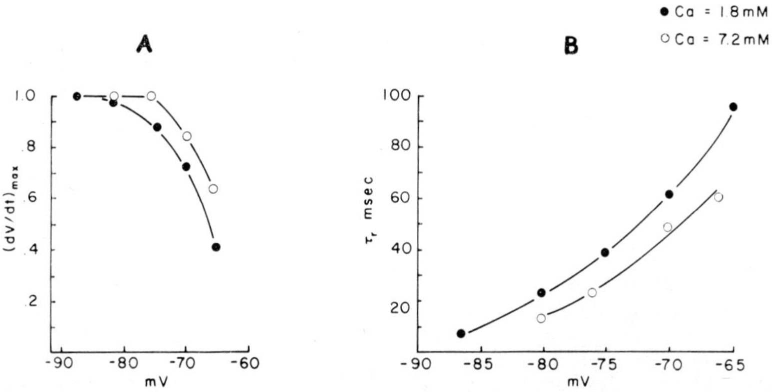

FIG. 11, 2A. Relation between maximal upstroke velocity, $(dV/dt)_{max}$ of the ventricular action potential (guinea pig heart) and membrane potential. Abscissa: membrane potential from where the respective action potentials were elicited; ordinate: normalized $(dV/dt)_{max}$ of action potentials at slow (0·5/sec) driving rates (=steady state). Results were obtained with two different calcium concentrations in the Tyrode's solution: 1·8 mM Ca (filled circles); 7·2 mM Ca (open circles).
B. Relation between time constant of recovery (Tr) of $(dV/dt)_{max}$ from inactivation and membrane potential.

inactivation curve (Fig. 11, 2A) and, in the same fibre, on the curve relating the reactivation time constant (τr) to the membrane potential (Fig. 11, 2B). As expected from earlier studies, the steady state curve is shifted along the voltage axis in the depolarizing direction when the Ca concentration is increased. In addition, the τr-membrane potential curve is similarly shifted by an equal amount.

The clinical implications of our observations are of some interest. The prolonged recovery times of the Na system indicate that the rate of depolarization in early premature responses will be dependent on time as well as on the membrane potential from which the premature action potentials arise. Therefore, the rate of depolarization may be decreased in early premature responses arising from the normal resting potential. This slowing of depolarization will be even more pronounced in premature responses arising from partially depolarized (or incompletely repolarized) fibres, and may contribute to the development of re-entrant arrhythmias. Furthermore, the studies indicate that changes in conduction and refractoriness, such as those induced by antiarrhythmic drugs, may result from changes in the kinetic properties as well as changes in the steady state properties of the Na system.

In addition to the results on I_{Na} we obtained further information about the behaviour of the slow inward Ca current which is responsible for the plateau of the cardiac action potential.[2]

Figure 11, 3 illustrates the results of a double step voltage clamp experiment carried out with a single microelectrode impalement in

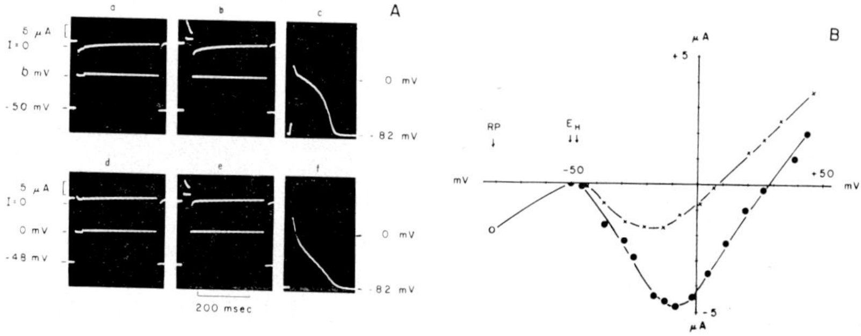

FIG. 11, 3A. Effect of La on the slow inward current and the plateau of the action potential measured in a pig ventricular trabeculum. a-c: controls in Tyrode's solution; a, b: double step voltage clamps from a holding potential of −50 mV (I_{Na} inactivated); upper traces: membrane current, lower traces: clamp potential; first step (30 msec) to 0 mV produces inward current (a), first step to +60 mV produces outward current (b); second clamp step always to +3 mV; note slowly decaying tails of inward current at the second clamp steps and the marked plateau of the action potential (c). d-f: Tyrode's solution containing 0·4 mM/l La Cl_3; same experimental procedure as in a-c; note marked decrease of the inward current tails at the second clamp step (d, e) and reduction of the plateau (f).

B. Current voltage relations of the slow inward current in the absence (filled circles) and presence (crosses) of 0·4 mM/l La Cl_3. The open circle indicates the current required to displace the membrane potential from the resting potential (RP) to constant holding potentials (E_H) at −50 mV in the absence and at −48 mV in the presence of La in order to inactivate I_{Na}. Plotted are maximum inward or minimum outward currents flowing during single step voltage clamps.

a pig ventricular trabeculum. Panels a, b and c are the controls without lanthanum (La) in the solution. In a and b the holding potential was set to −50 mV in order to inactivate I_{Na}. In a first clamp step (V_1) the membrane potential was either displaced for 30 msec, to 0 mV which produced inward current (panel a) or to +60 mV (panel b) which was above the reversal potential of this current and hence produced outward current. The second clamp step (V_2) in a and b was to +3 mV and elicited exponentially decaying tails of inward current. These inward currents are due to the inflow of Ca ions into the fibre (I_{Ca}). The plateau of the action potential (panel c) is obviously due to this slowly decaying inward current. Panels d, e and f were recorded after 20-25 min exposure to La-containing solution. The voltage clamp steps in d and e are the same as in a and b. The inward or outward currents at the first clamp steps were greatly reduced as were the tails of inward current at the second clamp steps. Correspondingly, the action potential had lost its plateau in the La-containing solution. A plot of the current-voltage relations of the slow inward current measured in the absence and presence of La in the solution showed a marked inhibition of this current component by La (Fig. 11, 3B). In contrast to this effect of La an increase in Ca in the bathing solution increases this current component. Simultaneously measured contractions decreased concomitantly with the inhibition of the slow inward current by La. Similar results were obtained with 3 other preparations. We also observed that La inhibited the Ca-dependent regenerative depolarizations during constant current pulses applied to preparations bathed in Na-free solution. In addition, ^{45}Ca uptake was measured in 8 paired sheep ventricular preparations stimulated at a constant rate of 0·5/sec. When one group of preparations was preincubated for 10 min in La-containing inactive solution and afterwards loaded for 15 min in La-containing radioactive solution ^{45}Ca uptake was reduced by $30 \pm 4{\cdot}6$ per cent (mean ±SE) as compared to the control group without La.

All these results reinforce the earlier interpretation[2] that the slow inward current in mammalian cardiac preparations is predominantly carried by Ca ions.

The rapid initial I_{Na} in cardiac muscle seems to be similarly influenced by La as in other excitable tissues. The sigmoid curve relating membrane potential and the maximum upstroke velocity of the action potential (as a measure of $I_{Na}{}^{1}$) was shifted along the voltage axis in the depolarizing direction by La, an effect similar to that of Ca (Fig. 11, 2A). In Figure 11, 3F $(dV/dt)_{max}$ and the maximum height of the action potential were unaffected by La at a time when the plateau was abolished.

These results provide additional evidence that in mammalian cardiac muscle I_{Na} and I_{Ca} are separate current systems. Though they have similar effects on I_{Na}, La and Ca have opposite effects on I_{Ca}.

ACKNOWLEDGMENT

This work was supported by the Swiss National Science Foundation (Grant 3.91.69).

REFERENCES

1 WEIDMAN, S. (1955). Effect of calcium ions and local anaesthetics on electrical properties of Purkinje fibres. *Journal of Physiology* **129,** 568-582.
2 BEELER, G. W. JR. & REUTER, H. (1970). Membrane calcium current in ventricular myocardial fibres. *Journal of Physiology* **207,** 191-209.

DISCUSSION

Durrer. This role of calcium during the depolarization phase of the action potential is an important observation.

Henderson. Dr Reuter, in the presence of lanthanum you showed that the action potential became triangular, having lost its plateau but that it did not become a simple spike. Do you attribute this to the incomplete action of the lanthanum in blocking the calcium current or to some residual sodium contribution? Secondly I believe I am right in saying that adrenaline shortens the action potential. Could you help me by explaining how this might come about?

Reuter. The persisting long duration of the action potential around -60 to -40 mV in 3+ lanthanum-containing solution could be due to the decrease of the outward conductance (inward-going rectification) occurring in this potential range in combination with a residual inward current. The effect of adrenaline on the action potential duration is variable, e.g. in a solution with a low calcium concentration the duration may even increase.

Parratt. If the plateau phase is due to the influx of calcium, then you would expect it to be shortened by drugs that inhibit this effect and this is what you have shown with lanthanum. Now I think Fleckenstein has shown that using drugs like iproveratril and the new Bayer compound 1040, he could prevent the contractile response following a stimulus without changing the plateau phase of the action potential. If these are both due to the influx of calcium how do you explain this finding?

Reuter. According to newer data from Fleckenstein's group, these substances greatly depress Ca inward current in the mammalian heart as well as the plateau phase.

Parratt. In the earlier work he used low concentrations of the drugs and showed that there was no effect on the action potential. There was a dose range where he could abolish the contractile response without changing the action potential.

Reuter. I cannot comment further on these findings since there are contradictory results.

Oliver. Is it the case then that any system which can be used to bind calcium such as EDTA will shorten action potential? Calcium soaps may form in the presence of excess unbound free fatty acids and make it less available.

Reuter. This is not so because external calcium also affects the permeability of the membrane to other ions. This complicates the analysis of its action.

Kurien. Could you relate the inotropic effect of digoxin and its arrhythmogenic effect to this new finding?

Reuter. We did not find an effect of cardiac glycosides on the calcium inward current. It is likely that these glycosides act by a different mechanism.

Wallace. The action potential of the normal cells of the AV node, particularly the upstroke, tends to be insensitive to tetrodotoxin and very sensitive to acetylcholine which is just the opposite of ventricular muscle and Purkinje fibres. Do you believe that would permit one to conclude that the upstroke of the action potential in AV nodal cells is generated by some mechanism other than sodium?

Reuter. Too little is known about the ionic dependence of the pacemaker—and action potentials in the AV node to answer this question. This tissue is particularly difficult to investigate.

CATION GRADIENTS IN THE ISCHAEMIC HUMAN MYOCARDIUM WITH OBSERVATIONS ON TISSUE AND PLASMA CATECHOLAMINES

P. I. TAGGART AND J. D. H. SLATER
In collaboration with MALCOLM CARRUTHERS

INTRODUCTION

Part I

ALTHOUGH many factors are involved in determining action potential characteristics, potassium (K) and sodium (Na) and catecholamines are of particular interest since they are measurable and can be influenced clinically. Arrhythmias and low output states remain the major complications and cause of death following both cardiac surgery and myocardial infarction. There is ample evidence that potassium and catecholamines are important to both these situations. For example, arrhythmias are commonly associated with a serum K outside the normal range and particularly with low serum K.[1 2] Many arrhythmias respond at least temporarily to the administration of intravenous K.[3] However, intravenous K may be effective not only when the serum K is low but also when it is normal or even slightly raised.[3] Therefore this relationship is complex.

Arrhythmias following coronary artery occlusion in the experimental animal are accentuated by infusion of catecholamines[4 5] and stellate ganglion stimulation,[6] but decreased by beta adrenergic blockade[7] or cardiac denervation.[8 9] There is a clinical correlation between the incidence of arrhythmias and increased sympathetic activity in man following myocardial infarction.[10 11] However, this relationship is also complex.

Much of this complexity probably results from the multiplicity of variable factors, particularly with regard to the different behaviour of specialized cell groups,[12] the interplay between alterations of one factor upon another,[12] and the many possible mechanisms by which aberrant rhythms may be produced.[13]

We present some observations which may be relevant.

Part II
In a preliminary unpaired study we compared atrial biopsies taken before and after cardiopulmonary bypass surgery with respect to their content of potassium, sodium and water expressed on a fat free wet weight (F.F.W.W.) basis (Fig. 12, 1). The potassium content after bypass was 3·21 (±0·74 SD) mEq/100 g F.F.W.W. compared with 6·06 (±0·76 SD) mEq/100 g F.F.W.W. before the procedure. The sodium content increased from 9·8 (±1·18 SD) mEq/100 g F.F.W.W. before bypass to 10·39 (±0·19 SD) mEq/100 g F.F.W.W. after the procedure.

	BEFORE (n=9)		AFTER (n=9)		
	MEAN	S.D.	MEAN	S.D.	P
POTASSIUM mEq/100g	6.06	±0.76	3.21	±0.74	<0.001
SODIUM mEq/100g	9.80	±1.18	10.39	±0.19	<0.05
WATER%	79.92	±0.75	81.86	±1.13	<0.001

UNPAIRED STUDY OF BIOPSIES REMOVED BEFORE AND AFTER BYPASS. (FAT FREE WET WEIGHT BASIS)

FIG. 12, 1. Sodium, potassium and water content of atrial biopsies taken from one group of patients immediately prior to cardiopulmonary bypass and a second group at the end of bypass.

Total water content showed only a small change, increasing from 79·92 (±0·75 SD) ml per cent F.F.W.W. before bypass to 81·86 (±1·13 SD) ml per cent F.F.W.W. in the samples taken after bypass. The apparent discrepancy between the potassium loss and sodium gain requires explanation. While the potassium content of the tissue biopsies is almost entirely intracellular, the sodium content would be expected to be largely extracellular in the pre bypass biopsies and to a lesser extent in the post bypass samples. It is therefore necessary to postulate a loss of extracellular fluid in the 'late' samples. Since the total water content remains virtually constant, this would imply a shift of extracellular fluid (E.C.F.) into the intracellular compartment (I.C.F.). If, for example, the E.C.F. were to contain 140 mEq/1 of sodium, and the E.C.F. and I.C.F. volumes were 40 ml/100 mg F.F.W.W. of tissue, then a shift of 10 ml from E.C.F. to I.C.F. would, assuming perfusion of the E.C.F., effectively reduce the total sodium content of the biopsy by 1·4 mEq (per 100 g F.F.W.W.). In other words, this amount, together with the 0·59 mEq, being the increase in tissue content noted between the before and after samples, may have entered the cells. A shift of water of the magnitude would also have an important effect on the K concentration gradient as a consequence of dilution of the intracellular K. It therefore becomes mandatory to determine the distribution of water between I.C.F. and E.C.F. compartments.

We therefore performed a second study taking paired biopsies from 12 patients undergoing aortic valve replacement. The technique of intermittent cross clamping of the aorta was used, which allowed us to take biopsies both before and after timed periods of coronary artery occlusion. The biopsies were analysed for potassium, sodium, chloride, total H_2O, E.C.F. and catecholamines, together with plasma concentrations of K, Na, Cl and catecholamines.

Methods

The methods used for analysis of tissue K, Na, Cl, total H_2O and E.C.F. have been described elsewhere.[14] Plasma catecholamines were estimated by a method also previously described.[15] Full validation of the method used for estimation of tissue catecholamine content will shortly be presented.[16]

Results

The potassium content of the atrial biopsies is presented in Figure 12, 2. The linear regression line indicates a fall of from a mean value of 5·8 mEq/100 g F.F.W.W. before coronary artery occlusion to a mean value of 2·9 mEq/100 g F.F.W.W. after 152 min occlusion, the rate of loss being 0·078 mEq/100 g F.F.W.W./min. While the total water content showed only a slight increase, comparable with the preliminary study, an initial and impressive cellular swelling was apparent. After longer periods of coronary artery occlusion a shift of water distribution in the opposite direction was observed with ultimate cell shrinkage (Fig. 12, 3). The tissue catecholamine content of these samples is presented in Figure 12, 4. The computed

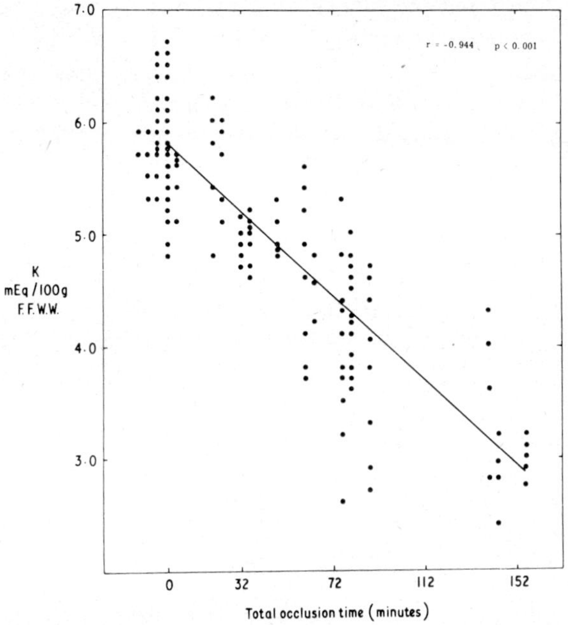

FIG. 12, 2. The potassium content of atrial biopsy specimens removed after specified periods of coronary artery occlusion followed by 3 minutes subsequent reflow.

regression line relating tissue content to the period of coronary artery occlusion indicates a rapid depletion followed by a slower progressive depletion. The plasma catecholamine concentrations at the times of these biopsies is presented together with the values in the tissue biopsies in Figure 12, 5.

Discussion

The loss of tissue potassium in our second study confirms our preliminary observations, though it is perhaps greater than one might have anticipated. The initial cell swelling that we observed supports our explanation for our preliminary results. The apparent subsequent shift of water from I.C.F. to E.C.F (Fig. 12, 3), presents a separate challenge.

We have used the computed regression lines relating to loss (Fig. 12, 2) and distribution of H_2O (Fig. 12, 3) to total coronary artery occlusion time, and the total H_2O content of the tissue biopsies to calculate the intracellular K concentration [K_1]. We have used the Nernst equation as an approximation to calculate the Resting Membrane Potential (R.M.P.) for two arbitrary values of extracellular K concentration [K_0] namely 3 mEq/1 and 6 mEq/1.

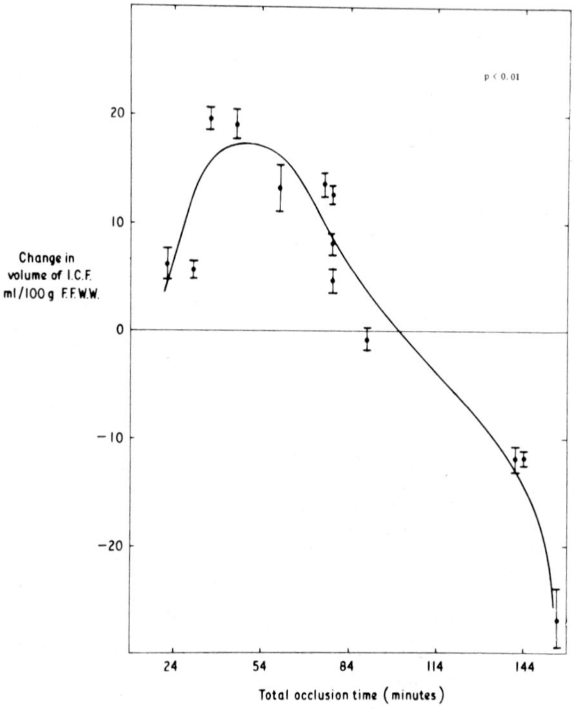

FIG. 12, 3. Computed regression line relating the change volume of intracellular fluid (I.C.F.) to timed periods of coronary artery occlusion.

Diagrammatic representation of phase 4/phase 0 of the action potential (A.P.) is presented in Figure 12, 6 for different periods of coronary artery occlusion. The reduction in gradient $\frac{[K_1]}{[K_0]}$ results from loss of intracellular K together with dilution of the remaining (K_1) due to shift of water from E.C.F. to I.C.F.

Our finding of an apparent reversal in the redistribution of water after longer periods of occlusion with shift from I.C.F. to E.C.F.

requires explanation. It is possible that the initial cell swelling results in rupture of the membrane of some cell groups such that the interior of these cells effectively becomes continuous with the surrounding E.C.F. If this is the case, then the surviving cells in fact continue to swell further, rather than shrink. Alternatively, if a genuine shift of I.C.F. to E.C.F. does occur, then the ultimate cellular dehydration would actually increase the gradient $\frac{[K_1]}{[K_0]}$ despite further losses of (K_1). As may be seen from Figure 12, 6,

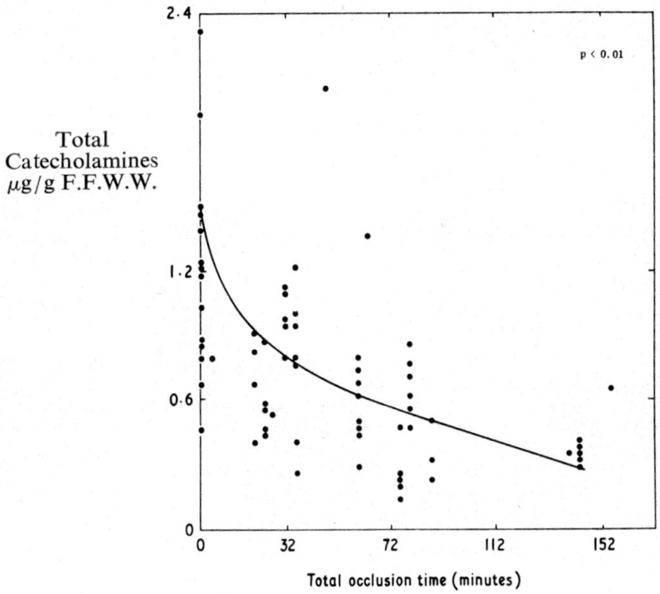

FIG. 12, 4. Computed regression line relating the biopsy catecholamine content to total coronary occlusion time.

the R.M.P. when calculated for a [K_0] of the order of 5 mEq/1 approximates to the expected normal value of −90 mv. Initial periods of occlusion result in incomplete repolarization, though this is less so for low [K_0] values. Disregarding small changes in the value of the threshold potential (T.P.) that would be expected to occur under these circumstances, it is apparent that after periods of ischaemia of intermediate duration the R.M.P. remains close to a value of about −60 mv at which activation of pacemaker fibres occurs.

While the intracellular sodium content (Na_1) increased in a manner not dissimilar from the (K_1) loss, the initial increase in I.C.F. resulted in little change in intracellular sodium concentration [Na_1]). If H_2O subsequently moves in the opposite direction [Na_1] increases progressively. We have calculated the Na equilibrium potential (E_{Na}) using the Nernst equation and similar criteria as described

		ATRIUM µg/g FFWW	PLASMA µg/l		
		N + A	N + A	N	A
BEFORE	MEAN	1.46	2.17	1.39	0.78
	RANGE	(+0.74 +2.92)	(+1.21 +3.74)	(+0.90 +1.90)	(+0.10 +2.12)
AFTER	MEAN	0.75	3.57	1.62	1.95
	RANGE	(+0.34 +2.03)	(+1.32 +8.12)	(+1.04 +2.91)	(+0.28 +6.59)
% CHANGE	MEAN	-51.9	73.2	25.8	278.2
	RANGE	(-13.1 -73.1)	(-19.8 +214.0)	(-25.3 +223.3)	(-9.2 +1030.01)

NORADRENALINE (N) AND ADRENALINE (A) VALUES IN ATRIAL BIOPSIES AND PLASMA SAMPLES TAKEN AT THE SAME TIME.

FIG. 12, 5. Noradrenaline (N) and Adrenaline (A) values in atrial biopsies taken before and after an unspecified period of coronary artery occlusion: together with plasma catecholamine content at the time of sampling. A loss of atrial N+A is apparent with an increase in both circulating N and A (Normal Ranges for plasma by method employed: $N=0{\cdot}6\pm0{\cdot}15$ $\mu g/l$, $A=0{\cdot}1\pm0{\cdot}1$ $\mu g/l$).

for K, for an extracellular Na concentration [Na_0] of 130 mEq/l. The use of E_{Na} as an approximation for the 'spike' or 'overshoot' amplitude clearly results, as perhaps should be expected, in considerable overestimation (Fig. 12, 7). The implied decrease in the slope of the upstroke of the AP in Figure 12, 7 is not derived from our data, but represents the expected pattern as a result of increased [Na_1].

Before considering the possible clinical relevance of our findings, it is important to draw attention to the question of trapped extracellular ions. If an area of muscle is rendered totally ischaemic and unperfused then as potassium is lost from the cell it will accumulate at the outside surface of the membrane. Similarly sodium leaving the E.C.F. and entering the cell will result in a low [Na_0] in that tissue. Figure 12, 8 illustrates the findings in two patients from whom biopsies were taken at the end of a period of occlusion and again after 3 minutes of reflow. While it is premature to dwell at length on results from two patients only, certainly as far as K is concerned, there is an apparent decrease in the tissue content of the second biopsies. It is therefore tempting to suggest that this K

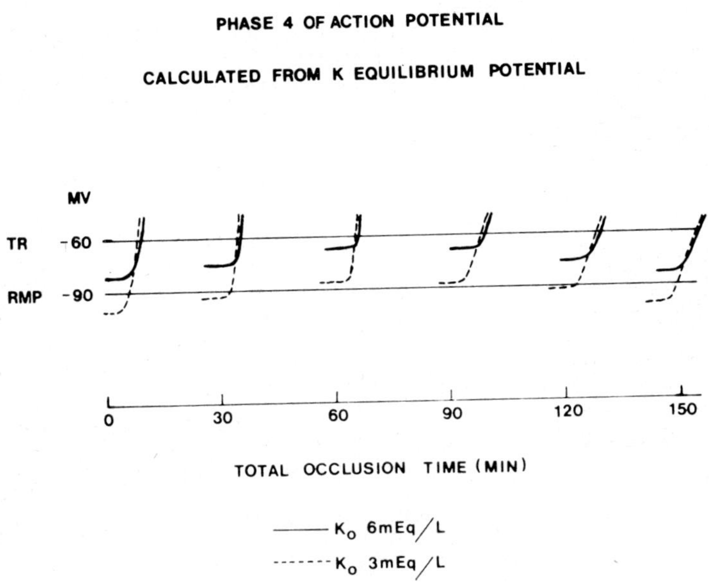

FIG. 12, 6. Phase 4 of action potential calculated from our data using the Nernst equation. TR=Region of threshold potential, RMP=Resting Membrane Potential).

had been washed from the E.C.F. on commencement of reperfusion. If extracellular trapping occurs to an appreciable extent in poorly perfused areas, it will materially affect the gradients of the ions concerned. Furthermore, recovery or reperfusion may be associated with an initial deterioration of the gradient[17] and this may be triggered by restoration of the ion concentrations in the E.C.F. towards normal. It is also important to remember that the distributions of ions in the E.C.F. may be non-uniform as suggested by the demonstration of a K diffusion barrier in the T system.[18]

In the majority of healthy fibre groups which have not been exposed to ischaemia, a [K_0] value of close to 5 mEq/1 probably results in an R.M.P. approximating to the optimum value of about −90 mv. Raising or lowering the serum potassium on the basis of the Nernst equation would be expected to result in depolarization

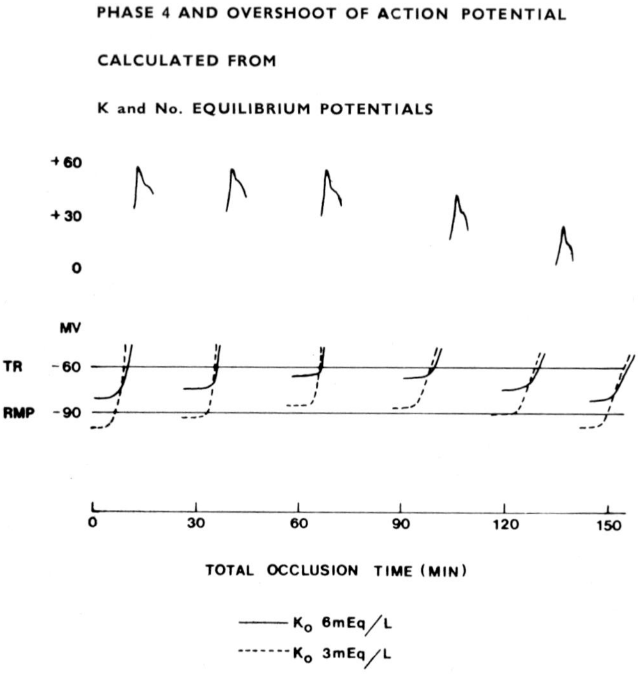

FIG. 12, 7. The calculated amplitude of the 'spike' of the action potential derived from our data using the sodium equilibrium potential and superimposed on Figure 12, 6.

or hyperpolarization. At low levels of [K_0] the R.M.P. is strongly influenced by the effect of [K_0] on permeability. Consideration of our data on the basis of the Nernst equation must therefore be limited to [K_0] values close to the normal range.

Depolarization results in the R.M.P. approximating closer to the TP, at which point pacemaker fibres or even latent pacemaker fibres may assume spontaneous activity. However, the slope of phase 0 is likely to be reduced and a weak AP results with a poor propagated wave of excitation. This in turn may terminate by decremental conduction and unidirectional block. If the fibre groups involved constitute an ectopic focus they are unlikely to capture the rhythm directly, but by leaving an area of myocardium refractory in front of the oncoming excitation wave from the normal focus may disorganize the rhythm or encourage re-entrant arrhythmias. If the normal focus is similarly affected, the converse may apply in that the normal wave of activation may be self limiting and allow the dominance of a potential ectopic focus.

			mEq/100g F.F.W.W.		
			K	Na	Cl
C.K.	before	mean	4.6	7.8	5.8
		S.D.	±0.2	±0.3	±0.4
	after	mean	3.5	8.6	6.4
		S.D.	±0.3	±0.6	±0.5
B.C.	before	mean	3.4	8.9	6.6
		S.D.	±0.5	±0.6	±0.5
	after	mean	2.7	9.4	6.8
		S.D.	±0.2	±0.5	±0.2

FIG. 12, 8. Sodium, potassium and chloride contents of atrial biopsies from two patients removed both at the end of a period of coronary artery occlusion immediately before the onset of reflow (before) and again after 3 min reflow (after).

Hyperpolarization, on the other hand, increases the slope of phase 0, tending to increase the rate and strength of the propagated impulse. An ectopic focus behaving in this manner may well compete successfully with the normal rhythm and even 'capture' it completely.

AP recordings obtained by micro-electrodes suggest that a reduction in the rate of rise of phase 0 occurs early in response to ischaemia, probably much earlier than we have implied in Figure 12, 7. If this is so, then the propagated impulse may behave decrementally at all levels of serum K after relatively short periods of ischaemia.

Catecholamines exert their principal effect on the action potential by increasing the slope of phase 4 in pacemaker fibres, and encouraging latent pacemakers to assume pacemaker activity. This increased rate of spontaneous diastolic depolarization results in the R.M.P. reaching the TP in a shorter time and so increasing the rate of firing. While this is operative in normal fibres its effect would be expected to be particularly pronounced in tissues exposed to moderate ischaemia.

Our data suggests a rapid depletion of catecholamine stores (noradrenaline) while the plasma levels of both noradrenaline and adrenaline are greatly elevated. The depleted myocardial stores would be expected to protect against arrhythmias, although encouraging low output states. The heart may under these circumstances depend on circulating catecholamines for augmentation of contractility. However, in addition to the possibly advantageous high plasma noradrenaline concentration, there is the powerfully arrhythmogenic high plasma adrenaline concentration.

Summary

Coronary artery occlusion during bypass surgery results in a loss of intracellular potassium and a gain in intracellular sodium in myocardial biopsies. Little change in total water content is apparent, but a shift of extracellular fluid into the cell occurs. There is uncertainty as to whether longer periods of ischaemia result in rupture of some cell groups or cell shrinkage.

A loss of myocardial noradrenaline occurs with an elevation of both plasma adrenaline and noradrenaline concentrations.

We have used the Nernst equation as an approximation to calculate the resting membrane potential and the ‘ spike ’ amplitude of the action potential from our data.

Certain generalizations are made with regard to the possible relevance of our findings to alterations of myocardial excitability and contractility.

REFERENCES

1 LEVINE, H. D., MERRILL, J. P. & SOMERVILLE, W. (1951). Advanced disturbances of cardiac mechanism in potassium intoxication in man. *Circulation* **3,** 889-905.

2 SURAWICZ, B. (1968). Role of electrolytes in etiology and management of cardiac arrhythmias. *Progress in Cardiovascular Diseases* **8,** 364-386.

3 BETTINGER, J. E., SURAWICZ, B., BRYFOGLE, S. W., ANDERSON, N. & BELLET, S. (1956). Effect of intravenous administration of potassium chloride on ectopic rhythms, ectopic beats and disturbances in A-V conduction. *American Journal of Medicine* **21,** 521-533.

4 CEREMUZYNSKI, L., STASZEWSKA-BARCZAK, J. & HERBACZYNSKA-CEDRO, K. (1969). Cardiac rhythm disturbances and the release of catecholamines after acute coronary occlusion in dogs. *Cardiovascular Research* **3,** 190-197.

5 MALING, H. M. & MORAN, M. C. (1957). Ventricular arrhythmias induced by sympathomimetic amines in unanaesthetized dogs following coronary artery occlusion. *Circulation Research* **5,** 409-413.

6 HARRIS, A. S. (1966). Potassium and experimental coronary occlusion. *American Heart Journal* **71,** 797-802.

7 SHANKS, R. G. & DUNLOP, D. (1967). Effect of propranolol on arrhythmias following coronary artery occlusion in dogs. *Cardiovascular Research* **1,** 34-41.

8 SCHAAL, S. F., WALLACE, A. G. & SEALY, W. C. (1969). Protective influence of cardiac denervation against arrhythmias of myocardial infarction. *Cardiovascular Research* **3,** 241-244.

9 EBERT, P. A., VANDERBEEK, R. B., ALLGOOD, R. J. & SABISTON, D. C. JR. (1970). Effect of chronic cardiac denervation on arrhythmias after coronary artery ligation. *Cardiovascular Research* **4,** 141-147.

10 MCDONALD, L., BAKER, C., BRAY, C., MACDONALD, A. & RESTIEAUX, N. (1969). Plasma-catecholamines after cardiac infarction. *Lancet* **II,** 1021-1023.

11 JEWITT, D. E., MERCER, C. S., REID, D., VALORI, C., THOMAS, M. & SHILLINGFORD, J. P. (1969). Free noradrenaline and adrenaline excretion in relation to the development of cardiac arrhythmias and heart failure in patients with acute myocardial infarction. *Lancet* **I,** 635-641.

12 HOFFMAN, B. F. & CRANEFIELD, P. F. (1960). In *Electrophysiology of the Heart*. New York: McGraw-Hill.

12A HOFFMAN, B. F. (1968). The genesis of cardiac arrhythmias. *Progress in Cardiovascular Diseases* **8,** 319-329.

14 TAGGART, P. & SLATER, J. D. H. (1971). Significance of potassium in genesis of arrhythmias in induced cardiac ischaemia. *British Medical Journal* **4,** 195-198.

15 CARRUTHERS, M., TAGGART, P., CONWAY, N., BATES, D. & SOMERVILLE, W. (1970). Validity of plasma-catecholamine estimations. *Lancet* **II,** 62-68.

16 CARRUTHERS, M. E., TAGGART, P. & SLATER, J. H. D. Criteria for the measurement of catecholamines and lipid in cardiac muscle. (In preparation.)

17 JENNINGS, R. B., SOMMERS, H. M., KALTENBACH, J. P. & WEST, J. J. (1964). Electrolyte alterations in acute myocardial ischemic injury. *Circulation Research* **14,** 260-269.

18 LANGER, G. A. (1968). Ion fluxes in cardiac excitation and contraction and their relation to myocardial contractility. *Physiological Reviews* **48,** 708-757.

DISCUSSION

Oliver. You showed a linear regression between loss of potassium and the time of occlusion and said that this was unaffected by the frequency with which occlusion was applied or relaxed. Yet you also indicated that with every relaxation of occlusion and episode of reflow there was potassium washout. Could you put these two points together, please?

Taggart. What I meant was not that the relative periods of occlusion and reflow were unimportant but that the manner in which our data has been assembled and presented does not take this factor into account. As yet we have not sufficient data to attempt to analyse it from this point of view, although clearly this is an important observation from the practical surgical point of view.

Oliver. But if you analyse those where there was intermittent occlusion and reflow, was there a different statistical relationship?

Taggart. We have not done that as yet.

Oliver. What changes occur in plasma noradrenaline and adrenaline during the open heart procedure when there is no occlusion of the aorta, or impairment of coronary artery flow?

Taggart. We have data on 14 patients undergoing closed mitral valvotomy. A small increase in both plasma adrenaline and noradrenaline concentrations was observed but it was nothing like the magnitude of change we found following cardiopulmonary bypass. We have not so far attempted to differentiate between the catecholamine release seen following aortic occlusion with intermittent coronary artery perfusion. I think from the data we have so far it is unlikely that there will be much difference between the two techniques. It is probable that the majority of the increased circulating catecholamines are liberated from extracardiac sources and reflect the peripheral perfusion.

Jennings. I would like to support Dr Taggart's observations in general. We have done similar studies in left ventricular muscle. The first thing that stands out is that simple tissue analysis does not tell you where the electrolytes are in an area of severe permanent ischaemia. For example, in the papillary muscle you cannot detect changes in total tissue potassium or any other electrolyte at 60 min because our assay techniques simply measure potassium in the tissue and don't tell you whether it is intracellular or extracellular. Changes in potassium don't become apparent until diffusion washes extracellular K from the area. On the other hand, if one allows periods of reflow to irreversibly injured cells then the changes in potassium concentration develop very quickly. Tissue water, sodium, chloride, and calcium increase; magnesium and potassium decrease. It is interesting that if the cells are reversibly injured by 15 minutes of ischaemia and you then allow a period of two to three minutes of reflow you cannot detect changes in electrolyte concentration. I interpret these data as an indication that the metabolic pumps must be adequate to re-accumulate potassium and pump out sodium and water if they indeed have changed during this period of time. Thus it is very important to use either total permanent ischaemia or a defined period of reflow at the end in order to better interpret the data. Another finding of interest that Eugene Grachowski, Charles Ganoli and I have recently made is relative to the effect of incubation of tissue slices in the cold on electrolytes and intracellular water. If one places a slice of muscle in the cold, metabolism is inhibited. It swells to an enormous extent, potassium leaks to the medium and sodium and water enter the cell. If you warm the tissue to 37°C, the water returns to 78 per cent. These are not new observations, I learned of this cold swelling through the studies of Mudge on kidney slices in the late 1940s. The point is that energy is required to maintain electrolyte and water balance once the water and sodium are pumped out, and the slice water concentration comes back to the same concentration the tissue exhibited prior to slicing. However, if you put it in the cold again, it doesn't swell up as much. This phenomenon should be taken into account in incubating atria.

Wallace. Several years ago Dr Ebert compared the potassium content of atrial biopsies obtained from patients in normal sinus rhythm with those in chronic atrial fibrillation. There was a striking difference, the patients with chronic atrial fibrillation having very low potassium. What is the rhythm of the atrium during this period of occlusion in your patients and does the presence or absence of sinus rhythm influence your results? We used aortic cross clamp in the dog for electrophysiological studies and cannulated the coronary sinus and collected coronary sinus blood in small aliquots immediately following reperfusion. We obtained extremely high potassium concentrations in the early samples from the coronary sinus following reperfusion. This was abolished if we pretreated the animal with Tris buffer prior to putting them on bypass. I wonder whether Tris buffer was used in your perfusions? Tris will dramatically effect the potassium flux electrophysical consequences and survival of the heart during periods of coronary occlusion.

Taggart. No specific buffer was used; the pumps were primed either with 5 per cent dextrose or with Hartmanns solution.

Durrer. What was the concentration of Tris buffer, Dr Wallace?

Wallace. I don't recall the concentration, but I do remember that we raised the animal's pH to 7·7 with Tris buffer prior to the time of the aortic occlusion. We also used the same amount of Tris and buffered it to a pH of 7·4 so that there was no change in the arterial pH. We still got the protective effect. Dr Nahas and others interpreted these results as consistent with an alteration of intracellular pH because Tris is supposedly a very good intracellular buffer and moves much more easily into the intracellular space than bicarbonate. As a matter of fact with sodium bicarbonate, the CO_2 flows into the cell and creates intracellular acidosis, if you can believe in methods of measuring intracellular pH.

Taggart. We chose patients with aortic valve disease and none of them had atrial fibrillation prior to operation. We avoided mitral valve disease because it is such a peculiar entity in its own right and includes the problem of atrial fibrillation. The technique used was that of ischaemic arrest. I do not have any particular data on people who are or have been for some time in chronic atrial fibrillation.

Reuter. I would like to comment on your calculation of the potassium equilibrium potential on the basis of the Nernst equation. Of course in the equation you don't have only the intracellular but you also have extracellular potassium concentration. Now, provided your intracellular potassium estimations are reasonably correct, how correct are the estimations of extracellular potassium concentration?

Taggart. The problem is just how many extracellular spaces are there. To consider the distribution of water and ions across the cell membrane using a simple two-compartmental model is too naïve. It is likely that from a physiological point of view there are several zones of intermediate composition between the intra- and extracellular spaces. There is, for example, evidence to support the existence of a diffusion barrier for potassium in the T-tube system, which might very well result in a localized increased potassium concentration adjacent to the morphological cell membrane. Under these circumstances, it is quite remarkable that by applying the Nernst equation to our data we derive calculated resting potential to the order of 85 Mv for a theoretical serum potassium of 5 mEq/1, prior to occlusion. This is very much the sort of figure that one would expect had we used microelectrodes. Your point about the uncertainty of the extracellular fluid composition adjacent to the functional electrical membrane following ischaemia and particularly the influence of extracellular potassium on conductance is well made. Clearly both factors would modify our calculated values for the resting potential based on the Nernst equation. We did not use the Goldman type of equation since what we would gain from the use of the theoretically more correct mathematical interpretation, we would lose by being obliged to guess permeabilities.

Oliver. It is obvious that the interpretation of these results depends to a large extent on the extracellular space marker that you choose. Have you used anything other than radioactive inulin? For example, have you looked at ^{125}I albumin or any of the other standard ECF markers and if so, do they alter your conclusions? The advantage of an albumin marker is that any sequestration of albumin and resultant change in cell osmolarity could be taken into account.

Taggart. No, we have confined ourselves to using inulin and and chloride or, to be more precise, the ratio of the two. Measurement of the extracellular fluid volume is absolutely fraught with difficulty. One problem is that during the incubation process for *in vitro* determination the tissue changes composition enormously, gaining sodium and chloride and losing a large quantity of potassium. Therefore, after a period of incubation are we justified in saying that a space measured is representative of that tissue space prior to incubation? Furthermore, whatever tracer substance we use is going to, even assuming perfect conditions, give a different volume of distribution. We are therefore obliged to choose our marker rather according to where we wish to place our ‘ cell membrane ’. If we want to place it close into the cell, as it were, one would use something like chloride with its large volume of distribution, whereas if we wished to place it further back we would choose a large molecule like inulin. Possibly this matters less in studies conducted on a comparatively ' before ' and ' after ' basis as we have been doing, but as I say, this measurement is very much the 'Achilles heel ' of any studies of this type.

Jennings. Would you agree that atrium is a tissue which is less differentiated than left ventricular myocardium in the sense that it is not as dependent upon aerobic metabolism, works less hard, contains much more collagen and is less sensitive to the impact of ischaemia or anoxia than left ventricular myocardium?

Taggart. We are at the moment involved in repeating this study on ventricular muscle and the changes in composition are very considerably greater, both in terms of incubation of the extracellular fluid volume measurements and during the procedure itself, but these are based on only a few observations so far.

Allison. We studied the distribution of inulin and chloride *in vitro* in such samples as you describe. There is a differential rate of distribution through the extracellular space so that at any given time chloride may have equilibrated in the extracellular space and inulin is unevenly distributed through the muscle piece. From the point of view of extrapolating to the clinical applications of your findings, much metabolic change occurs during bypass; for instance, there is complete suppression of insulin released through high free fatty acid levels and these changes are abruptly reversed as the patient comes off bypass, there is an abrupt potassium fall at this time as well as a pH fall due to changes induced by ventilation. In addition a low plasma potassium as the patient comes off bypass, may precipitate arrhythmias due to digoxin hypersensitivity in patients with mitral valve disease.

SUBSTRATE UPTAKE IN EXPERIMENTAL MYOCARDIAL ISCHAEMIA. EVALUATION OF ROLE OF GLUCOSE, FATTY ACIDS AND GLUCOSE-INSULIN-POTASSIUM THERAPY

L. H. OPIE, A. LOCHNER, P. OWEN, K. BRUYNEEL,
D. WHITELAW, W. LUBBE and K. R. L. MANSFORD*

WE would like to examine the proposition that the provision of glucose as substrate may be 'good' for the survival of the ischaemic myocardium, while the provision of fatty acids (free fatty acids, FFA) may be 'bad'.

Historical background

The possibility that various sugars might be beneficial for the diseased heart is by no means new, and dates back to at least 1911 when Goulston[1] advocated cane sugar, taken orally, in the therapy of various cardiac disorders because 'dextrose is capable of nourishing the heart muscle in a most peculiar and wonderful manner'. In 1914 Büdingen[2] published a 45-page, carefully-argued article urging that increased provision of carbohydrate was good for the diseased heart. If he advocated the right thing, it was certainly for the wrong reason. He argued that glucose uptake occurred in isolated preparations and was increased by increased heart work. Furthermore, he reasoned that glucose was a precursor of glycogen, and glycogen was known to be decreased in various pathological conditions. Therefore, increased glucose could allow the heart to beat more strongly and build up the glycogen stores. Because glucose taken orally would be unlikely to provide a better sugar supply than the liver did, he recommended an intravenous infusion of sugar solution. He specifically commented on the desirability of high glycogen stores to cope with the decreased coronary blood flow found in some severe cases of 'atherosclerosis' and 'angina pectoris' of the heart. The sugar infusion would serve the heart in an emergency.

Büdingen suggested at least two possible modes of action: (1) Increased nourishment for the heart with increased provision of fuel for contraction; and (2) an osmotic effect of the infused sugar. He also presented eight cases in whom the infusion was thought to have benefited patients. Four of the patients appeared to have suffered from either severe angina pectoris or myocardial infarction. Two of these wrote to him later commenting on their wonderful intravenous therapy. In an additional patient, ventricular arrhythmias (pulsus bigeminus and trigeminus) were apparently cured by intravenous sugar. Unfortunately, however, the whole article reflects a state of affairs which has been characteristic of many articles also advocating glucose (or glucose-potassium-insulin) therapy. Theoretical hypotheses, apparently soundly based on laboratory work, have been associated with reports of spectacular improvement in some patients, but on the whole there have been no carefully controlled studies. These early theoreticians ignored substantial evidence suggesting that non-carbohydrate could sometimes be the major fuel for the heart even after glucose administration.[3]

When insulin became more widely available, the apparently logical combination of glucose and insulin was advocated in therapy of heart disease.[4-7] This early work is well-summarized in 1937 by Martin in 'Dextrose Therapy in Everyday Practice'.[8]

About this time, new physiological observations were being made to give different and apparently equally strong arguments for the use of dextrose in ischaemic heart disease. An important new observation was made by Evans and colleagues[9] who showed that during deprivation of oxygen, the heart took up more glucose and there was production of lactate instead of the normal lactate uptake. Basic biochemical observations had shown the importance of the conversion of glucose (and glycogen) to lactate as a source of energy during oxygen limitation.

The addition of potassium to glucose-insulin therapy came much later. The initial observations of Dennis and Moore in 1938[10] had shown increased coronary venous potassium concentrations in blood leaving the ischaemic myocardium after coronary artery ligation. In 1952 a decreased tissue potassium was found by Iseri *et al.*[11] There were indirect suggestions, from the data of Harris *et al.*,[12] that such losses of potassium ion could be contributing to the genesis of serious post-myocardial infarction arrhythmias. Also about the same time Selye, Bajusz, Raab and their colleagues[13 14] were stressing the possible role of the potassium loss in promoting heart cell necrosis. A further elaboration of this treatment by Laborit[15] was to give the potassium in the form of potassium aspartate.

It was attractive to postulate that replacement of potassium lost from the heart cell could lead both to a decreased incidence of arrhythmias and to lessened tissue necrosis. There was evidence that glucose and insulin administration promoted uptake of potassium by the cells of the body.[16] Hence there appeared to be a series of arguments for the use of glucose-insulin, together with potassium in acute myocardial ischaemia. As far as acute myocardial infarction is concerned, this therapy has been especially promoted by Sodi-Pallares and his ' polarizing ' regime was described in 1962.[17]

Today we should see where we stand in relation to glucose-potassium-insulin administration ten years later in 1972.

Use of glucose and potassium in well-perfused, anoxic heart

When the isolated perfused heart is deprived of oxygen and is totally anoxic, the major sources of energy are glucose and glycogen and lactate. The possibility of a minor contribution from mitochondrial anaerobic metabolism[18] is discussed elsewhere.[19] Each mole of glucose converted to lactate produces two moles of ATP; each mole of glucose-glycogen produces 3 moles of ATP. This contrasts with approximately 32 moles of ATP produced by aerobic metabolism through the Krebs' citrate cycle. However, by the Pasteur effect glycolysis is accelerated several-fold in the anoxic, perfused heart[20 21] with the result that the energy deficit is limited by the presence of added glucose, and some contractile activity may be maintained.[22] It is important to note several features of this glucose effect in anaerobic hearts:[21-23]

1. Maximal rates of anaerobic glycolysis are achieved with an extracellular glucose concentration of 10-20 mM.
2. The additional presence of insulin at these high glucose concentrations does not accelerate the rate of anaerobic glycolysis.
3. The isolated rat heart is a preparation in which there is an abnormally high perfusion rate; during anoxia the coronary perfusion rate rises even more.

4. The addition of glucose during severe oxygen restriction has been shown to have a beneficial effect on the survival and recovery of the isolated Langendorff-perfused heart, which contracts at abnormally low work-loads (usually about half-normal) even during normoxia. Thus the ATP deficit developing during anoxia was subnormal.

Theoretically the cessation of all contractile activity by the addition of potassium to the perfusion medium could reduce the oxygen demand to a level which could be satisfied by the maximum observed rates of anaerobic glycolysis during total anoxia. We studied the effect of increasing the potassium concentration in the perfusion fluid during a period of anoxia on the subsequent aortic output of the heart during reoxygenation. Langendorff (i.e. low work-load) hearts were subject to 15 min of total anoxia, with glucose in the perfusion medium; the potassium concentration was doubled. After 15 min of anoxia such hearts were suddenly switched to an atrial perfusion with normally oxygenated medium (' working hearts '). In this recovery period, hearts protected by a high potassium medium during anoxia developed within 10 min a cardiac output comparable to that of hearts which had not been anoxic at all (Table 13, 1). Anoxic hearts not protected by a high potassium concentration only partially recovered. Similarly, high-energy phosphates and other biochemical parameters at the end of the 15 min anoxic period were better preserved in hearts perfused with the high potassium medium (Table 13, 2). Potassium may act by causing more rapid arrest of the heart during the anoxic period and therefore lessening the demand on myocardial ATP.[24] The protective value of this beneficial potassium arrest of the anoxic heart has been known to cardiac surgeons for years.

In summary, a high extracellular glucose concentration (10 mM or more), by promoting maximal rates of anaerobic glycolysis in the totally anoxic but well-perfused heart, can aid survival and recovery during re-oxygenation. Added insulin may be of benefit by promoting glucose uptake when the circulating glucose concentration is lower. An increased potassium concentration confers additional protection, presumably by causing cardiac arrest. However, it would not be possible safely to double the plasma potassium in patients with acute myocardial infarction; hence this work on the isolated

Table 13, 1. *Effect of various procedures in anoxic perfusion period of 15 min on subsequent mechanical performance of the heart during reoxygenation and commencement of atrial perfusion ('working heart')*

PREPERFUSION			ATRIAL PERFUSION PERIOD						
Gas Phase	Substrate	K^+	AORTIC OUTPUT ml/min						
5% CO_2; balance			1	2	3	5	10	15	30 min
O_2	Glucose 11·1 mM	Normal K^+	—	38 ±8 (17)	—	—	—	38 ±2 (14)	38 ±2 (17)
N_2	Glucose 11·1 mM	Normal K^+	—	6 ±2 (19)	13 ±3 (18)	19 ±5 (14)	21 ±3 (11)	19 ±3 (7)	19 ±3 (7)
N_2	Glucose 11·1 mM	High K^+	—	29 ±4 (7)	28 ±5 (7)	29 ±5 (9)	36 ±5 (6)	36 ±5 (6)	—
N_2	No substrate	Normal K^+	—	—	—	11 (6)	16 ±4 (6)	20 ±4 (6)	26 ±4 (5)
N_2	Pyruvate 11 mM	Normal K^+		Poor and erratic recovery					
N_2	Lactate 11 mM	Normal K^+		No recovery in 4 hearts					

A dash (—) indicates absence of data.
Normal K^+=5·8 mEq/l; High K^+=11·6 mEq/l.
Mean values ±SEM (number of observations).

Table 13, 2. *Effect of various procedures in anoxic period on values of high-energy phosphates and intermediates at end of anoxic period*

Nature of Anoxic Perfusion:	*ATP*	*ADP* µMole/g	*AMP*	*PCr*	*Glycogen* µMoleC6/g	*G6P* nMole/g	*F6P* nMole/g	*FDP*	*Pyruvate* nMole/g	*Lactate* nMole/g	*Citrate* nMole/g	*Tissue* H_2O µl/g
Control: Normal O_2, K^+; Glucose 11.1 mM	3.33 ± 0.17 (10)	0.75 ± 0.03 (11)	0.14 ± 0.06 (11)	4.42 ± 0.22 (11)	13.6 ± 0.9 (27)	149 ± 10 (20)	34 ± 2 (20)	19 ± 2 (11)	30 ± 5 (12)	615 ± 63 (12)	161 ± 15 (10)	841 ± 10 (7)
Glucose 11.1 mM; Normal K^+, N_2	1.28 ± 0.12 (18)	0.79 ± 0.04 (18)	0.33 ± 0.03 (16)	0.66 ± 0.09 (18)	1.89 ± 0.32 (9)	106 ± 8 (13)	25 ± 3 (13)	32 ± 2 (8)	14 ± 1 (11)	1545 ± 164 (11)	88 ± 8 (17)	877 ± 5 (7)
Glucose 11.1 mM; High K^+, N_2	2.15 ± 0.13 (16)	0.85 ± 0.06 (16)	0.22 ± 0.02 (16)	1.53 ± 0.19 (16)	3.73 ± 0.53 (8)	157 ± 14 (8)	33 ± 4 (8)	21 ± 3 (8)	10 ± 1 (8)	1268 ± 104 (7)	180 ± 13 (8)	877 ± 3 (8)
Pyruvate 11 mM; Normal K^+, N_2	0.41 ± 0.10 (4)	0.66 ± 0.14 (4)	0.31 ± 0.13 (4)	0.35 ± 0.04 (4)	—	—	—	—	—	—	—	—
Substrate-free; Normal K^+, N_2	0.16 ± 0.03 (4)	0.57 (2)	1.44 (2)	0.25 ± 0.02 (4)	—	—	—	—	—	—	—	—
Lactate 11 mM; Normal K^+, N_2	0.25 (2)	0.23 (2)	0.78 (2)	0.31 (2)	—	—	—	—	—	—	—	—

Hearts perfused at 100 cm H_2O pr. for 15 min by Langendorff non-recirculation procedure, with Krebs-Henseleit bicarbonate at 37°, equilibrated with 95% N_2 + 5% CO_2.

Normal K^+ = 5.8 mEq/1; High K^+ = 11.6 mEq/1. At 15 min, hearts freeze-clamped. For analytical procedures, see Opie *et al.*(37) Mean values ± SEM (number of observations). PCr = phosphocreatine; G6P = glucose 6-phosphate; F6P = fructose 6-phosphate; FDP = fructose 1,6-diphosphate. N_2 = 95% nitrogen, balance CO_2. O_2 = 95% oxygen balance CO_2.

perfused rat heart is based on an extreme experimental situation not transferable to a human disease state.

The application of the above principles to the ischaemic and infarcting myocardium

A partially ischaemic preparation is one in which the coronary blood flow has been reduced to pathological levels, but not totally cut off.[23] Does the beneficial effect of glucose-insulin-potassium still hold? A major difference between the ischaemic under-perfused heart and the totally anoxic well-perfused heart lies in the magnitude of intracellular accumulation of hydrogen ions during ischaemia. These hydrogen ions, derived both from the breakdown of ATP and of glucose-glycogen to lactate, almost certainly accumulate within the cell during ischaemia. A major rate-limiting step in the control of glycolysis, the phosphofructokinase reaction, is very sensitive to hydrogen ion accumulation which sensitizes the enzyme to the normal inhibition by ATP.[25] Thus, it is important to distinguish between total ischaemia, where hydrogen ions accumulate intracellularly and phosphofructokinase becomes rate-limiting, and partial ischaemia where there is less intracellular accumulation of hydrogen ions and, presumably, less inhibition of phosphofructokinase. From this point of view it would be logical to add therapy aimed at normalizing the intracellular pH, e.g. by the additional use of a buffer, such as Tris, which can penetrate intracellularly.

If, for simplicity sake, we assume that the basic event in acute myocardial infarction is coronary artery occlusion, then there clearly must be a period of reversible myocardial damage or ischaemia developing before infarction occurs. If this is so, then theoretical considerations suggest that glucose-potassium-insulin therapy might help to alter the outcome of coronary artery occlusion. Initial observations, supporting this possibility, were made by Calva, Sodi-Pallares and co-workers[26] who found markedly improved mitochondrial function in the ischaemic area of hearts from dogs infused for 4 hrs or more with a glucose-potassium-insulin solution.

Because of the theoretical arguments in favour of the use of glucose-potassium-insulin in coronary artery occlusion, we were surprised to find that the study of Calva *et al.*[24] was the only fully reported one in which this regime had been shown to have a definite cellular metabolic effect in well-controlled experiments. We decide to reinvestigate this regime in acute experimental coronary artery occlusion.

We studied a subhuman primate, the baboon, which is developmentally far nearer to man than the dog or pig. Results are summarized in Table 13, 3. In the dose used by Calva *et al.*[24] this regime had no effect on mitochondrial metabolism although there was a

Table 13, 3 *Acute myocardial infarction in the baboon. Effects of infusion of potassium or glucose-insulin-potassium (GIK) 60 min after coronary artery ligation*

	CONTROL LIGATION	K^+ INFUSION	GIK LOW DOSE	GIK HIGH DOSE
Number studied	36	10	12	6
Incidence of ventricular fibrillation	high	low	intermediate	intermediate
ATP	20%	19%	*34%	17%
PCr	34%	23%	*30%	35%
Tissue K^+	88%	*95%	69%	—
Mitochondrial P/O ratio	50%	54%	45%	—
Mitochondrial O_2 uptake	83%	56%	67%	—

The above percentage values are (Area 1 value)÷(Area 4 value)×100, where area 1 is the most severely damaged tissue and area 4 apparently normal tissue (see Fig. 13, 1). Control values were: ATP 4·0 to 4·5 μmole/g wet wt; phosphocreatine 7·0 to 10·7 μmole/g wet wt; tissue potassium 61 to 67 μEq/kilo fresh wt (i.e. dry weight ×5); mitochondrial P/O ratio 2·4 to 2·5; mitochondrial O_2 uptake 4·9 to 5·9 μatoms/mg mitochondrial protein /22 min. Infusion rate: 0·18 ml/kg body wt/min for 60 min. Composition of infusion, per litre: K^+ infusion=K^+ 40 mEq; GIK low dose=dextrose 100g, high purity soluble insulin 20 units, K^+ 40 mEq; GIK high dose=dextrose 200 to 500 g, insulin 60 units, K^+ 60 mEq. *$p<·05$ for comparison between K^+ and GIK low dose infusion.

small effect in improving ATP and creatine phosphate levels in the centre of the infarcting area (Table 13, 3). We have not yet tested the effects of longer periods of infusion because the tissue metabolic changes after 1 hr indicate that severe tissue damage had already occurred (see Fig. 13, 1). There was no evidence that the regime had an important effect in altering the size of the infarction as delineated by epicardial ST-mapping or by the visible size of the infarction.

At the moment we believe that this disappointing result is because acute coronary artery occlusion in the baboon results in a very severe infarction. The collateral blood flow, as studied with

RELATION BETWEEN EPICARDIAL EGG
CHANGES AND TISSUE METABOLIC CHANGES

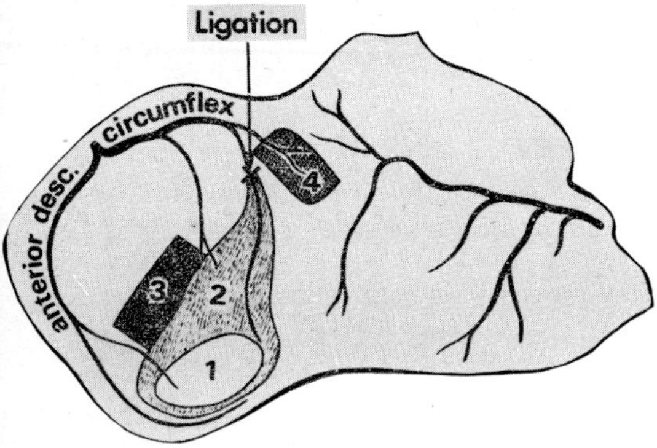

AREA 1: Centre infarct

AREA 2: Edge infarct

AREA 3: Edge non-infarct

AREA 4: Normal

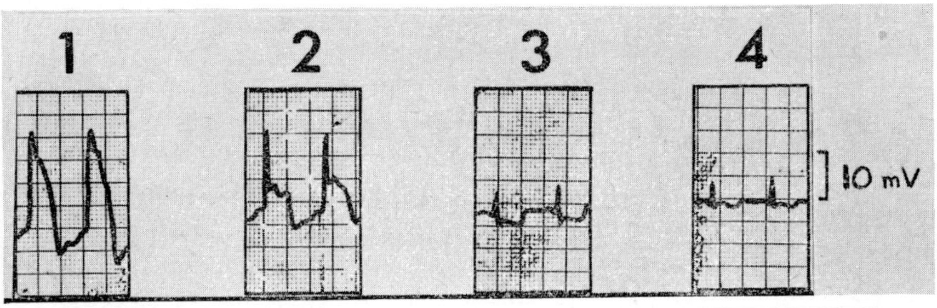

TISSUE pH	5·9	6·2	6·9	6·9
TISSUE K+ mEq/kilo	68	69	65	72
P/O RATIO	1·8	2·2	2·1	2·7

FIG. 13, 1. Example of tissue metabolic changes 60 min after circumflex artery ligation in a baboon infused with K^+. Areas 1 and 2 designate infarcting tissue with definite ST-segment elevation on the epicardial ECG; area 3 is non-infarcting tissue on the edge of the infarct, and with ST-segment depression; area 4 is apparently normal tissue far from the infarcting zone. Note maintenance of tissue K^+ in the infarcting tissue to near-normal values, but marked fall in homogenate pH and mitochondrial phosphorylation/oxidation ratio.

radioactive-microspheres, is extremely low being less than 10 per cent of the control value in the centre of the infarcting tissue even after 10 minutes, and only up to about 30 per cent of the control value at the edge of the infarction. If one is dealing with very severe infarction, then coronary blood flow will be very low and manipulation of the extracellular fluid will achieve relatively minor results. This does not mean that in less severe infarcts, as found in some dog preparations, the regime could not be beneficial. But for the moment we are forced to admit that, in the baboon at any rate, an infarct is an infarct and it cannot be changed very much.

Comparison of glucose-potassium-insulin with potassium therapy
As it is now held that up to 70 per cent of all deaths from coronary artery disease occur as a result of lethal arrhythmias before the patient even reaches the hospital, it would be most intriguing if we could give the general practitioner who first reaches the patient a simple metabolic procedure to use in addition to anti-arrhythmic drugs. The rationale of glucose-potassium-insulin therapy was precisely to replace potassium loss from the heart because it was held that this potassium loss could be instrumental in causing or promoting the serious arrhythmias. However, here we have a serious contradiction. Most serious arrhythmias occur within 1 hour of coronary artery occlusion, whereas the measured potassium loss in a dog heart infarction after 1 hour is only about 10 per cent.[27] In the baboon, too, potassium loss after 1 hour in the infarction area is also of this magnitude and our attempts to alter this K^+ loss by glucose-potassium-insulin infusion have not met with success (Table 13, 3). It may be that the potassium ion could move from one cell compartment to another or from within to without the cell without an overall tissue loss, or that the loss is greater in the conducting tissue or the mitochondria[26] than elsewhere.

Nevertheless, a glucose-potassium-insulin infusion appeared to decrease the incidence of ventricular fibrillation in the first hour following coronary artery ligation in our baboon experiments. An infusion of potassium by itself had an even more marked protective effect. The infusion rate corresponded to 30 mEq/hr for a 70 kg man and increased the blood arterial K^+ by 0·4 mEq/litre/hr. Tissue potassium fell less in the infarcting myocardium after K^+-infusion. There were no changes in the tissue contents of high-energy phosphate compounds or of lactate and α-glycerolphosphate. Mitochondrial phosphorylation/oxidation ratios were unchanged. However, mitochondrial oxygen uptake in all areas was about half that of non-treated or glucose-potassium-insulin treated hearts.

The link between these tissue metabolic effects of K^+-infusion and the decreased incidence of ventricular fibrillation is not clear. However, the K^+-infusion did prevent the fall in arterial K^+ otherwise found in the experimental animals. An infusion of glucose-potassium-insulin was less able to maintain plasma and tissue K^+ than a K^+ infusion by itself.

In man, Sodi-Pallares claims to have reduced the incidence of arrhythmias to a very low figure by the use of the glucose-potassium-insulin regime.[28] The more disappointing results of others[29] may be explained by their deviation from the details of Sodi-Pallares' regime or by a genuine failure of the regime to work. There is still much room for assessing the possible effects of this therapy by carefully controlled trials on an adequate number of patients. It should be noted that there are no clinical studies comparing the effects of glucose-potassium-insulin with glucose-insulin, glucose alone, or K^+ alone. The administration of glucose alone to man is perhaps likely to be of limited value because of the diminished rates of insulin secretion found in some patients.[30]

FFA 'toxicity' and glucose administration

We have been studying the possible toxic effects of an unphysiological fatty acid octanoate and the possible beneficial effect of glucose on the ischaemic isolated perfused rat heart. When normal rat hearts are perfused with octanoate in a concentration of 0·5 mM the heart rate is decreased. In higher concentrations there may be heart block.[31] The oxygen uptake is virtually unchanged and therefore the oxygen uptake per beat is increased. This is entirely compatible with the suggestion that free fatty acids may, in certain circumstances, 'uncouple' oxidative metabolism. During ischaemia hearts perfused with octanoate underwent more mechanical deterioration than those perfused with glucose. If, however, glucose was added to octanoate then there was considerable mechanical but only minimal biochemical improvement. In these instances, glucose did not appear to act by altering the rate of anaerobic glycolysis. An attractive possibility is that the presence of glucose helps maintain reactivity of the membrane ATPase.[32] Thus in this simple model of ischaemia we can indeed show that glucose is ' good ' and fatty acid is ' toxic '.

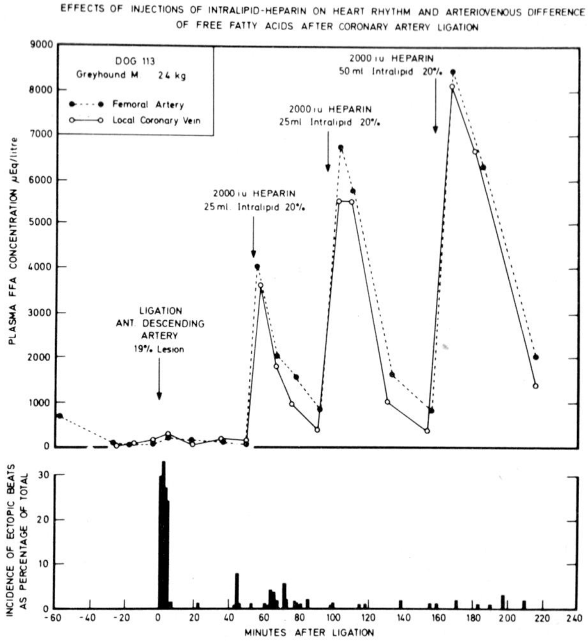

FIG. 13, 2. An example of repetitive elevation of plasma FFA concentrations (by injection of Intralipid-heparin) failing to increase the ectopic activity in an open-chest greyhound preparation. Taken from *Lancet* **2,** 818, 1971, by permission of authors and editor.

An important question is whether the glucose-potassium-insulin regime (or glucose by itself) could act on arrhythmias by decreasing the circulating blood free fatty acid concentration. This is an intriguing possibility which follows from the work of Dr Michael Oliver and colleagues.[33]

At the moment the evidence that free fatty acids are an important arrhythmogenic agent is still not settled.[34] Reasons for doubt include:

1. Experiments in the open-chest greyhound dog with coronary artery ligation showed that in this model extremely high free fatty acid concentrations were not by themselves arrhythmogenic[35] (Fig.

13, 2). The threshold for ventricular fibrillation is also not altered by high free fatty acid concentrations.[36]

2. Using closed-chest dogs in which myocardial infarction had been induced by an electrolytically-induced thrombus, we have been able to obtain a preparation in which there has been an extremely high incidence of ectopic beats, usually of the multi-focal variety, for about 6 to 72 hr after thrombosis. In this preparation infusion of triglyceride-heparin, with consequent elevation of blood free fatty acid values to very high values (in the presence of an average blood albumin value of only 1 gm per 100 ml) failed to provoke ventricular fibrillation on 4 occasions. When infusions were made within 4 hours of coronary thrombosis, increased ectopic activity appears in 3/7 experiments including ventricular fibrillation in one. Thus in a total of 11 infusions in close-chest dogs with coronary thrombosis, increased ectopic activity appeared in only 3. However, our experience with this model is limited to 14 dogs and we do not adequately know the natural history of the ectopic activity in these surviving dogs.

3. Thus far it has not been shown that patients with myocardial infarction and with serious arrhythmias have blood free fatty acid concentrations in the range shown to be toxic in some animal preparations.

Conclusions

1. In simplified experimental systems, such as the isolated perfused rat heart, it can be readily shown that glucose (with insulin and potassium) is 'good' and that free fatty acids are 'bad' for the survival of the hypoxic or anoxic myocardium.

2. It is more difficult to show similar clear-cut effects in models of acute myocardial infarction.

3. In an open-chest baboon model of acute myocardial infarction, a K^+-infusion for 1 hr had a more definite anti-arrhythmic effect than an infusion of glucose-potassium-insulin. The K^+-infusion also appeared to preserve the tissue K^+ value in the infarcting area, but reduced mitochondrial oxygen uptake in all areas.

4. An infusion of glucose-potassium-insulin did not conserve tissue K^+ in the infarcting myocardium but caused small increases in ATP and creatinine phosphate. Mitochondrial metabolism was unaltered.

5. Preliminary results in closed-chest dogs with coronary thrombosis suggest that a triglyceride-heparin infusion did not have a consistent effect in precipitating ectopic activity.

6. Metabolic manipulation of substrate level reaching the infarcting myocardium may be expected to influence the outcome of myocardial infarction most when the collateral blood supply is relatively good. Hence it may be that patients with severe infarction and little collateral blood flow may not respond well to substrate alterations.

ACKNOWLEDGMENTS

We thank the Chris Barnard Fund, the M.R.C. of the Republic of South Africa, and the Universities of Cape Town and Stellenbosch for financial support.

REFERENCES

1 GOULSTON, A. (1911). A note on the beneficial effect of the ingestion of cane sugar in certain forms of heart disease. *British Medical Journal* **1,** 615-617.

2 BÜDINGEN, T. (1914). Ueber die Möglichkeit einer Ernährungs behandlung des Herzmuskels durch Einbringen von Traubenzuckerlösungen in den grossen Kreislauf. *Deutsches Archiv für Klinische Medizin* **114,** 534-579.

3 EVANS, C. L. (1914). The effect of glucose on the gaseous metabolism of the isolated mammalian heart. *Journal of Physiology* **47,** 407-418.

4 MATHIEU, L., COLLESSON, L. & SIMONIN, J. (1931). Recherches électrocardiographiques chez des cardiaques traités par l'association insuline-glucose. *Comp. Rend Societe de Biologie* **107,** 365-366.

5 MARTIN, G. A. (1931). L'association sucre-insuline en thérapeutique cardiaque. *Montpellier Medicine* **53,** 391-396.

6 MASCHERONI, O. (1933). Considerazioni-sulla terapia ' glucosio-insulina ' nelle cardiopatie scompensate. *Riforma Medicina* **49,** 1929-1931.

7 SMITH, K. S. (1933). Insulin and glucose in treatment of heart disease, with special reference to angina pectoris. *British Medical Journal* **1,** 693-696.

8 MARTIN, E. (1933). In *Dextrose Therapy in Everyday Practice,* p. 240.

9 EVANS, C. L., GRAFF, A. C., KOSAKA, T., MACKENZIE, K., MURPHY, G. E., VACEK, J., WILLIAMS, D. H. & YOUNG, F. G. (1933). Utilization of blood sugar and lactate by heart-lung preparation. *Journal of Physiology* **80,** 21-40.

10 DENNIS, J. & MOORE, R. M. (1938). Potassium changes in functioning heart under conditions of ischemia and of congestion. *American Journal of Physiology* **123,** 443-447.

11 ISERI, L. T., ALEXANDER, L. C., MCCAUGHEY, R. S., BOYLE, A. J. & MYERS, G. B. (1952). Water and electrolyte content of cardiac and *Heart Journal* **43,** 215-227.
skeletal muscle in heart failure and myocardial infarction. *American*

12 HARRIS, A. S., BISTENI, A., RUSSELL, R. A., BRIGHAM, J. C. & FIRESTONE, J. E. (1954). Excitatory factors in ventricular tachycardia resulting from myocardial ischaemia. *Science* **119,** 200-203.

13 Bajusz, E. & Selye, H. (1960). The chemical prevention of cardiac necrosis following occlusion of coronary vessels. *Canadian Medical Association Journal* **82,** 212-213.

14 Raab, W. (1969). Myocardial electrolyte derangement: crucial feature of pluricausal, so called coronary heart disease. *Annals of the New York Academy of Science* **147,** 627-686.

15 Laborit, H. (1963). The treatment of cardiovascular insufficiency and myocardial infarct with the combination of insulin, hypertonic glucose and potassium salts. *Presse Médicale* **71,** 1-3.

16 Harrop, G. A. Jr. & Benedict, E. M. (1922). The relation of the diffusion content to mountain sickness. *Proceedings of the Society for Experimental Biology and Medicine* **20,** 279-282.

17 Sodi-Pallares, D., Testelli, M. R., Fishler, B. L., Bisteni, A., Medrano, G. A., Friedland, C. & De Micheli, (1962). Effects of an intravenous infusion of a potassium-glucose-insulin solution on the electrocardiographic signs of myocardial infarction. *American Journal of Cardiology* **9,** 166-181.

18 Penney, D. G. & Cascarano, J. (1970). Anaerobic rat heart. *Biochemical Journal* **118,** 221-227.

19 Opie, L. H. (1972 in press). *Acta biologica et medica germanica.*

20 Newsholme, E. A. & Randle, P. J. (1961). Regulation of glucose uptake by muscle. *Biochemical Journal* **80,** 655-662.

21 Morgan, H. E., Henderson, M. J., Regan, D. M. & Park, C. R. (1961). Regulation of glucose uptake in muscle I. *Journal of Biological Chemistry* **236,** 253-261.

22 Weissler, A. M., Kruger, F. A., Baba, N., Scarpelli, D. C., Leighton,
ture of anoxic myocardium. *Journal of Clinical Investigation* **47,** 403-416.
R. F. & Gallimore, J. K. (1968). Role of anaerobic capacity and struc-

23 Opie, L. H. (1972). In *Metabolism of the Hypoxic and Ischaemic Heart.* Edited: P. Moret and Z. Fejfar. Karger, Basel. Pp. 2-21.

24 Regen, D. M., Young, D. A. B., Davies, W. W., Jack, J. Jr. & Park, C. R. (1964). Adjustment of glycolysis to energy utilization in the perfused rat heart. *Journal of Biological Chemistry* **239,** 381-384.

25 Danforth, W. H. (1965). In *Control of Energy Metabolism,* p. 287. Edited: B. Chance and R. Estabrook and J. R. Williamson. New York: Academic Press.

26 Calva, E., Múјica, N., Núnezi, R., Aoki, K., Bisteni, A. & Sodi-Pallares, D. (1966). Mitochondrial biochemical changes and glucose-KCl-insulin solution in cardiac infarct. *American Journal of Physiology* **211,** 71-76.

27 Jennings, R. B., Kaltenbach, J. P. & Sommers, H. M. (1965). In *Electrolytes and Cardiovascular Disease,* p. 123. Edited by E. Bajusz. Basel: S. Karger.

28 Sodi-Pallares, D., Bisteni, A., Medrano, G. A., Testelli, M. R. & De Micheli, A. (1963). The polarizing treatment of acute myocardial infarction. *Diseases of Chest* **43,** 424-432.

29 M.R.C. Working Party Report (1968). Potassium, glucose, and insulin treatment for acute myocardial infarction. *Lancet* **II,** 1355-1363.

30 Taylor, S. H. & Majid, P. A. (1971). Insulin and the heart. *Journal of Molecular and Cellular Cardiology* **2,** 293-317.

31 Opie, L. H. (1970). Effect of fatty acids on contractility and rhythm of the heart. *Nature* **227,** 1055-1056.

32 Fedelsova, M., Dhalla, N. S., Balasubramanian, V. & Ziegelhöffer, A. (1972 in press). In *Heart Overloading.* Edited by P. Y. Hatt. Inter-European Symposium, Paris.

33 Kurien, V. A., Yates, P. A. & Oliver, M. F. (1971). The role of free fatty acids in the production of ventricular arrhythmias after acute

coronary artery occlusion. *European Journal of Clinical Investigation* **1,** 225-241.
34 Opie, L. H. (1972). Metabolic response during impending myocardial infarction. *Circulation* **45,** 483-490.
35 Opie, L. H., Norris, R. N., Thomas, M., Holland, A. J., Owen, P. & Van Noorden, S. (1971). Failure of high concentrations of circulating free fatty acids to provoke arrhythmias in experimental myocardial infarction. *Lancet* **II,** 818-822.
36 Kostis, J. & Horstmann, E. (1972). Fatty acids and ventricular fibrillation threshold. *Lancet* **I,** 961-962.
37 Opie, L. H., Mansford, K. R. L. & Owen, P. (1971). Effects of increased heart work on glycolysis and adenine nucleotides in the perfused heart of normal and diabetic rats. *Biochemical Journal* **124,** 475-490.

Discussion

Henderson. I wonder whether it was quite fair to produce evidence in support of what you call the toxic fatty acid hypothesis using a concentration of octanoate which was pretty high and I guess without albumin, in which case it really was extremely high.

Opie. The octanoate concentration used in recent experiments was 0·5 mM. There was no albumin present. I used octanoate as an unphysiological fatty acid deliberately to get fatty acid toxicity and to try and elucidate the cellular mechanisms involved.

Maseri. What is the rationale of giving a potassium solution in acute myocardial infarction or necrosis? It is quite clear that injured cells leak potassium, creating a reduction of the concentration gradient across the membrane. If you are able to get potassium back into the cells, then it is understandable but the plasma concentration you achieve might serve only to reduce further the potassium gradient across the membrane. There is, after all, very little flow in your system and it probably would take a long time to get there.

Reuter. May I try to answer Dr Maseri's question about the infusion of potassium? If you add potassium then the potassium conductance of the cell membrane increases and this definitely counteracts the development of arrhythmias. Therefore I feel it is reasonable to infuse potassium in myocardial ischaemia. In addition it is well known that potassium outside activates the sodium pump so this may help to increase potassium concentration in cells where there has been potassium loss. But potassium moves inward not because the external potassium concentration is higher but because of activation of sodium pump due to increasing external potassium concentration.

Maseri. The problem that still bothers me after your comment is that I would expect, in the ischaemic zone compared with the normal, there to be a higher extra-cellular potassium concentration if the cells are leaking potassium. This is the problem of cells in the phase of transient ischaemia. Maybe the increased potassium concentration in extra-cellular fluid is beneficial in some way to healthy muscle.

Reuter. I think that accumulation of potassium outside the infarcted region may not be sufficient to depolarize the cell membrane. But it may actually create ectopic beats because of the decrease in potassium conductance in conjunction with depolarization. You can overcome this by adding additional potassium at the outside because the decrease in potassium conductance is less severe.

Opie. With potassium infusion it is the venous and not the arterial potassium concentration that is elevated. If the cellular uptake is determined in some way by a concentration difference then one might expect an effect from altering the arterial potassium. One doesn't know, however, whether a change in the arterial potassium means a change in the venous potassium.

Mjøs. Together with Dr Kjekshus, we also failed to induce arrhythmias in open chested dogs after coronary artery ligation with the infusion of Intralipid/heparin. So we agree with you using the same preparation and we agree with you in demonstrating no increase in average S-T segment elevation by Intralipid/heparin. On the other hand, if we pre-treated the dogs with an antilipolytic agent like nicotinic acid and then infused Intralipid/heparin i.v. at the same dosage, then we got an increase in the average S-T segment elevation, following coronary artery occlusion.

Carlson. What systemic reaction did your baboons have to the glucose insulin infusion with regard to glucose, insulin and free fatty acid levels in the blood? Did you measure glucose and fatty acid uptake in the heart during these conditions? I do not think that you should only look at a-v differences..

Opie. The arterial free fatty acid values were usually low at the start of the experiment and only rose slightly. We have not measured uptake of glucose or free fatty acids.

Oliver. I am sure that you did not really mean to say that you infused fatty acids. Using Intralipid/heparin to raise free fatty acids may produce a different tissue response. I do not think it is a wise idea to look for an increased incidence of arrhythmias at times when there is already a chaotic state. It is difficult enough to know what is going on in the myocardium at that time and interpretation of the effects of raising free fatty acids may be impossible. May we have more details of your closed-chest preparation—where do you place the catheter, which artery it occludes, which part of the myocardium is infarcted and to what extent is it myocardium infarcted?

Opie. You are quite right we did infuse Intralipid/heparin and not FFA. We have also found it difficult to be sure about this chaotic rhythm, but ventricular fibrillation is not precipitated and this would be the final disastrous event. Our closed-chest technique is simply a modification of the Regan technique. We have only studied 14 animals to date and passed the catheter fairly far down either the anterior descending or circumflex artery of the dog. The thrombus occludes the artery and a wedge shape infarct results.

Kurien. I think if Dr Opie wanted to study the FFA hypothesis in a dog in which there is 100 per cent arrhythmia, he should have used an antilipolytic agent. If an antilipolytic agent could reduce arrhythmia to 50 per cent or so, it might give indirect support to the fatty acid hypothesis. Secondly, the system of balloon occlusion of the coronary artery is very similar to Harris' three stages in the production of arrhythmias. There is an initial stage, followed by three hours of complete quiescence followed at about four to six hours by completely chaotic rhythm. You should really use that two to three hours of quiescent phase to test the hypothesis. We originally showed that when ectopics had fallen to a frequency of no more than 3 per minute, you could really demonstrate the effect of intralipid and heparin in increasing arrhythmia.

Opie. Perhaps we should have been keener on using antilipolytic agents. We have studied two dogs in this early arrhythmia-free period and found no effect.

Randle. Is there any evidence that this fall in pH is of significance? The only way in which I can think that one could manipulate the fall in pH is to attempt to alter the cardiac glycogen concentration before interrupting the coronary circulation, because presumably if the glycogen is low the pH fall should be less because there would be less glycolysis. The second question I wanted to ask you is whether there are any manipulations in the life of man or animal which influence the glycolytic potential of cardiac muscle? Is the maximum rate of glycolysis dependent on exercise, previous dietary history and so on, because this might influence pH and also ATP production?

Opie. This touches on the whole very interesting question of adaptability of the heart, which is by no means worked out. Scheuer increased the glycogen content of rat and then found that the hearts survived longer during hypoxia. Concerning pH, the key enzyme of glycolysis is phosphofructokinase and it is pH-sensitive. A low concentration relieves the inhibitory effect of a low pH. In the centre of the baboon heart infarction, the whole tissue pH ranges 6·2 and 6·5. To allow any phosphofructokinase activity at all then the ATP must be very low. Thus any therapy raising the cellular ATP may inhibit glycolytic flow. It would be desirable if possible to change intracellular pH to regulate the glycolytic flow rate.

Randle. Yes, but my question is whether in fact it is the diminished glycolytic flux and ATP synthesis which is harmful to this injured muscle or whether it is the pH fall itself. Would this piece of infarcted muscle really do better if it had less glycolysis and a higher pH rather than having increased glycolysis and a lower pH?

Opie. During glucose-potassium-insulin infusions we found no change in tissue lactate or pH in the centre of the infarction. Yet we found a significant, albeit small, increase in ATP and phosphocreatinine suggesting that an alteration in glycolytic rate was not the important thing but that some other mechanism was involved.

Carlson. One way of testing this would be the pre-treatment of animals with nicotinic acid. Then you could deplete glycogen stores quite considerably and later induce the ischaemic event.

THE NATURE AND CONTROL OF MYOCARDIAL SUBSTRATE METABOLISM IN HEALTHY MAN

B. W. LASSERS, L. A. CARLSON, L. KAIJSER, AND M. WAHLQVIST

THE myocardium has a continual demand for energy which is normally satisfied by the oxidation of substrates ultimately derived from the blood. Investigations of the nature of these substrates and of the regulation of their supply were first made using isolated perfused heart preparations. Early studies established that the myocardium could take up and catabolize glucose, lactate, pyruvate, fatty acids and ketone bodies.[1,2] Subsequent studies with the isolated heart have indicated the importance of substrate concentrations, hormones, and free fatty acids (FFA) in the control of substrate utilization by the heart.[3,4]

The introduction of the technique of coronary sinus catheterization with the measurement of arterio-venous differences in concentration across the heart allowed the investigation of these problems in the intact animal including man. During the past 25 years much has been learned about the nature of the substrates extracted by the heart from the blood in healthy subjects or patients at rest.[4] However, relatively little is known about the effect of physiological changes such as exercise on the pattern of myocardial substrate utilization. In addition, although it has been recognized for some time that intracellular or endogenous substrate stores are an important source of energy in exercising skeletal muscle, there is virtually no information about their role in the human myocardium. Furthermore, little has been done to establish the role in man of factors which have been found to control substrate utilization by isolated hearts, apart from the demonstration of a general relationship at rest between substrate concentration and myocardial extraction.

The purpose of this communication is to review those aspects of our own studies in healthy fasting men[5-11] which are concerned with (a) the pattern of utilization of blood substrates at rest and during prolonged exercise, (b) the role of endogenous substrate in myocardial energy metabolism and (c) the control of substrate uptake.

Material and methods

The subjects were 42 healthy men each of whom had been fasting overnight. Seventeen of them were studied only at rest; the other 25 were investigated both at rest and during approximately 2 hours of supine leg exercise. In order to examine the effect of lowering plasma FFA on the pattern of substrate metabolism, ten of the latter group received a continuous intravenous infusion of nicotinic acid throughout the study (Fig. 14, 1). The details of these studies, the catheterization and sampling techniques, analytical methods and calculations have been described.[6 8 9]

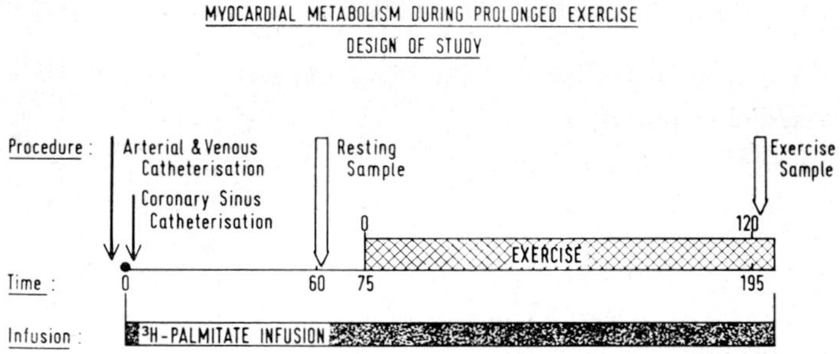

FIG. 14, 1. Design of studies of myocardial metabolism during prolonged exercise. After insertion of arterial and venous catheters a constant infusion of ^{3}H-palmitate was begun as an FFA tracer. The coronary sinus was catheterized and at 60 min resting samples were collected. The subjects then performed two hours of supine leg exercise and further samples were collected during the final minutes of this period. The design of the nicotinic acid investigation was identical except that the subjects received a constant intravenous infusion of nicotinic acid throughout the study.

The pattern of substrate utilization at rest and during prolonged exercise

The pattern of substrate utilization (as assessed by calculation of the oxygen extraction ratios of the various substrates[6]) which we found in our subjects at rest is shown in Table 14, 1. This pattern only differs substantially from that found by other workers[4] in that we were able to demonstrate a significant extraction of plasma triglycerides.[5] Prolonged exercise was accompanied by a decrease in the relative contribution of glucose to myocardial energy metabolism, a concomitant increase in the contribution of lactate and no significant change in that of FFA or triglycerides (Table 14, 1). Thus there was no difference between rest and prolonged exercise in the relative importance of total blood lipid and total blood carbohydrate as fuel for myocardial energy metabolism. In this respect prolonged exercise would appear to differ from short periods of submaximal exercise. The marked rise in the arterial concentration of lactate and the fall in that of FFA which occur in the first half hour or so of exercise enhance the contribution of lactate to myocardial energy metabolism and decrease that of FFA. Hence, during this period, carbohydrate is a quantitatively more important source of energy for the heart than it is either at rest or when exercise has been prolonged.[8 12]

The role of endogenous substrate as a source of energy for myocardial metabolism

A considerable proportion of the energy requirements of exercising skeletal muscle is derived from the metabolism of endogenous glycogen and triglycerides.[13 14] Endogenous substrates are also metabolized by the isolated perfused heart and changes in the glycogen and triglyceride content of the intact rat heart are known to occur with physiological changes such as ageing, exercise, and dietary alterations and with the administration of drugs such as nicotinic acid. However, because it is difficult to obtain biopsy material from the human heart, the significance of these stores in myocardial energy metabolism in man is not clear. Nevertheless, inferences about the stores can be drawn from data on oxygen extraction ratios, and for the endogenous glyceride pools, from measurement of arterial coronary sinus differences in free glycerol concentration.

It can be seen from Table 14, 1 that at rest, both with and without nicotinic acid, the total oxygen extraction ratio for blood substrates did not differ significantly from 100 per cent. Measurements of substrate extraction by the heart obviously do not indicate whether a substrate is immediately oxidized or stored for catabolism later, but as the total oxygen extraction ratio was very close to 100 per cent it follows that in the resting fasting state there is little change in

Table 14, 1. *The relative contribution of various blood substrates to myocardial oxidative metabolism as assessed by their oxygen extraction ratios at rest and during prolonged exercise in: (A) a control group of 15 subjects not receiving nicotinic acid and: (B) a group of 10 subjects receiving a continuous intravenous infusion of nicotinic acid. FFA = free fatty acids; TGFA = triglyceride fatty acids.*

SUBSTRATE	OXYGEN EXTRACTION RATIO %							
	A. CONTROL GROUP				B. NICOTINIC ACID GROUP			
	REST		EXERCISE		REST		EXERCISE	
FFA	49 ± 4	64 ±6	49 ± 2	58 ±4	11 ± 3	22 ±7	4 ± 10	2 ±10
TGFA	15 ± 5		9 ± 3		11 ± 6		−2 ± 3	
Glucose	25 ± 5		13 ± 2		48 ± 5		35 ± 4	
Lactate	8 ± 2	33 ±5	16 ± 3	30 ±5	22 ± 2	72 ±5	30 ± 4	67 ±6
Pyruvate	0 ± 1		1 ± 0		2 ± 1		2 ± 0	
TOTAL	97 ± 8		88 ± 6		94 ± 9		69 ± 12	

(mean ± SEM)

the total energy content of endogenous myocardial substrate pools, although shifts between the various pools could, of course, occur.

During prolonged exercise the average total oxygen extraction ratio for the control group fell to 88 per cent. This fall was not significant, and the total ratio does not in fact differ significantly from 100 per cent. Nevertheless, it does raise the possibility that during prolonged exercise energy is being derived from sources other than the blood substrates which were measured. It seems very unlikely that other blood metabolites such as ketone bodies or amino acids are a significant source of energy in this circumstance[8] and, therefore, it could be that there is a net decrease in the total energy content of endogenous substrate pools. On the other hand, it is clear from the magnitude of the contribution of blood substrate that if the myocardium does indeed derive energy from endogenous pools during exercise, it is very much less dependent on them than is skeletal muscle which may obtain as much as 70 per cent of its energy from intracellular stores.[14]

In the case of the nicotinic acid group during prolonged exercise, the total oxygen extraction ratio of 69 per cent was significantly less than 100 per cent. Again it is unlikely that this deficit can be accounted for by other blood metabolites, and it is probable that there has been a reduction in the total energy content of endogenous myocardial substrate pools.[9] Evidence that the substrate is in fact lipid stems from a comparison of estimates of the relative utilization of carbohydrate and lipid derived in two different ways: from the oxygen extraction ratio data, and from the myocardial RQ's (Table 14, 2). In both the control and nicotinic acid groups at rest and in

Table 14. 2. *The relative contribution of blood carbohydrate (CHO) and lipid to myocardial oxidative metabolism as assessed by the oxygen extraction ratios (OER), compared with the contribution predicted from the average myocardial RQ's (RQm) (given in brackets)*

	CONTROL		NICOTINIC ACID	
	OER	RQm	OER	RQm
REST		(0·76)		(0·91)
Lipid	64 ± 6%	82%	22 ± 7%	31%
CHO	33 ± 5%	18%	72 ± 5%	69%
TOTAL	97 ± 8%	100%	94 ± 9%	100%
EXERCISE		(0·81)		(0·91)
Lipid	58 ± 4%	65%	2 ± 10%	31%
CHO	30 ± 5%	35%	67 ± 6%	69%
TOTAL	88 ± 6%	100%	69 ± 12%	100%

(mean ± SEM)

the control group during prolonged exercise the percentage participation of carbohydrate and lipid as measured by the oxygen extraction ratios are in good agreement with those predicted by the average myocardial RQ's. In the nicotinic acid group during prolonged exercise, the two methods give concordant estimates for carbohydrate, whereas in contrast, for lipid there is a considerable discrepancy between the oxygen extraction ratio value of 2 per cent and the RQ one of 31 per cent. This implies that in this rather extreme condition of prolonged exercise combined with inhibition of FFA mobilization, lipid is the principal type of endogenous substrate from which the heart is deriving energy.[9]

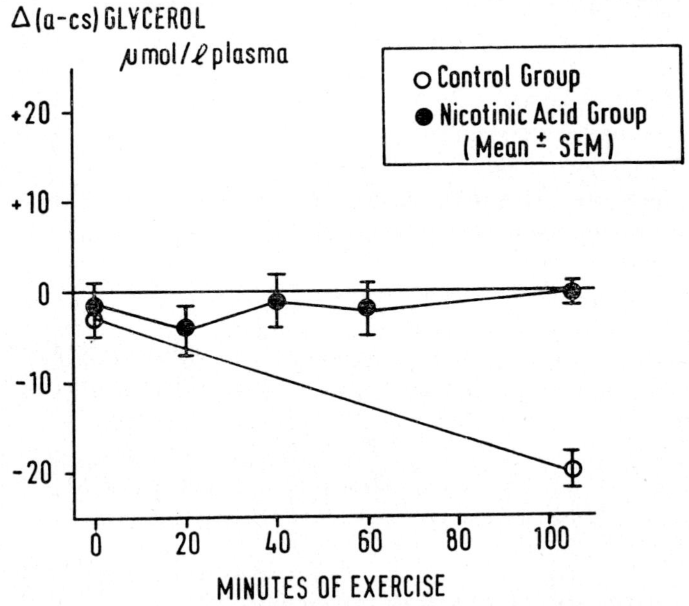

FIG. 14, 2. Arterial-coronary sinus differences in free glycerol concentration ($\Delta_{(a\text{-}cs)}$ Glycerol) at rest and during prolonged exercise in the control and nicotinic acid groups. Positive differences indicate myocardial extraction of glycerol and negative differences the release of glycerol into the coronary sinus blood.

Further evidence that endogenous lipid pools are metabolically active in man comes from measurement of arterial-coronary sinus differences in free glycerol concentration (Fig. 14, 2). At rest, in both the control and nicotinic acid groups, there was no evidence of either myocardial uptake of free glycerol or release of it into the coronary sinus. However, during prolonged exercise there was marked efflux of glycerol into the coronary sinus blood in the control group, but not in the nicotinic acid one. For a number of reasons it seems that the most likely source of free glycerol entering the coronary sinus is endogenous myocardial glycerides.[8 9] Thus it would appear that during prolonged exercise without nicotinic acid, in contrast to the situation at rest or during exercise with nicotinic acid, the rate of glyceride hydrolysis has exceeded the capacity of the myocardium to reutilize glycerol. On the other hand, when nicotinic acid was administered, prolonged exercise was not accompanied by an efflux of glycerol from the heart. These somewhat paradoxical results present a problem of interpretation. However, if glycerol release reflects the turnover of endogenous glycerides rather than changes in actual pool size, then these findings could be consistent with the oxygen extraction ratios. As described above, these suggested that during prolonged exercise without nicotinic acid there was very little, if any, depletion of endogenous energy stores, but that with the combination of nicotinic acid and exercise there was net utilization of intracellular lipid pools. Thus, in the normal circumstance in which exercise is accompanied by increased plasma FFA concentrations, the turnover rate of endogenous glycerides could exceed the myocardial capacity for reutilization of glycerol while in the situation of exercise with very low FFA concentrations, and therefore, possibly a reduced rate of synthesis of endogenous glycerides, the rate of utilization of endogenous lipid may have been greater than the rate of its formation without being sufficiently great to exceed the ability of the heart to metabolize glycerol.

The control of myocardial substrate uptake

In intact man, the investigation of factors affecting or controlling myocardial substrate uptake is dependent on inferences made from the relationships found between substrate and hormone concentrations and substrate extraction by the heart which do not, in themselves, imply a causal relationship. The inability to make precise measurements of coronary blood flow severely restricts the examination of these relationships under different physiological circumstances. Thus, although valid information about substrate uptake (extraction × flow) can probably be obtained by comparing extractions among healthy individuals at rest when coronary flow rates are likely to be very similar, a comparison of resting and exercising extractions could be misleading. Similarly, since there may well be substantial differences among individuals in coronary flow during exercise—even when they are performing similar work loads in relation to their physical fitness[6]—it is difficult in this circumstance to make inferences about control of substrate uptake which are quantitatively meaningful from measurements of substrate extractions alone.

For example, one factor known to be of importance in the uptake of many substrates is the arterial concentration. Thus we found, like other workers, that at rest there is a significant linear relationship between extraction and arterial concentration of FFA but that during exercise this was not so (Fig. 14, 3). One interpretation of

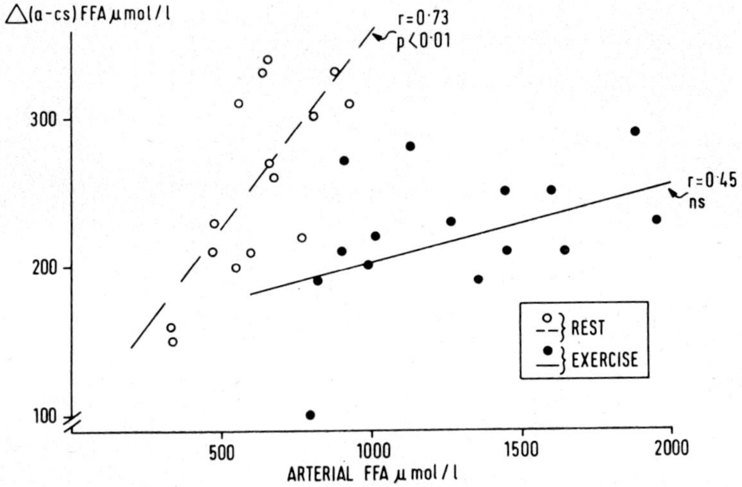

FIG. 14, 3. The relationship, both at rest and during prolonged exercise, of myocardial FFA extraction ($\Delta_{(a\text{-}cs)}$ FFA) and arterial FFA concentration.

these data is that, at the higher FFA concentrations found during prolonged exercise, FFA uptake had become saturated and no longer dependent on concentration. On the other hand, if those individuals with the higher FFA concentrations during exercise also had higher coronary flow rates, then uptake could still be dependent on arterial concentration.

For glucose similarly a close linear relationship was found at rest, but not during exercise (Fig. 14, 4). However, in this instance the exercising values all lie close to or above the regression line for the relationship at rest. Since coronary flow was probably two to three times greater during exercise of the type performed by our subjects,[8] this implies that the rate of myocardial glucose uptake must be considerably greater for a given arterial glucose concentration during exercise. This acceleration of glucose uptake occurred despite the fact that arterial insulin concentration had fallen[11] and FFA concentrations had risen.[8] This observation suggests that exercise may, in fact, augment glucose uptake in man in a manner analogous to that found when the isolated perfused rat heart is made to perform at increased work loads.[15]

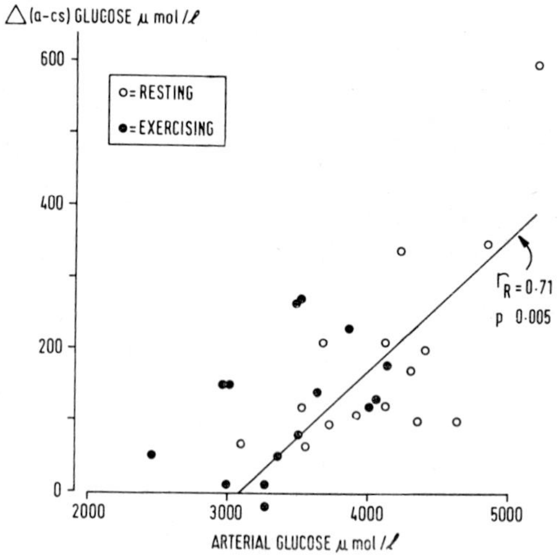

FIG. 14, 4. The relationship at rest and during prolonged exercise between myocardial glucose extraction ($\Delta_{(a\text{-}cs)}$ glucose) and arterial glucose concentration. Since the variables were not significantly correlated during exercise, the regression line has been drawn for the resting points only (r_R=correlation coefficient for resting points).

Studies with the isolated perfused rat heart have also shown that FFA may inhibit glucose utilization[16, 17] and our investigations in man support this idea.[6, 7, 9, 10] We found that there were significant, negative correlations between arterial FFA concentration and myocardial extraction of glucose, lactate and pyruvate: as FFA concentration increased, extractions of these substrates fell, and in the case of pyruvate there was net efflux from the heart at higher

FFA concentrations. This inhibition disappeared when FFA concentrations were reduced with nicotinic acid. Not only do these findings support the general concept of an inhibiting effect of fatty acids on myocardial glucose utilization, but the observation of pyruvate efflux also supports the idea that at least in part this inhibition may occur at the level of pyruvate dehydrogenase.[18]

An additional relationship between FFA concentrations and

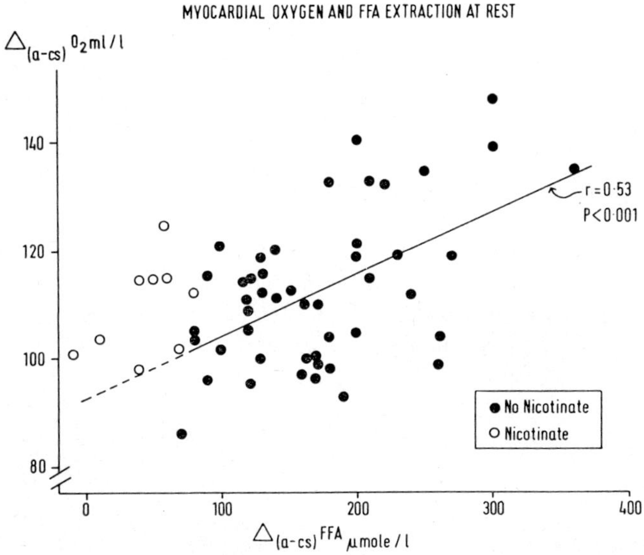

FIG. 14, 5. The relationship at rest between myocardial oxygen ($\Delta_{(a\text{-}cs)}$ O_2) and FFA ($\Delta_{(a\text{-}cs)}$ FFA) extractions. The regression line has been drawn only for the measurements in subjects not receiving nicotinic acid.

myocardial metabolism is seen in Figure 14, 5. Here, there is a significant correlation between the myocardial extractions of FFA and oxygen.[10] Thus, increased FFA extraction by the heart is associated with increased myocardial oxygen utilization—unless there has been a concomitant fall in coronary blood flow. On the other hand, it can also be seen that lowering FFA extraction below the normal range by decreasing FFA concentrations with nicotinic acid is not associated with a parallel decrease in oxygen extraction.

One possible explanation for this association between FFA and oxygen extraction is that fatty acid metabolism increases myocardial oxygen requirements in man as it appears to do in the isolated rat heart[19] and in the intact dog.[20] An alternative explanation is that some third factor such as catecholamines has increased myocardial oxygen utilization but not coronary blood flow and at the same time has produced increased plasma FFA concentrations.

The inter-relationships between the various factors affecting myocardial uptake of blood substrates is obviously complex. It is always possible that the apparent relationship between two variables is really a function of some third variable or a number of other variables (for example, as discussed above for oxygen and FFA extractions). Conversely, it is also possible that a genuine relationship may be obscured by the interaction of other factors.

Table 14, 3. *Various factors which were found on partial correlation analysis to be significant determinants of glucose extraction. The magnitude of their effect is illustrated in the table by showing the predicted effect on glucose extraction of a 10 per cent increase in each variable, the remaining variables being held constant.*[10]

10% INCREASE IN:	EFFECT ON GLUCOSE EXTRACTION:
Arterial insulin	24% increase
FFA extraction	17% decrease
Arterial glucocorticoid	13% decrease

Thus, for example, although glucose extraction and arterial insulin concentration were not directly correlated with each other at rest, when the effect of other variables was allowed for by multiple regression and partial correlation analysis, extraction was found to increase with insulin concentration. At the same time, however, the significant relationship between glucose extraction and concentration disappeared.[10] Table 14, 3 summarizes the factors which were found to be significant determinants of glucose extraction in resting fasting man.

Summary

1. Prolonged exercise is associated with a decrease in the contribution of glucose, and an increase in the contribution of lactate to myocardial energy metabolism. However, there is no change in the relative importance of blood lipid and carbohydrate as sources of energy for the heart in this circumstance.

2. Neither at rest nor during prolonged exercise, do endogenous myocardial energy stores appear to be important net sources of energy for the heart. Only in the rather extreme situation of prolonged exercise and low FFA concentrations produced by nicotinic acid infusion is there any indication of net depletion of endogenous myocardial energy pools: under these circumstances it is probable that the heart derives energy from intracellular lipid.

3. At rest myocardial extraction of FFA and glucose increased with their respective arterial concentrations. A negative correlation between glucose extraction and arterial FFA concentration supports the contention that FFA can inhibit glucose uptake. The observation that myocardial oxygen extraction increased with increasing FFA concentration is consistent with the hypothesis that fatty acid metabolism increases myocardial oxygen requirements.

Acknowledgments

This work was supported by grants from the Swedish Medical Research Council (No's. 19x—204—06 and 07). B. W. L. was a recipient of a Wellcome Swedish Travelling Fellowship and M. L. W. of a Life Assurance Medical Research Fund of Australia and New Zealand Overseas Research Fellowship.

REFERENCES

1 Cruickshank, E. W. H. (1936). Cardiac metabolism. *Physiological Reviews* **16,** 597-639.

2 Evans, C. (1939). The metabolism of cardiac muscle. *Advances in Physiology* **6,** 157-215.

3 Opie, L. H. (1968). Metabolism of the heart in health and disease. I. *American Heart Journal* **76,** 685-698.

4 Opie, L. H. (1969). Metabolism of the heart in health and disease. II. *American Heart Journal* **77,** 100-122.

5 Carlson, L. A., Kaijser, L., Lassers, B. W. (1970). Myocardial metabolism of plasma triglycerides in man. *Journal of Molecular and Cellular Cardiology* **1,** 467-475.

6 Lassers, B. W., Kaijser, L. & Carlson, L. A. (1972). Myocardial lipid and carbohydrate metabolism in healthy, fasting men at rest. *European Journal of Clinical Investigation* **2,** 348-358.

7 LASSERS, B. W., WAHLQVIST, M. L., KAIJSER, L. & CARLSON, L. A. (1971). Relationship in man between plasma free fatty acids and myocardial metabolism of carbohydrate substrates. *Lancet* **II,** 448-462.
8 KAIJSER, L., LASSERS, B. W., WAHLQVIST, M. L. & CARLSON, L. A. (1972). Myocardial lipid and carbohydrate metabolism in fasting men during prolonged exercise. *Journal of Applied Physiology* **32,** 847-858.
9 LASSERS, B. W., WAHLQVIST, M. L., KAIJSER, L. & CARLSON, L. A. (1972). Effect of nicotinic acid on myocardial metabolism in man at rest and during exercise. *Journal of Applied Physiology* **33,** 72-80.
10 CARLSON, L. A., KAIJSER, L., LASSERS, B. W. & WAHLQVIST, M. L. (1972 in press). Fatty acids as a determinant of myocardial substrate and oxygen metabolism in man at rest and during prolonged exercise. *Acta Medica Scandinavica.*
11 WALQVIST, M. L., KAIJSER. L., LASSERS, B. W., LÖW, H. & CARLSON, L. A. (1972 in press). The role of fatty acid and of hormones in the determination of myocardial carbohydrate metabolism in healthy fasting man. *European Journal of Clinical Investigation.*
12 KEUL, J. (1971). Myocardial metabolism in athletes. In *Muscle Metabolism During Exercise*, p. 447. Edited by B. Pernow and B. Saltan. New York and London: Plenum Press.
13 HULTMAN, E. (1967). Studies on muscle metabolism of glycogen and active phosphate in man with special reference to exercise and diet. *Scandinavian Journal of Clinical Laboratory Investigation* **19, suppl. 94,** 1-63.
14 CARLSON, L. A., EKELUND, L.-G., FRÖBERG, S. (1971). Concentrations of triglycerides, phospholipids and glycogen in skeletal muscle and free fatty acids and beta-hydroxybutyric acid in blood in man in response to exercise. *European Journal of Clinical Investigation* **1,** 248-254.
15 CRASS, M. F., MCCASKILL, E. S. & SHIPP, J. C. (1969). Effect of pressure development on glucose and palmitate metabolism in perfused heart. *American Journal of Physiology* **216,** 1569-1576.
16 SHIPP, J. C., OPIE, L. H. & CHALLONER, D. (1961). Fatty acid and glucose metabolism in the perfused heart. *Nature* **189,** 1018-1019.
17 RANDLE, P. J., GARLAND, P. B., HALES, C. N. & NEWSHOLME, E. A. (1963). The glucose fatty acid cycle. Its role in insulin sensitivity and the metabolic disturbances of diabetes mellitis. *Lancet* **I,** 785-789.
18 GARLAND, P. & RANDLE, P. J. (1964). Control of pyruvate dehydrogenase in the perfused rat heart by the intracellular concentration of acetylcoenzyme A. *Biochemical Journal* **91,** 6c-9c.
19 CHALLONER, D. R. & STEINBERG, D. (1966). Effects of free fatty acids on the oxygen consumption of perfused rat heart. *American Journal of Physiology* **210,** 280-286.
20 MJØS, O. D. (1971). Effect of free fatty acids on myocardial function and oxygen consumption in intact dogs. *Journal of Clinical Investigation* **50,** 1386-1389.

DISCUSSION

Mjøs. You measured glycerol in some of your experiments both during rest and exercise. Did you see any output of glycerol from the myocardium? When patients were pretreated with nicotinic acid and then exercised, did they then show any release of glycerol from the myocardium? Is it possible to inhibit myocardial lipolysis by nicotinic acid?

Lassers. Figure 14, 2 of the text shows the arterial coronary sinus difference in concentration of free glycerol at rest and during exercise in the control group of subjects (open circles). You will see that, although there was no significant extraction or release of glycerol in the control group during rest, there was a marked efflux of glycerol from the heart during exercise. For a number of reasons we think that the most likely source of this glycerol was endogenous myocardial glyceride and that this efflux probably reflects increased turnover of this pool rather than its net depletion. Now, when nicotinic acid was administered continuously throughout the study, glycerol release was completely inhibited. These observations may seem paradoxical in view of the oxygen extraction ratio and RQ predictions which suggested that endogenous glycerides are being utilized. The answer may be that the glycerol release reflects rates of turnover of endogenous glyceride pools and that, in the nicotinic acid group, this has not exceeded the capacity of the myocardium for reutilization of the glycerol. In the control group, on the other hand, the rate of glycerol production may have exceeded the rate of reutilization without any change in pool size.

Carlson. It is unfortunate that the myocardium in contrast to adipose tissue has an active glycerokinase. This means that glycerol made available during lipolysis of myocardial triglycerides does not necessarily need to be released into plasma but could be reutilized by the heart.

Randle. We have recently reported (Neely, Denton, England and Randle, *Biochem. J.* (1972), **128,** 147) the results of a study of the effects of cardiac work on the regulation of the citrate cycle in rat hearts and this is relevant to Dr Carlson's observations on the utilization of myocardial triglyceride. In these studies we increased cardiac work acutely by raising the perfusion pressure abruptly from 50-120 mmHg in rat hearts perfused (a) with glucose + insulin and (b) with glucose + insulin + acetate. The hearts were thus deprived of exogenous sources of long chain fatty acids. The experimental period employed involved an 8 min period of perfusion at either 50 mmHg followed by a further 12 min of perfusion at either 50 mmHg or 120 mmHg. At low perfusion pressure, rates of oxygen consumption were essentially constant at 25 μmol/min/g dry heart with glucose and 29 μmol/min/g dry heart with glucose

+ acetate (the higher rates with acetate are attributed to the lower P : O ratio for oxidation of this substrate as compared to glucose). Increasing the perfusion pressure led to an abrupt increase in oxygen consumption to a new steady state level (2·5 times) within 2 min.

The most striking change in substrate utilization was in the oxidation of fatty acids derived from muscle glyceride. This increased ninefold in perfusions with glucose and tenfold in perfusions with glucose+acetate. This was shown in two ways (a) by measurement of the concentration of muscle glycerides and (b) by calculation of the fraction of the oxygen consumption which was not accounted for by the oxidations of glucose or of glucose + acetate. The two methods of calculation showed close agreement. Other changes noted were a twofold increase in glycolytic rate with glucose or glucose acetate; and a twofold increase in oxidation of glucose with glucose alone but no increase when glucose and acetate were present. In the latter situation there is little if any oxidation of glucose by the heart. The rate of acetate oxidation showed little change on increasing cardiac work. These studies indicate that work stimulates lipolysis of muscle glycerides and are in general agreement with Dr Carlson's *in vivo* findings. They also indicate that an apparently abundant supply of certain fuels (in this study glucose and acetate) may not be adequate to support increased cardiac work and to prevent utilization of endogenous triglyceride. Consequently, it may be unwise in the clinical situation to assume that glucose can substitute for long chain fatty acids when lipolysis is inhibited with nicotinate or other antilipolytic drugs. It might be advisable to consider supplying other substrates such as ketone bodies. The rates of oxidation of endogenous glycerides that we have seen in the rat heart could only continue for about 15 to 30 min at the most and by this time the triglyceride stores would have been utilized.

Lassers. It does seem that at least *in vivo,* unless there is a profound stress such as nicotinic acid and prolonged exercise, control mechanisms are such that other substrates become available : for example, lactate concentrations rise and lactate is taken up, or glucose concentrations rise. It seems that even during very prolonged exercise the heart still derives adequate energy from circulating substrates.

Allison. Working in Professor Randle's department, we have studied the dog heart *in vivo* and have shown striking effects of elevating free fatty acids by using Intralipid and heparin on the inhibition of uptake of lactate and pyruvate. Furthermore, we have studied the effects of two substances—bromostearate which has to be bound to albumin, and the water soluble sodium dichloracetate. Both block the oxidation of free fatty acids and cause a striking reversal of the inhibition of pyruvate, lactate and glucose uptake caused by free fatty acids. These results add further confirmation to the glucose fatty acid cycle *in vivo*.

A COMPARISON OF SUBSTRATE METABOLISM OF THE HUMAN HEART IN THE FASTING AND FED STATES

L. A. Carlson, L. Kaijser, B. W. Lassers, S. Rössner
and M. L. Wahlqvist

Available information about the metabolism of the human heart deals almost exclusively with the fasting state. Furthermore in the few non-fasting studies only glucose has been administered.[1 2] During most of the day the human heart is perfused by blood which from the substrate and hormonal point of view is quite different from that perfusing the heart in the fasting state. This report deals with two questions related to the substrate uptake of the human heart in the fed state.

1. Are exogenous plasma triglycerides extracted by the human heart and if so, what is the quantitative importance of that extraction compared to the extraction of endogenous plasma triglycerides?
2. Does the extraction of FFA and glucose differ in the fed and fasted states?

This report is based on data from several studies in our laboratories on the metabolism of the human heart.[3 4 5 6]

Material and methods

The general procedures for catheterization of the coronary sinus and the physiological and biochemical methods have been described elsewhere.[3 4 5 7] All catheterizations were started at about 8 a.m., when the young healthy male subjects reported to the laboratory. An *oral* fed state was induced by eating 200 ml of cream (40 per cent fat), 15 g cheese and 50 g of bread. An *intravenous* fed state was created by the infusion of Intralipid-S[1] (containing sorbitol instead of glycerol as in Intralipid) and glucose. The advantage of the intravenous fed state is that fairly steady blood levels of exogenous triglycerides and of glucose can be reached.

Results

The human heart extracted exogenous triglycerides when they were present in blood either as chylomicrons or Intralipid emulsion (Table 14a, 1). Earlier studies have shown that the kinetics for

Table 14a, 1 *Arterial (A) concentration and arterial-coronary sinus difference (A-Cs) of exogenous plasma triglycerides and oxygen extraction ratio (OER) for the extracted exogenous triglycerides*

	ORAL FED STATE	INTRAVENOUS FED STATE
	μmol per l	μmol per l
A	1190 ± 160	2580 ± 160
A-Cs	70 ± 20	80 ± 20
OER (per cent)	51 ± 14	43 ± 17

Mean ± SEM of 6 determinations in 3 subjects (one determination at 3 hr and one at 4 hr after the meal for the oral fed state and of 38 determinants in 12 subjects for the intravenous fed state.

removal of Intralipid[R] from blood are identical to those for chylomicrons and that the elimination below a certain plasma concentration (C) is a first order reaction and above this concentration it is a zero order reaction.[8] The value for C is usually around 1000 μmoles of exogenous triglycerides per litre plasma. Above that concentration, removal follows zero order kinetics, which means that a constant amount of exogenous triglyceride is cleared from blood per unit time regardless of the plasma level of triglycerides. This kinetic

[1] Kindly supplied by Dr Ivàn Håkuonsson, AB Vitrum, Stockholm, Sweden.

behaviour with an apparent saturation of the removal mechanism above 1000 μmol/l may explain why the same amount of exogenous triglyceride was extracted by the heart in the two fed state conditions (Table 14a, 1) despite the fact that the plasma level of exogenous triglycerides was about twice as high in the intravenous as in the oral fed state.

The mechanism for the uptake of exogenous triglycerides by the human myocardium has been discussed in detail elsewhere.[5] The significant production of glycerol by the heart in the fed state, which does not occur in the fasting state (Table 14a, 2), suggests that hydrolysis of the exogenous triglycerides had occurred. If certain assumptions are made, it can be calculated from these glycerol

Table 14a, 2. *Comparison of myocardial extraction of FFA, glucose and glycerol in the oral fed state, the intravenous fed state and the fasting state*

		FFA	GLUCOSE	GLYCEROL
		μmol per 1 plasma	μmol per 1 blood	μmol per 1 plasma
Oral fed n=3	A	1070±70	4370±80	47±23
	A-Cs	170±50	70±70	−17±8
	OER (%)	31±7	10±4	
I.v. fed n=12	A	720±40^{ns}	8330±330^{xxx}	100±14^{xxx}
	A-Cs	80±10^{xxx}	280±60^{ns}	−26±3^{xxx}
	OER (%)	24±3^{xxx}	29±8^{ns}	
Fasting n=15	A	620±50	4110±140	46±4
	A-Cs	170±20	190±40	−3±2
	OER (%)	49±4	25±5	

ns and xxx indicate that the difference between the i.v. fed and fasting groups are not significant ($p>0{\cdot}05$) and significant ($p<0{\cdot}001$) respectively.

values that at least about 50 per cent of the exogenous triglycerides taken up by the heart had been completely hydrolyzed (presumably by lipoprotein lipase) to fatty acids and glycerol before the triglyceride fatty acids were extracted.[5]

The quantitative importance of the exogenous triglycerides to myocardial energy balance is apparent from the fact that their oxygen extraction ratio (OER) was about 50 per cent (Table 14a, 1). In our two fed state conditions, exogenous plasma triglycerides were the substrate with the highest OER (Table 14A, 2), and this was just as high as the OER for FFA in the fasting state (Table 14a, 2). In the fasting state, the OER for endogenous plasma triglycerides is about 15 to 20 per cent.[4 7]

In the intravenous fed state, the uptake of plasma FFA by the human heart was significantly less than in the fasting state in spite of the fact that the arterial levels of FFA were quite similar (Table 14a, 2). That the reduced extraction was not due to release of triglyceride fatty acids is evident from the fact that the uptake of ^{3}H-palmitate was also decreased.[6] In the fasting, resting state we, as others, have observed a positive linear relationship between the extraction of FFA and the arterial FFA level (Table 14a, 3). Such a relation was not present in the fed state (Table 14a, 3). One possible

Table 14a, 3. *Linear correlation coefficient (r) between the extraction of FFA and arterial FFA concentration in the fasting and the fed state.*

STATE	FASTING	FASTING	I.v. FED
r	0·57^{xx}	0·66^{xx}	0·28^{ns}
n	30	15	38
Ref no.	(8)	(3)	(5)

n=number of observations; ns=not significant ($p>0·05$); xx=significant ($p<0·01$). Ref no=Reference number.

explanation for this change in the relationship between FFA extraction and concentration from the fasting to the fed state is competition between triglyceride fatty acids and FFA. In the fasting state 170 μmoles of FFA were extracted per litre plasma by the heart and at the same time 50 μmoles of triglyceride fatty acids were extracted.[3 4] In the intravenous fed state the corresponding figures were (Table 14a, 1 and 2) 80 and 240. Comparing FFA uptake in the fasting and in the oral fed state, FFA extraction was the same in both despite the fact that arterial FFA were twice as high in the oral fed state. Thus, in the oral as in the intravenous fed state, the relationship between FFA concentration and extraction is altered from that found in the fasting state. Glucose concentration would not seem to be an important factor in the depressed FFA extraction associated with feeding, since it occurred not only in the intravenous fed state but also in the oral fed state when glucose concentration was not significantly different from that found during fasting (Table 14a, 2).

Glucose extraction was not significantly different in the intravenous fed and in the fasting state in spite of the fact that arterial glucose and insulin levels had doubled. As in the fasting state,[4] glucose extraction was negatively correlated (r−0·50) with the arterial concentration of FFA. It is likely that the exogenous triglyceride fatty acids as well as FFA have had an influence on glucose uptake, since chylomicra reduce glucose uptake in the isolated, perfused rat heart.[9]

It is interesting to see that in the fasting and in the fed states, when both lipid and carbohydrate are available, lipid appears to be the preferred substrate. In the fasting state, FFA were the dominant substrate for the human heart; in our fed states, however, exogenous triglycerides appeared on the stage as the dominant substrate for the energy supply of the human heart. It is clear that if one would like to lower the extraction of fatty acid by the heart, in certain clinical situations, restriction of FFA mobilization from adipose tissue and of the supply of exogenous triglycerides need to be considered.

Summary

We have compared the extraction of lipid and carbohydrate substrates for the normal human heart in the fasting and in the fed state.

In the fed state, the heart extracts exogenous triglycerides in amounts sufficient to cover about 50 per cent of the heart's energy requirement. The release of glycerol, which does not exist in the resting fasting state, suggests that at least half of the triglycerides removed by the heart are completely hydrolyzed before extraction.

In the fed state less FFA is extracted by the heart at a given FFA level than in the fasting state, possibly because of the pronounced uptake of exogenous triglyceride fatty acids.

Glucose extraction did not differ significantly between the fasting and fed states, although both glucose and insulin levels had doubled.

In both the fasting and fed states, lipid appears to be the dominant substrate for the human heart.

ACKNOWLEDGMENT

Supported by grants from the Swedish Medical Research Council (19x–204).

REFERENCES

1 BING, R. J., SIEGEL, A., VITALE, A.. BALBONI, F., SPARKS, E., TAESCHLER, M., KLAPPER, M. & EDWARDS. S. (1953). Metabolic studies on human heart *in vivo*; studies on carbohydrate metabolism of human heart. *American Journal of Medicine* **15**, 285-296.

2 GOODALE, W. T., OLSON, R. E. & HACKEL, D. B. (1959). The effect of fasting and diabetes mellitus on myocardial metabolism in man. *American Journal of Medicine* **27**, 212-220.

3 KAIJSER, L., LASSERS, B. W., WAHLQVIST, M. L. & CARLSON, L. A. (1972). Myocardial lipid and carbohydrate metabolism in fasting men during prolonged exercise. *Journal of Applied Physiology* **32**, 72-80.

4 LASSERS, B. W., KAIJSER, L. & CARLSON, L. A. (1972). Myocardial lipid and carbohydrate metabolism in healthy, fasting men at rest. *European Journal of Clinical Investigation* **2**, 348-358.

5 CARLSON, L. A.. KAIJSER, L., RÖSSNER, S. & WAHLQVIST, M. L. (1972 in press). *Acta Medica Scandinavica.*

6 WAHLQVIST, M. L., RÖSSNER, S., KAIJSER, L. & CARLSON, L. A. *To be published.*

7 CARLSON, L. A., KAIJSER, L. & LASSERS, B. W. (1970). Myocardial metabolism of plasma triglycerides in man. *Journal of Molecular and Cellular Cardiology* **1**, 467-475.

8 CARLSON, L. A. & HALLBERG, D. (1963). Studies on the elimination of exogenous lipids from the blood stream. *Acta Physiologica Scandinavica* **59**, 52-61.

9 ONTKO, J. A. & RANDLE, P. J. (1967). Inhibition of glucose utilization by perfusion with chylomicrons in rat heart. *Biochemical Journal* **104**, 43C-44C.

DISCUSSION

Opie. Data suggesting that triglyceride can substantially inhibit glucose metabolism have been obtained in rat heart studies.

Do your experiments really mimic the fed state?

Carlson. Yes, for the oral fed state but of course not for the intravenous when the gastrointestinal tract is bypassed. But the increase in exogenous triglycerides corresponds closely to what you see with alimentary lipaemia. The purpose of the intravenous route of administration was to achieve a steady state in arterial levels of triglycerides.

Wallace. You both discuss the metabolism of the heart. You, Dr Carlson, have plotted on the vertical axis the arterial coronary sinus difference for various substrates and then used the term uptake. It seems to me that in the absence of a knowledge of flow, you cannot use that term. Dr Lassers, you showed that the AV difference for glucose decreased in proportion to the free fatty acid concentration in arterial blood. Can we draw any interpretation from that without knowledge of what the coronary flow was?

Lassers. Obviously one cannot measure rates of uptake unless one knows flow. On the other hand, I think one can compare extractions among healthy individuals at rest. All of our subjects were of similar physical fitness and in a similar dietary state and had been resting for an hour: the differences in coronary flow rates among such a group are probably relatively small. I have tried to avoid the word ' uptake ' when I mean ' extraction '. It is, as you point out, an extremely important point since rate of uptake is a different variable.

Carlson. I agree entirely. There are, however, two valid comments: (1) You may talk about ' uptake ' if you consider the uptake (disappearance) from the blood per unit volume. (2) You can avoid the need to measure flow when you study, at the same time, the relation between uptake of two different blood substrates—then flow cancels out.

Wallace. Do you have any idea about changes in coronary blood flow during your nicotinic acid experiments?

Lassers. Coronary blood flow has not been measured in man after nicotinic acid administration. But we do know that the haemodynamic variables such as heart rate and blood pressure, which are of importance in determining coronary flow, return to basal values after about 30 min of continuous infusion of nicotinic acid.

Maseri. Were you measuring the arteriovenous difference of free fatty acids from radioactive palmitate?

Lassers. In all the data presented, we determined arterial-coronary sinus differences in FFA from chemical estimates: these are, therefore, net differences. Our radioisotope data suggest that there is efflux of unlabelled FFA into the coronary sinus blood. If this is the case, then there is both extraction and release of FFA during passage of blood across the heart.

Maseri. Yes, that is exactly the point I wanted to make. When you measure the concentration difference between the artery and coronary sinus you are measuring something that takes into account both uptake and release, whereas if you inject labelled palmitate and measure initial extraction of palmitate you only take release into account.

Lassers. Net extraction is what is required in order to calculate the oxygen extraction ratio.

Maseri. Did you infuse C^{14} palmitate during exercise following nicotinic acid?

Lassers. Yes, ^{3}H-palmitate actually. If you follow the time course of change in the specific activity of fatty acids in the artery and coronary sinus in the control group, the activity in coronary sinus blood gradually approaches that in arterial blood. However, during prolonged exercise, there continues to be a difference in the two specific activities and this difference is greater in the nicotinic acid than in the control group.

Maseri. Does this mean that the isotope infusion was started too early to allow calculation of the net extraction? The data seem to suggest that during exercise in the presence of nicotinic acid, there is a greater extraction of labelled palmitate.

Lassers. The differences in specific activities indicate an *apparent* increase in the extraction of labelled FFA. In fact, this is due to the entrance of unlabelled fatty acid into the coronary sinus from some pool with a lower specific activity. As time proceeds and this pool becomes labelled, the difference decreases.

SUBSTRATE UPTAKE BY THE ISCHAEMIC HUMAN HEART DURING ANGINA INDUCED BY ATRIAL PACING

L. KAIJSER, L. A. CARLSON, B. EKLUND, E. R. NYE, S. RÖSSNER AND M. L. WAHLQVIST

IN healthy man the myocardial uptake of carbohydrate substrates has been shown to decrease with increased arterial concentration of free fatty acids (FFA)[1 2 3 4] in accordance with the 'glucose-fatty acid cycle' hypothesis of Randle and coworkers.[5] For a given amount of oxygen, less energy is liberated by lipid than by carbohydrate oxidation[6] and evidence has recently been presented indicating that the myocardial oxygen requirement at a given level of work increases with increased FFA uptake.[3 7 8] Thus the role of arterial FFA concentration as a determinant of myocardial substrate and oxygen metabolism might be especially important under ischaemic conditions.

The relationship between myocardial carbohydrate and fat metabolism is of interest for another reason. Normally the heart extracts lactate but, rendered hypoxic, it can liberate energy by anaerobic glycolysis. In this situation NADH accumulates and lactate is produced. Since the demonstration of lactate production can be of diagnostic value[9 10 11 12], it seems important to establish whether fatty acids affect lactate metabolism in the hypoxic heart. In the present study the myocardial extraction of substrates and oxygen was measured in patients with coronary heart disease at rest and during episodes of angina pectoris induced by atrial pacing. The effect of pacing was also studied under normal fasting conditions and after the infusion of nicotinic acid which decreased the arterial FFA concentration.

SUBJECTS

Twelve male patients with symptoms of ischaemic heart disease of more than two years duration were studied. Seven of them had been hospitalized for myocardial infarction 5 to 12 months before the study: the remaining five had moderate or severe angina pectoris on exertion and a typical ECG of myocardial ischaemia during an exercise test.[13 14 15] Each subject underwent an exercise test on a bicycle ergometer[13 14] a few days before the study. Patients who could tolerate more than 500 kpm/min without angina were not included in the study. Known diabetics were excluded. No selection was made on the basis of serum lipid values.

PROCEDURE

Treatment with anticoagulants, β-blockers and antilipolytic drugs was stopped 3 to 7 days before the study; glyceryl trinitrate was not taken on the day of the study. The patients were studied in the supine position without premedication after 15 hr fasting. Catheters were inserted percutaneously into the right brachial artery and the coronary sinus for blood sampling and arterial pressure recording. The coronary sinus catheter was kept patent by a continuous infusion of 0·5 per cent citrate at a rate of about 50 ml/hr; heparin was not administered. A bipolar electrode catheter (US Catheter and Instrument Corp., Glensfalls, N.Y.) was inserted percutaneously from the right femoral vein to the right atrium, and connected to an Elema Schönander, Model EM 145, external pacemaker unit. In those patients who were to receive an infusion of nicotinic acid. a catheter was inserted into another arm vein.

Each study started with blood sampling from the artery and coronary sinus, ECG recording (Leads CR_5 and CR_7) and arterial pressure measurements at rest. During continuous ECG and blood pressure recording, the heart rate was then increased every min by 10 beats/min by pacing up to a heart rate of 10 beats/min below the rate at which angina had developed during exercise. Thereafter the heart rate was increased every 2 min by 5 beats/min until the patient experienced angina of a moderate degree. Blood sampling from the coronary sinus and the artery was begun when 2 min had elapsed at that heart rate. Pacing was continued at the same rate until all sampling was completed about 3 min later. In 6 of the patients, sodium nicotinate was infused at a rate of 400 mg/hr for 90 min after a bolus injection of 200 mg. Thereafter a second period of pacing was carried out according to the same schedule as the first pacing. The remaining 6 patients served as controls to determine the effect of repeated pacing on myocardial metabolism and were rested for 90 min without nicotinic acid before the second pacing period.

Two patients developed heart block as pacing rate was increased; this is not uncommon during atrial pacing in healthy, young subjects (own observations). Once the block had developed the pacing was stopped, 0·5 mg atropine was given intravenously and about 15 min later pacing was recommenced.

Treatment of Samples and Analytic Methods

Paired samples of atrial and coronary sinus blood were drawn into unheparinized plastic syringes. Samples for the estimation by enzymatic methods of blood glucose,[16] lactate[17] and pyruvate[18] were deproteinized immediately with perchloric acid. Samples for plasma FFA determinations were immediately transferred from the collection syringes to heparinized test-tubes, placed in iced water and centrifuged at 4° C within 1 hour.[19]

Oxygen saturation was measured spectrophotometrically.[20] Oxygen tension was measured with a polarographic electrode (Instrumentation Laboratory, Mod. 113). Oxygen content was calculated from the saturation and the haemoglobin concentration. For the estimation of the RQ of the myocardium, the oxygen and carbon dioxide content of arterial and coronary sinus blood were determined with the van Slyke technique.

Results

At rest

No patient had an arterial pressure above 170/95 mmHg. All subjects had normal arterial oxygen saturation. The average coronary sinus oxygen saturation was $28{\cdot}8 \pm 0{\cdot}9$ (S.E.) per cent, which is slightly lower than in healthy subjects,[21] and the oxygen tension was 22·7 mmHg.

The arterial FFA concentration was higher than in the above mentioned group of healthy subjects, and so was the arterial-coronary sinus difference in FFA concentration (FFA extraction). Myocardial FFA extraction was significantly and positively correlated with arterial FFA concentration and the regression line was not significantly different from that found in normal subjects (Fig. 15, 1).

Pyruvate extraction, but not lactate extraction, was significantly and positively correlated with its arterial concentration and significantly and negatively related to the arterial FFA concentration. At a given arterial concentration, lactate extraction was in many patients smaller than in healthy subjects (Fig. 15, 2).

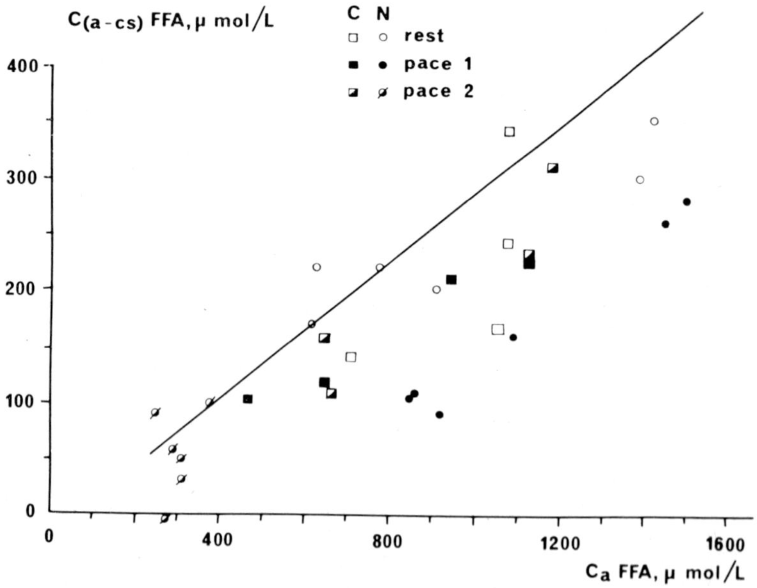

FIG. 15, 1. FFA extraction in relation to arterial FFA concentration. Symbols as in Figure 15, 2. The regression line is for healthy subjects at rest.[21]

The myocardial extraction of glucose was the same as that in normal subjects. It was neither significantly correlated with its own arterial concentration nor with the arterial FFA concentration.

The oxygen extraction ratio (OER) for FFA was 57·5 per cent, for glucose 21·4 per cent, for lactate 10·9 per cent, and for pyruvate 1·0 per cent—the total OER for these substrates was 90·8 per cent (Fig. 15, 3). Myocardial RQ was 0·78.

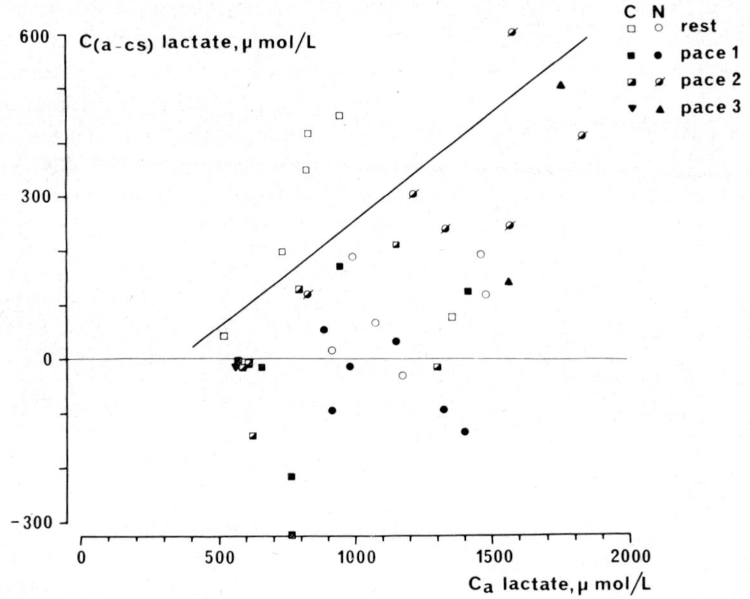

FIG. 15, 2. Lactate extraction in relation to arterial lactate concentration. C denotes patients not given nicotinate, N patients given nicotinate during their second pacing period. Pace 3 is the third pacing period at a higher heart rate in those patients who experienced less pain during pacing with than without nicotinate. The regression line for healthy subjects at rest and during exercise[22] is given for comparison.

During pacing

Chest pain, heart rate, arterial pressure. In all patients it was possible to increase the heart rate so as to produce moderate angina and keep the heart rate at that level for the time needed for blood sampling. During this time most patients experienced a slight increase in the degree of anginal pain. The average heart rate was 127 beats/min. For most patients the angina threshold was about 10 beats/min higher during pacing than during the exercise test. In all patients arterial mean pressure increased during pacing.

When pacing was repeated after 90 min rest without nicotinic acid, five out of six patients experienced the same degree of angina at the same heart rate, whereas one subject experienced less pain. This patient also had a lower arterial mean pressure before and during the second pacing, whereas the other five had approximately the same pressures during the first and the second pacing period.

Nicotinate infusion initially decreased the arterial pressure, which gradually increased again and in four of the six patients it had reached the preinfusion level by the start of the second pacing period. On pacing during the infusion of nicotinate, three out of six patients developed angina of approximately the same degree as during the first pacing period (without nicotinate), whereas one had angina of a milder degree and two felt no pain at all. After blood

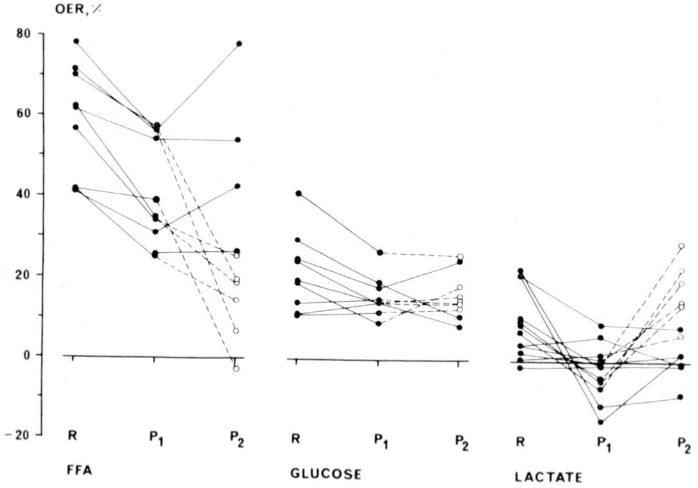

FIG. 15. 3. Oxygen extraction ratios for FFA, glucose and lactate for the individual patients at rest (R), during the first (P_1) and the second (P_2) pacing period. Filled circles: without nicotinate, unfilled circles connected with dashed lines: during nicotinate infusion.

sampling was completed, the heart rate was increased in the latter two subjects by 25 and 10 beats/min, respectively, to produce moderate angina. The arterial mean pressure during pacing was lower with than without nicotinate. This might be either the cause for or an effect of the reduced chest pain.

Oxygen extraction. Pacing did not change the coronary sinus oxygen saturation or tension or myocardial oxygen extraction, either without or with nicotinate infusion.

Lactate and pyruvate. During pacing, myocardial lactate extraction decreased in almost all patients and in 8 of them it changed from extraction to production (Figs 15, 2, 3). When pacing was repeated after nicotinate infusion, lactate was invariably extracted and in all subjects the extraction was greater than during the first pacing. The increased lactate extraction could partly be explained by increased arterial lactate concentration. But it was greater than expected from the lactate concentration increase according to the relation between extraction and arterial concentration in normal subjects at rest and during exercise.[22] If observations during pacing with and without nicotinate are considered, the lactate extraction was correlated with its arterial concentration ($r=0{\cdot}50$, $p<0{\cdot}05$) as well as the arterial FFA concentration ($r=0{\cdot}75$, $p<0{\cdot}001$) and the FFA extraction ($r=0{\cdot}74$, $p<0{\cdot}001$). In the patients who were not given nicotinate infusion, lactate metabolism did not differ systematically during the first and the second pacing. Pyruvate extraction was not changed by pacing alone, but increased when pacing was repeated after nicotinic acid. This increase could be explained by an increased arterial pyruvate concentration since the pyruvate extraction was significantly and positively correlated with its arterial concentration; and the regression line was not different from that calculated at rest or that described for healthy subjects.[22] For observations at rest, during the first and the second pacing combined, the correlation coefficient was 0·61 ($p<0{\cdot}001$). The pyruvate extraction during pacing (without or with nicotinate) was correlated with the arterial FFA concentration ($r=0{\cdot}75$, $p<0{\cdot}001$) and the FFA extraction ($r=0{\cdot}64$, $p<0{\cdot}01$).

Glucose. The average myocardial glucose extraction remained unchanged during pacing and was not significantly smaller than in normal resting and exercising subjects. The glucose extraction did not change during nicotinate infusion.

FFA. During pacing, FFA extraction decreased in all patients, and was smaller in relation to its arterial concentration than in normal resting subjects. After nicotinate infusion, FFA extraction decreased further. In this situation the extractiin was the same as in normal subjects, in relation to arterial FFA concentrations (Fig. 15, 3). Considering all the observations in relation to pacing, FFA extraction was correlated with arterial FFA concentration.

OER, RQ. During the first pacing period the OERs for FFA were 41·6, for glucose 21·4, for lactate 0·6 and for pyruvate 0·6 per cent; the total was 63·0 per cent. The myocardial RQ was 0·78. When pacing was repeated during nicotinate infusion, the OER:s for FFA were 9·4, for glucose 17·1, for lactate 18·1 and for pyruvate

2·2 per cent; the total was 46·8 per cent. The myocardial RQ was 0·93.

Discussion

At rest, the patient group was characterized by a slightly lower coronary sinus oxygen saturation, a slightly higher FFA extraction (which was normal in relation to its arterial concentration), and a lower lactate extraction than in normal subjects: glucose and pyruvate extractions were the same as in normal. The sum of the OERs for the substrates studied was 90·8 per cent. Since triglycerides[23] and ketone-bodies[24] might contribute 10 to 15 per cent, the extracted substrates seem to cover the energy requirements. Since it was possible almost to double the heart rate by pacing in all patients, it is not likely that any major part of the myocardium was hypoxic at rest, and hence differences in myocardial metabolism between the patients and normal subjects are probably not attributable to oxygen lack *per se*.

When the heart rate was increased above the angina threshold, coronary sinus oxygen saturation did not decrease. This is surprising in view of the nature of the disease and the finding in normal subjects of decreasing saturation when the heart rate is increased by exercise.[22] However, the angina patients had a coronary sinus oxygen saturation which was at rest already as low as that found in normal subjects during exercise with a heart rate of about 145 beats/min. Furthermore, the heart muscles of the patients probably were unevenly perfused and, since the coronary sinus drains both well perfused and less well perfused myocardial areas, blood with extremely low oxygen saturation would be mixed with normally oxygenated blood. This is, at present, an insurmountable difficulty in the study of substrate and oxygen extraction in a heart with coronary disease.

When the myocardium was rendered hypoxic by pacing to the point of angina, lactate extraction was decreased or even changed into lactate production.[8 9 10 11] At the same time, FFA extraction was decreased. Apparently the hypoxic myocardium does not readily take up fatty acids. It must be pointed out, though, that the FFA uptake might have been unchanged or even slightly increased, since the coronary blood flow was presumably increased. For comparison, in normal subjects the myocardial extraction of FFA in relation to its arterial concentration is smaller during exercise than at rest.[22] In our patients, the decreased FFA extraction was not compensated for by an increased glucose extraction, and since lactate extraction decreased, the total OER of carbohydrate substrates decreased. With a total OER for all substrates studied of 63·0 per cent, the substrate extraction was smaller than the total substrate oxidation. This is not seen in normal subjects except under extreme conditions, such as prolonged exercise, with reduced availability of FFA by nicotinic acid.[2 25] Apparently, coronary insufficiency is characterized not only by an insufficient oxygen supply to the myocardium, but also by an inability to extract substrates in amounts to match the oxidative capacity, and hence myocardial substrate stores must be utilized. Both the unchanged RQ (compared with resting conditions) and the unchanged relation between the OERs for fat and carbohydrates suggest that some of the stored carbohydrate and fat must have been oxidized. Lactate production presupposes carbohydrate breakdown and the lactate produced might to a substantial degree derive from extracted glucose as proposed by Most and coworkers,[26] who recently described a positive correlation between lactate production and glucose extraction in ischaemic human hearts. Such a relationship was not found in the present group of patients and seems unlikely unless the arterial FFA concentration is the same in the subjects studied, since both glucose and lactate extraction are positively correlated with FFA concentration,[1 2 3 4] and this would tend to produce a positive correlation between lactate *extraction* and glucose extraction. In our patients, the breakdown of myocardial glycogen seems to have contributed to the lactate production.

The present data do not answer the question as to why the total OER is reduced in the ischaemic heart. The availability of pyruvate dehydrogenase, held responsible for the interaction between fat and carbohydrate metabolism in the normal heart,[5] cannot be shown to be crucial since pyruvate extraction is unaffected by the pacing-induced ischaemia.

The decrease in FFA concentration produced by nicotinate infusion further reduced the uptake of FFA. However, the availability of FFA and not the capacity of the myocardium to metabolize it seem to limit its extraction, since the FFA extraction is the same in relation to its arterial concentration as in normal resting subjects.[21] In this situation, lactate is invariably taken up. It is also taken up after nicotinic acid in patients whose heart rate was increased to a higher level during pacing. One important conclusion from this finding is that if lactate production is used as a diagnostic sign of myocardial hypoxia, it must be considered in relation to the arterial FFA concentration as well as its own arterial concentration.

REFERENCES

1. LASSERS, B. W., WAHLQVIST, M. L., KAIJSER, L. & CARLSON, L. A. (1971). Relationship in man between plasma free fatty acids and myocardial metabolism of carbohydrate substrates. *Lancet* **II,** 448-462.
2. LASSERS, B. W., WAHLQVIST, M. L., KAIJSER, L. & CARLSON, L. A. (1972). Effect of nicotinic acid on myocardial metabolism in man at rest and during exercise. *Journal of Applied Physiology* **32,** 72-80.
3. CARLSON, L. A., KAIJSER, L., LASSERS, B. W. & WAHLQVIST, M. L. (1972, in press). *Acta Medica Scandinavica.*
4. WAHLQVIST, M. L., KAIJSER, L., LASSERS, B. W., LÖW, H. & CARLSON, L. A. (submitted). *European Journal of Clinical Investigation.*
5. RANDLE, P. J., GARLAND, P. B., HALES, C. N. & NEWSHOLME, E. A. (1963). The glucose fatty acids cycle. Its role in insulin sensitivity and the metabolic disturbance of diabetes mellitus. *Lancet* **I,** 785-789.
6. DOCUMENTA GEIGY (1962). In *Scientific Tables,* p. 627. Edited by K. Diem. Basel, Switzerland: Geigy Pharmaceuticals.
7. CHALLONER, D. R. & STEINBERG, D. (1966). Effect of free fatty acids on the oxygen consumption of perfused rat heart. *American Journal of Physiology* **210,** 280-286.
8. MJØS, O. D. (1971). Effect of free fatty acids on myocardial function and oxygen consumption in intact dogs. *Journal of Clinical Investigation* **50,** 1386-1389.
9. COHEN, L. S., ELLIOTT, W. C., KLEIN, M. D. & GORLIN, R. (1966). Coronary heart disease. *American Journal of Cardiology* **17,** 153-168.
10. PARKER, J. O., CHIONG, M. A., WEST, R. O. & CASE, R. B. (1969). Sequential alterations in myocardial lactate metabolism, S-T segments, and left ventricular function during angina induced by atrial pacing. *Circulation* **40,** 113-131.
11. PARKER, J. O., WEST, R. O., CASE, R. B. & CHIONG, M. A. (1969). Temporal relationship of myocardial lactate metabolism, left ventricular function, and S-T segment depression during angina precipitated by exercise. *Circulation* **40,** 97-111.
12. SCHEUER, J. (1967). Myocardial metabolism in cardiac hypoxia. *American Journal of Cardiology* **19,** 385-392.
13. SJÖSTRAND, T. (1961). *Acta Medica Scandinavica Suppl.* **196,** 1018.
14. WAHLUND, H. (1948). Determination of physical working capacity; physiological and clinical study with special reference to standardization of cardiopulmonary functional tests. *Acta Medica Scandinavica Suppl.* **215,** 1-78.
15. ÅSTRAND, I., et al. (1967). The ‘Minnesota code’ for ECG classification. *Acta Medica Scandinavica Suppl.* **481,** 42-78.
16. HJELM, M. (1966). Enzymatic determination of hexoses in blood and urine. *Scandinavian Journal of Clinical & Laboratory Investigation* **18,** *Suppl.* **92,** 85-98.

17 LUNDHOLM, L., MOHME-LUNDHOLM, E. & VAMOS, N. (1963). Lactic acid assay with L(+) lactic acid dehydrogenase from rabbit muscle. *Acta Physiologica Scandinavica* **58,** 243-249.
18 BÜCHER, T., CZOK. R.. LAMPRECHT, W. & LATZKO, E. (1962). In *Metoden der enzymatischen Analyse.* p. 253. Edited by E. Pyruvat. Weinheim: Verlag Chemie.
19 TROUT, D. L., ESTES, JR. E. H. & FREIDBERG, S. J. (1960). Titration of free fatty acids of plasma: a study of current methods and a new modification. *Journal of Lipid Research* **1,** 199-202.
20 HOLMGREN, A. & PERNOW, B. (1959). Spectrophotometric measurement of oxygen saturation of blood in the determination of cardiac output. *Scandinavian Journal of Clinical & Laboratory Investigation* **11,** 143-149.
21 LASSERS, B. W., KAIJSER, L. & CARLSON, L. A. (1972). Myocardial lipid and carbohydrate metabolism in healthy, fasting men at rest. *European Journal of Clinical Investigation* **2,** 348-358.
22 KAIJSER, L., LASSERS, B. W., WAHLQVIST, M. L. & CARLSON, L. A. (1972). Myocardial lipid and carbohydrate metabolism in fasting men during prolonged exercise. *Journal of Applied Physiology* **32,** 847-858.
23 CARLSON, L. A., KAIJSER, L. & LASSERS, B. W. (1970). Myocardial metabolism of plasma triglycerides in man. *Journal of Molecular and Cellular Cardiology* **1,** 467-475.
24 KEUL, J., DOLL, E., STEIN, H., FLEER, U. & REINDELL, H. (1965). Uber den Stoffwechsel des menschlichen Herzen. *Pflügers Archive* **282,** 43-53.
25 LASSERS, B. W., KAIJSER, L., WAHLQVIST, M. L. & CARLSON, L. A. *This symposium.*
26 MOST, A., GORLIN, R. & SOELDNER, S. (1972). Glucose extraction by the human myocardium during pacing stress. *Circulation* **45,** 92-96.

DISCUSSION

Opie. It would be wrong to leave the meeting here with the feeling that there is not an increased glucose arteriovenous difference

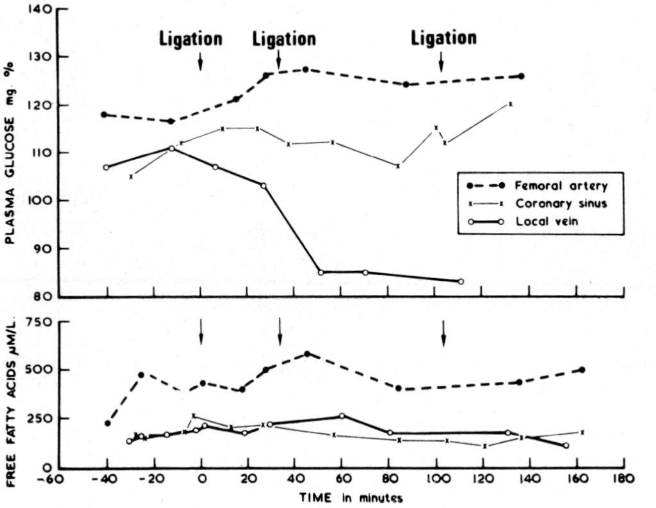

FIG. 15, 4

during ischaemia. This is a finding which has been shown by Dr Thomas and myself and co-workers, using an open-chest greyhound in which the blood going from the ischaemic area was sampled.

After arterial ligation there is a very distinct widening of the arterio-venous difference of glucose (Fig. 15, 4). The coronary sinus glucose value is unchanged during ischaemia. Arteriovenous difference for free fatty acids across the ischaemic section shows a small decrease, while the arterio-coronary sinus difference shows no decrease. We have attempted to increase the circulating free fatty acids by infusing Intralipid and heparin and then still find that there is increased glucose arteriovenous difference and still lactate output (see Table 15, 1).

Table 15, 1 *Effect of plasma free fatty acid concentration on arteriovenous difference of glucose across ischaemic myocardium*

In 8 starved greyhounds, glucose arteriovenous differences (using local vein sampling techniques) were measured 5 min before and 20 min after coronary artery ligation. Thereafter, circulating FFA was elevated by an infusion of Intralipid-heparin. Mean values ±SEM (number of observations).

EXPERIMENTAL CONDITION	ARTERIAL-LOCAL VENOUS PLASMA GLUCOSE DIFFERENCE: mg per 100 ml	ARTERIAL FREE FATTY ACID CONCENTRATION: mEq/litre
Pre-ligation (8)	12·6±3·5	519±122
Post-ligation (8)	25·6±3·7	689±110
Infusion of Intralipid-heparin (9)	22·3±2·2	2900±424

Our experimental work would fit in very nicely with the work from Dr Gorlin's group, using selective coronary sinus catheterization, showed an increased arteriovenous difference for glucose during human myocardial ischaemia at the same time as there was lactate output.

Mjøs What was the local arteriovenous flow in your preparation during coronary occlusion?

Thomas. The coronary sinus has, of course, a mixed flow from many areas. As the heart responds to any increase in demand, the percentage of blood flow in the coronary sinus from non-ischaemic areas will become greater due to relative reduction of flow from ischaemic areas. This effect will become most marked with angina, unless there is some generalized change in coronary vasculature. Therefore, under high stress situations, the contribution of blood from ischaemic areas is not easy to detect in terms of A.V. differences.

Kaijser. In the coronary sinus, we sample mixtures of blood from better and from less well perfused parts of the myocardium and this is one of the major difficulties in metabolic studies of this kind. It seems likely that under conditions of increased myocardial oxygen demand, such as pacing, blood flow will increase in the less diseased areas. However, in most patients, coronary heart disease is not localized to a small area, but widespread, and hence coronary sinus blood represents blood from the ischaemic myocardium. In our patients this is quite evident, since all patients decrease their lactate extraction on pacing. Furthermore, data from patients, not presented here, whose chest pain increased profoundly on pacing, showed a successively increasing negative arterial-coronary sinus lactate difference.

Thomas. Goulding's group showed that regional sampling gives a very different answer if you place your catheter selectively. If samples are taken from the coronary sinus, they will represent a heterogenous area of the myocardium.

Livesley. I would like to take up Dr Thomas' point since it is my experience that selective coronary venous catheterization has little value.

I think that Dr Kaijser has been extremely fortunate in choosing, for investigation, patients who have developed angina as a result of the tachycardia during effort, since their symptoms can be readily produced by fast atrial pacing. In my own study, of more than seventy cases of patients with angina on effort, pacing-induced angina has always been coincidental with myocardial lactate production. I have also observed that fast atrial pacing has neither induced angina nor increased myocardial lactate production in patients whose angina occurred predominantly at rest. However, these patients have experienced angina during recorded attacks of bradycardia. These observations have both clinical and biochemical importance, since patients may have to be divided into sub-groups if conflicting results are to be avoided in the biochemical study of ischaemic heart disease.

ENDOCRINE CHANGES ASSOCIATED WITH MYOCARDIAL ISCHAEMIA

S. P. ALLISON

I WOULD first like to review the endocrine changes associated with myocardial ischaemia, secondly to consider the metabolic consequences of such changes, and lastly to discuss the possible clinical relevance of these findings.

I have considered myocardial ischaemia as occurring in two situations; in association with myocardial infarction where, peripheral to the infarct, there may be a zone of potentially recoverable ischaemic tissue; and secondly, during periods of coronary insufficiency or ' pre-infarction syndrome '.

Dr Chamberlain and I have studied changes in insulin secretion associated with myocardial infarction.[1 2] We performed a standard 25 gram intravenous glucose tolerance test within 12 hours of the onset of symptoms and repeated the test 1 to 2 weeks later. Estimations of blood sugar, plasma insulin and plasma free fatty acids were carried out on venous blood samples. Basal samples were taken followed by samples at 2, 5, 10, 20, 30, 40, 50 and 60 min after the injection of glucose. Figures 16, 1 to 3 show results which were typical of the whole group studied.

In the acute phase there was impaired glucose tolerance, failure of insulin secretion and a high level of FFA. In the follow-up studies there was often persistent impairment of glucose tolerance associated with high insulin levels suggesting insulin resistance at this stage. Of the twelve patients studied, four were suffering from cardiogenic shock. This group had significantly higher blood sugars at all times and significantly lower plasma insulins at 2, 5 and 10 min than the group with the less severe clinical picture. My colleague, Dr Rowe, has studied a group of patients with acute coronary insufficiency of whom half went on to develop infarction. He has kindly given me permission to quote his results which, though very variable, are qualitatively similar to our own if much less marked in degree. We have made similar observations in other patients subjected to acute illness, notably burn injury, and have concluded that

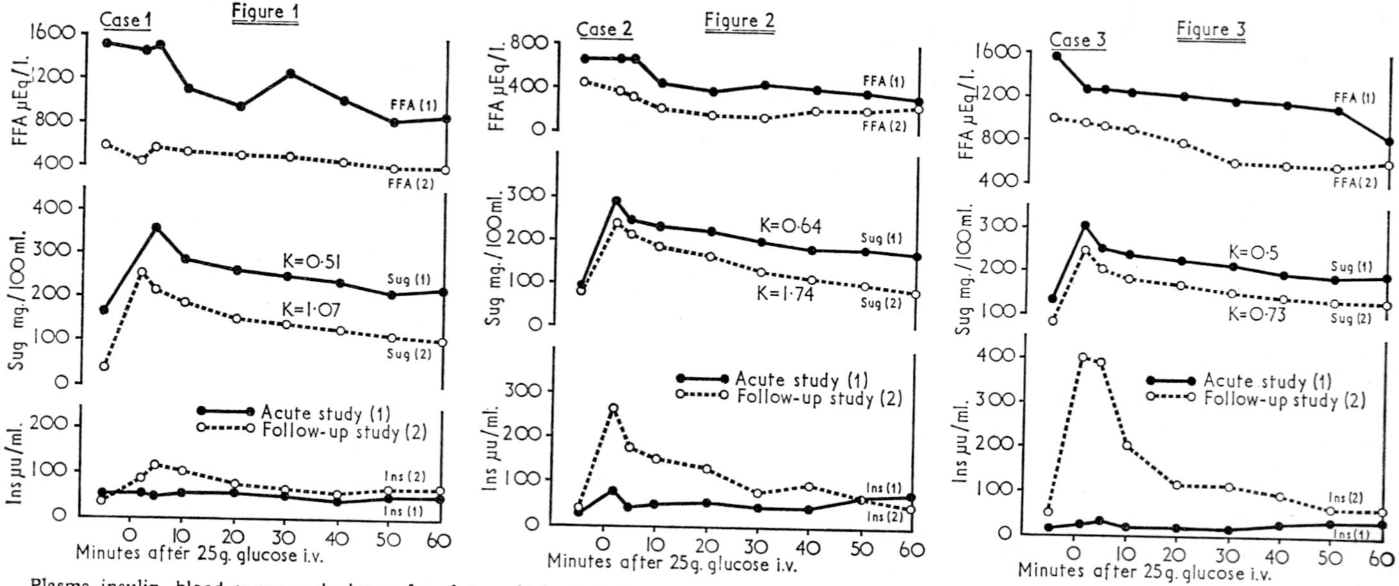

Plasma insulin, blood sugar, and plasma free fatty acid levels before and after 25 g. of glucose intravenously in three patients with myocardial infarction. The values in the acute study (×——×) are compared with those in the follow-up study (O——O). Case 1, man aged 67. Case 2, man aged 38. Case 3, man aged 52.

FIG. 16, 1-3

suppression of insulin secretion in the acute phase of illness, followed by a period of insulin resistance, is a non-specific effect of stress rather than a phenomenon peculiar to myocardial ischaemia. Similar observations have been made by Taylor *et al.*[3]

It seems likely that the suppression of insulin release in the acute phase is related to the increase in catecholamine secretion which occurs after myocardial infarction.[4] Coore and Randle[5] showed that the insulin secretion from pancreatic tissue slices could be diminished by adrenaline. Porte *et al.*[6] also showed that adrenaline infusion into normal human subjects could suppress the insulin response to a glucose load. Furthermore he showed that this was an α-adrenergic effect, being blocked by phentolamine. The cause of the insulin resistance seen subsequently in these patients is not known.

Other workers have studied changes in the secretion of adrenal cortical hormones. Logan and Murdoch[7] have shown that, as following other forms of injury, there is an increase in cortisol secretion following myocardial infarction. Lebovitz and his colleagues[8] showed that growth hormone secretion is elevated under these circumstances. Dr Unger, I hear, has shown that glucagon secretion is increased in other forms of injury and I think it is a safe presumption that a similar change occurs after myocardial infarction.

To summarize, therefore, the endocrine changes associated with myocardial ischaemia and infarction are:—

1. Failure of insulin secretion in the acute phase of myocardial ischaemia or infarction, followed by a period of insulin resistance.
2. An increase in the secretion of:—
   (a) catecholamines
   (b) cortisol
   (c) growth hormone
   (d) probably glucagon.

These changes are not specific to myocardial ischaemia, being non-specific effects of stress.

Metabolic Effects of Endocrine Changes

How do the metabolic effects which we might predict from these endocrine changes match up to those actually observed? Insulin opposes the action of the other hormones mentioned throughout intermediary metabolism. There is an opposing action of insulin and cortisol on the activity and induction of enzymes which govern the irreversible steps of glycolysis and gluconeogenesis, such that glycolysis is enhanced and gluconeogenesis is inhibited by insulin and the reverse effects are promoted by cortisol. The effect of insulin on glucose transport is well known. Catecholamines enhance the breakdown of glycogen to glucose. Growth hormone and glucagon also have diabetogen effects. It is not surprising, therefore, to find high blood sugar and glucose intolerance associated with myocardial infarction.

Insulin enhances the synthesis of triglyceride and opposes lipolysis in adipose tissue, whereas the reverse effects are produced by catecholamines, growth hormone, and glucagon. The high levels of FFA observed after myocardial infarction are therefore predictable.

Protein breakdown for gluconeogenesis is promoted by cortisol and glucagon whereas the transport of amino-acids into cells and their incorporation into protein is enhanced by insulin. Protein catabolism is perhaps seen more strikingly following major injury, such as burning, rather than after myocardial infarction.

Clinical Applications

To discuss the possible clinical relevance of these changes is to enter on controversial, not to say thorny, ground.

Owen *et al.*[9] have shown that the ischaemic myocardium is dependent on glycolysis for its energy and have suggested that it may be important for the ischaemic myocardium to be supplied plentifully with glucose to enable it to survive: Weissler *et al.*[10] demonstrated the protective effect on the anoxic isolated perfused rat heart of glucose. Austen *et al.*[11] showed a similar effect on the ischaemic dog heart, although the concentrations of glucose used in these last experiments were extraordinarily high. None of these experiments have exactly reproduced the situation in human myocardial ischaemia where there are not only limitations to the supply of glucose substrate to the eschaemic myocardium owing to loss of perfusion, but also an inadequate rate of removal of toxic products such as lactate. If there were an advantage in improving the supply of glucose to the ischaemic myocardium it could be argued that a further beneficial effect might be expected with insulin. Against this, I would question whether the effect of anoxia on improving glucose transport and on increasing the rate of glycolysis through the Pasteur effect could be significantly enhanced by insulin.

To bring fatty acids to Edinburgh is like taking a certain other substrate to Newcastle. Dr Oliver's work on the toxic effects of fatty acids on the heart's action will, I am sure, be discussed fully elsewhere at this meeting. Another possible effect of fatty acids may be that described by Professor Randle with whom I had the good fortune to work for two years. Glycolysis is inhibited by the oxidation of free fatty acids because of the build up of citrate and acetyl CoA which inhibit phosphofructokinase and pyruvate dehydrogenase. We have confirmed this effect on the dog heart *in vivo* and Lassers *et al.*[13] have shown the same in the human heart. Both insulin and glucose would have the effect of lowering fatty acid levels and therefore removing the possible toxic effects of these on the ischaemic heart.

Sodi-Pallares and his colleagues[14] put forward their potassium, insulin and glucose regime as a treatment of myocardial infarction and, ever since then, there have been conflicting reports of its efficacy from workers who have used widely different selection of patients, doses of insulin and routes of administration. The treatment has therefore fallen into disrepute. I feel entirely uncertain in my own mind about it as a treatment of myocardial ischaemia. I have no doubt, however, that it does have an effect on the failing heart in some patients.

Flear and his colleagues[15] have shown that in both anoxic and failing heart muscle cells, there is an impairment of the sodium pump mechanism such that Na^+, Cl^- and water accumulate within the cells, K^+ is lost and the resting potential is diminished. This leads to an impairment of contractile force.

Zierler[16] has shown *in vitro* that in skeletal muscle insulin not only causes an increased passage of potassium into cells but also an increased extrusion of Na^+ ions.

We have studied the effect of high doses of insulin and glucose (500 to 1000 ml of 50 per cent glucose/day containing 100 to 120 units of soluble insulin/litre, and 100 to 300 mEq of KCl/litre according to the patient's plasma K^+ level) in six patients with severe congestive heart failure. The only criterion of selection was that they should have been referred by other physicians who considered that conventional treatment had failed and had nothing more to offer. In two patients there was no effect and death occurred within a few days. In 4 patients there was a striking effect. The

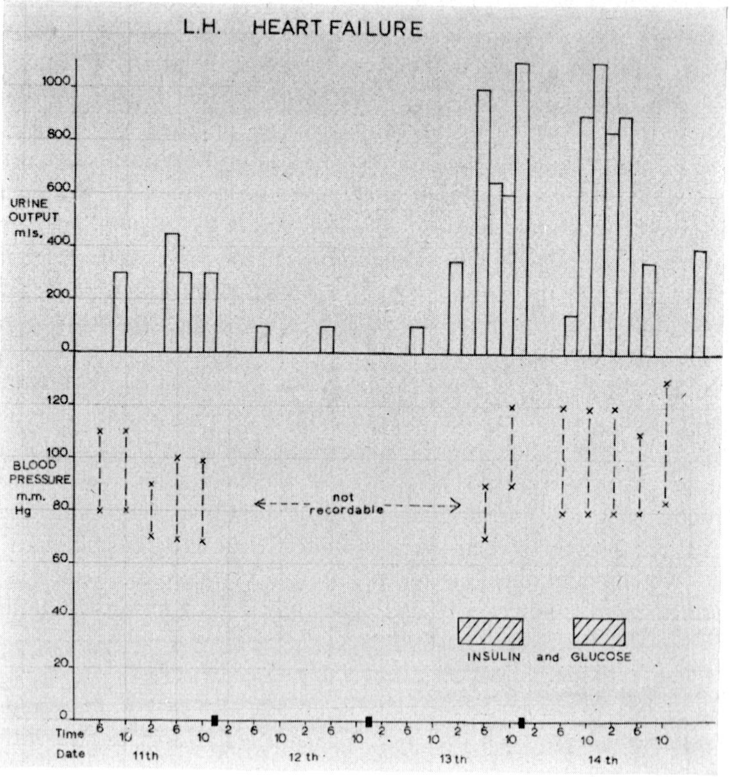

FIG. 16, 4

results in one of these is illustrated in Fig. 16, 4. This man with mitral incompetence had been admitted for surgery, but his downhill course was so rapid that he became unfit for operation. Despite digoxin, frusemide and ethacrynic acid he accumulated oedema, and became more breathless. Eventually he became oliguric, his blood pressure became unmeasurable by the cuff method and he fell into semi-coma. Within an hour of starting insulin and glucose, not only did his blood pressure rise to normal, but having been in atrial fibrillation for at least five years he went into sinus rhythm. His urine output rose to 600 ml/hr. When the treatment was stopped for the first time he had an anti-diuresis, but continued to pass large amounts of urine with a high sodium content (see Fig.

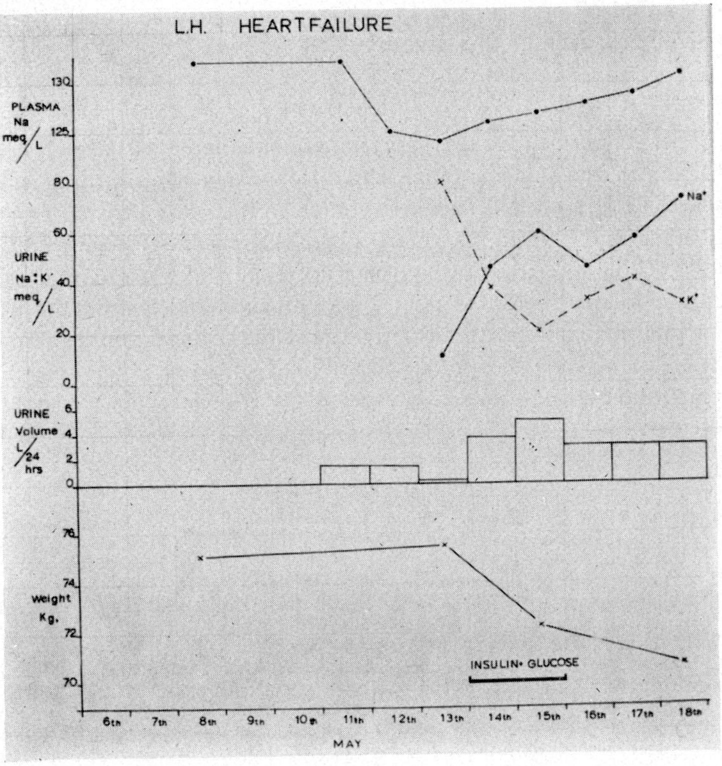

FIG. 16, 5

16, 5) as soon as the treatment was resumed. Twenty-four hours later the treatment was stopped and his improvement was maintained. Two weeks later he had a successful mitral valve replacement.

All of the patients studied showed hyponatraemia and in the four successful cases there was a rise in plasma sodium level after treatment. In two of these, the change was so abrupt that the rise in concentration could not be explained by water losses (as judged by weight change over a few hours). It must be presumed, therefore, that the sodium came from some other space, probably the intracellular space. From these results, it is conceivable that the use of insulin in ischaemic heart disease may be worth re-examining. One cannot pretend that the dosage used is in any way physiological, nor perhaps that the cell membrane changes in abnormal heart muscle are caused by insulin lack. However, insulin may be a useful pharmacological agent in this situation.

Summary

The endocrine changes associated with acute ischaemic heart disease are the same as those which follow any other form of acute illness, i.e. diminished insulin secretion in the acute phase, followed by a period of insulin resistance. There is an increase in the secretion of catecholamines, cortisol, growth hormone and possibly glucagon. This endocrine pattern is associated with catabolic changes throughout intermediary metabolism. The possible clinical implications of these findings have been discussed and although many of these remain matters of conjecture, they present a hopeful field for further research.

REFERENCES

1 Allison, S. P., Prowse, K. & Chamberlain, M. J. (1967). Failure of insulin response to glucose load during operation and after myocardial infarction. *Lancet* **I,** 478-481.

2 Allison, S. P., Chamberlain, M. J. & Hinton, P. (1969). Intravenous glucose tolerance, insulin and free fatty acid levels after myocardial infarction. *British Medical Journal,* **4,** 776-778.

3 Taylor, S. H., Saxon, C., Majid, P. A., Dykes, J. R. W., Ghosh, P. & Stoker, J. B. (1969). Insulin secretion following myocardial infarction with particular respect to the pathogenesis of cardiogenic shock. *Lancet* **II,** 1373-1378.

4 Valori, C., Thomas, M. & Shillingford, J. P. (1967). Urinary excretion of free noradrenaline and adrenaline following myocardial infarction. *Lancet* **1,** 127-130.

5 Coore, H. G. & Randle, P. J. (1964). Regulation of insulin secretion studied with pieces of rabbit pancreas incubated in vitro. *Biochemical Journal* **93,** 66-78.

6 Porte, D., Graber, A. L., Kuzuya, T. & Williams, R. H. (1966). The effect of epinephrine on immunoreactive insulin levels in man. *Journal of Clinical Investigation* **45,** 228-236.

7 Logan, R. W. & Murdoch, W. R. (1966). Blood levels of hydrocortisone, transaminases and cholesterol after myocardial infarction. *Lancet* **II,** 521-524.

8 Lebovitz, H. E., Shultz, K. T., Mathews, M. E. & Scheele, R. (1969). Acute metabolic response to myocardial infarction: changes in glucose

utilisation and secretion of insulin and growth hormone. *Circulation* **30,** 171-181.
9 OWEN, P., THOMAS, M. & OPIE, L. H. (1969). Relative changes in free fatty acid and glucose utilisation by ischaemic myocardium after coronary artery occlusion. *Lancet* **I,** 1187-1190.
10 WEISSLER, A. M., KRUGER, F. A., BABA, N., SCARPELLI, D. C., LEIGHTON, R. F. & GALLIMORE, J. K. (1969). Role of anaerobic metabolism in the preservation of functional capacity and structure of anoxic myocardium. *Journal of Clinical Investigation* **47,** 403-416.
11 AUSTIN, W. G., GREENBERG, J. J. & PICCININI, J. C. (1965). Myocardial function and contractile force affected by glucose loading of the heart during anoxia. *Surgery* **57,** 839-845.
12 RANDLE, P. J., GARLAND, P. B., HALES, C. N. & NEWSHOLME, E. A. (1963). The glucose fatty acid cycle, its role in insulin sensitivity and the metabolic disturbances of diabetes mellitus. *Lancet* **I,** 785-789.
13 LASSERS, B. W., WAHLQVIST, M. L., KAIJSER, L. & CARLSON, L. A. (1971). Relationship in man between plasma free fatty acids and myocardial metabolism of CHO substrates. *Lancet* **II,** 448-462.
14 SODI-PALLARES, D., TESTELLI, M. R., FISHLER, B. L., BISTENI, A., MEDRANO, G. A., FRIEDLAND, C. & DE MICHELI, A. (1962). Effects of an intravenous infusion of potassium—glucose—insulin solution on the electrocardiographic signs of myocardial infarction. A preliminary clinical report. *American Journal of Cardiology* **9,** 160-181.
15 SINGH, C. M., FLEAR, C. T. G. & ROSS, D. (1970). Anoxic arrest during heart surgery: its effects on water and electrolyte contents of the human heart, p. 31. *Annual Meeting of the International Study Group for Research in Cardiac Metabolism.* Milan.
16 ZIERLER, K. L. (1966). Possible mechanisms of insulin action on membrane potential and ion fluxes. *American Journal of Medicine* **40,** 735-739.

DISCUSSION

Kurien. What were the levels of free fatty acids and glucose in these patients before treatment was started?

Allison. We didn't measure these. We have of course found in patients with severe congestive heart failure a similar picture—that is one of high blood sugar, glucose intolerance, low insulin secretion and high free fatty acids, so one can only presume that this was also the case in these patients.

Oliver. Is there a clear inverse relationship between elevated blood cortisol and insulin depression in the first 48 hours? What affect does hydrocortisone have on insulin levels in patients with acute myocardial infarction?

Allison. Unfortunately we didn't measure any other hormonal levels in these particular patients but we know that cortisol levels tend to be high in proportion to the severity of illness and that the degree of insulin suppression is probably also in proportion to the severity. I know of no evidence of the effect of cortisol on insulin secretion, except that secondarily of course it will cause hyperinsulinaemia as in patients with Cushing's syndrome.

Wallace. One advantage of the mini-pig model is that it undergoes a series of hormonal changes in response to primary occlusion similar to those in man, including suppressed insulin secretion and paradoxical growth hormone rise. The suppressed insulin secretion during the first 3 or 4 days after myocardial infarction in the pig may be preventable with phentolamine, which would suggest to me that it is due to catecholamine response.

Carlson. There are two other changes in response to myocardial infarction and in response to other trauma which could be of interest. The fall in cholesterol is well known and there is also an increase in oxygen uptake. We had hoped to find a correlation between the free fatty acid rise and oxygen uptake, but there was none. We have studied this in burned patients. There were dramatic falls in plasma cholesterol from 250 to 100 mg/100 ml and increases in oxygen consumption around 100 per cent. There was an extremely good correlation between the fall in cholesterol and the increase in oxygen consumption, perhaps suggesting that thyroid hormones should be integrated into this whole picture. I think it would be very interesting for instance to measure T_3, T_4 and T.S.H. levels in response to acute trauma.

Fitzgerald. Dr Harland in Glasgow has been studying prealbumin-bound thyroxine in patients undergoing surgery. There seems to be a remarkable reduction in bound and an increase in free thyroxine. Is it worth speculating a little about the non-cardiac actions of potassium, glucose and insulin in respect to vascular smooth muscle? Could there be marked vasodilatation with unloading of the ventricle? What happens to peripheral vascular resistance?

Oliver. It is always tidy to have a unitarian hypothesis and I presume therefore that the increased free thyroxine is due to competition by FFA for binding sites on albumin?

Thomas. As a rider to Dr Fitzgerald's comments, are you asking us to accept that insulin and glucose had an effect on the heart alone, or on other organs as well—such as the kidney? When you stopped the infusion, the diuresis stopped too and it seemed that the patient was improving in parallel with the diuresis. There are several ways in which these changes can be linked of course.

Allison. It must have an effect on the heart because of the abrupt change in rhythm. You can show the same effect in burned patients who have the same electrolyte changes.

Opie. Did you calculate the osmolarity of the blood during these procedures? Osmolarity is known to affect left ventricular function and Dr Regan has suggested that glucose might act at least in part through an osmotic effect.

Allison. A large change in blood sugar levels would be required to alter osmolarity. We were deliberately keeping the blood sugar of these patients as near to normal as possible, certainly below 180 mg per cent, so I don't think this could have significantly altered osmolarity.

Opie. Even immediately after your infusion?

Allison. Urine excretion of glucose was less than $\frac{1}{4}$ per cent over a short period of time and we were taking hourly urine volumes and it is unlikely that the blood sugar rose to a substantial extent immediately after infusion. If it had done, we would have had marked glycosuria.

Burges. I wonder if Dr Allison would care to speculate about the reported beneficial action of glucagon in cases of cardiac failure. How does this fit when glucagon has an opposite action to insulin in most of its metabolic effects?

Allison. I don't know. Glucagon is an unpleasant drug to give and its effect in patients with heart failure after infarction is not encouraging.

Oliver. Surely one of the most important effects of glucagon is to facilitate the transference of calcium ions into myocardial cells?

Allison. Glucagon has an effect in increasing sodium and potassium excretion, while insulin causes a rise in sodium and a fall in potassium excretion.

Maseri. How many patients did you treat with this solution and how often did you make biochemical measurements?

Allison. Six patients. I used dextro-stix but it is a very crude estimation although sufficient for these purposes. We do a finger prick estimation of glucose at the end of each hour before giving the next infusion. Once a patient is given the correct dose of insulin in relation to his glucose concentration, you can go on for several days without difficulty.

Maseri. How about potassium concentrations?

Allison. We watched the ECG very carefully and we estimated serum potassium twice a day. We have never had any potassium problems. Providing you give insulin and glucose, you can keep patients normokalaemic for a long time with this mixture.

Taggart. How much was the effect due to the insulin and how much due to the glucose?

Allison. We don't have controlled data to check this in cardiac patients. The retention of sodium in burned patients is not affected by hypertonic glucose alone, but as soon as you introduce insulin, a diuresis occurs. In this situation therefore insulin is essential.

MYOCARDIAL HYPOXIA AND MECHANICAL PERFORMANCE

A. H. HENDERSON AND D. L. BRUTSAERT

BEFORE attempting to describe the changes in mechanical performance of heart muscle induced by hypoxia, the problems inherent in any analysis of heart muscle mechanics must first be considered. In the last decade, the principles of muscle physiology derived from skeletal muscle studies[1] have been usefully applied to cardiac muscle,[2 3] although the situation is then complicated by a number of factors including the need to consider the time course of contraction, since cardiac muscle functions normally by twitch contractions rather than by tetanic contractions. In particular, the characteristic inverse relationship between force and peak velocity, which constitutes such a fundamental property of muscle, has been shown to be generally applicable also to heart muscle. This force-velocity relationship has been used to measure, and indeed to define, contractility. However, in recent years, there has been growing criticism of the validity of force-velocity relations measured in heart muscle,[4 5] based mainly on the possible limitations imposed by time, on the influence of initial muscle length, and on the need to employ one or other of several possible muscle models, as well as on the conceptual grounds that observed changes in peak velocity at comparable low loads might be attributable to the presence of an unrecognized internal load.[6] The results of some more recent studies have gone far to elucidate these problems[7-10] and a new experimental approach has evolved which is thought to offer a means of measuring valid force-velocity relations in isolated heart muscle preparations.[11] It is in the light of these developments and with these new techniques that the influence of hypoxia on heart muscle mechanical performance has been re-evaluated.[12]

Isolated cat right ventricular papillary muscles (cross-sectional area less than 1·2 mm^2) were suspended in bicarbonate buffer containing 5 mM glucose, at 29° C., pH 7·4, and were stimulated at a frequency of 12/min. After stabilization, they were studied during well oxygenated conditions (buffer equilibrated with 95 per cent O_2:

5 per cent CO_2 gas mixture to pO_2 c. 600 mmHg) and during anoxic conditions (buffer equilibrated with 95 per cent N_2: 5 per cent CO_2 gas mixture to pO_2 c. 30 mmHg) as described in more detail elsewhere.[8 11 12]

The relationship between muscle length and both resting and developed force was first obtained. The resting force (preload) applied to the muscle was then maintained at that which resulted in maximum developed force; the muscle was thus held at the peak of its active length-force relationship at a resting length, l_{max}, where ultrastructural studies indicate that sarcomere length is about 2·2μ (the physiological range being between 2·2 and 1·8μ) corresponding to optimal overlap of the myofilament cross-bridges.[13] During anoxia, isometric force declined, but maximum force was developed at the same muscle length and no change in either resting or active length-force relationships occurred. Other isolated heart muscle preparations have been shown to exhibit a reversible change in resting length-force relations during hypoxia[14] and this may be a general phenomenon which occurs also clinically during acute ischaemia.[15] It suggests that the maintenance of resting tension may be partly an active process and further work on this is needed. Ischaemic contracture may be analogous to rigor mortis.

Isometric contractions present only an incomplete picture of the mechanical capability of the muscle, however, and it is necessary to consider muscle shortening for a more complete analysis. Shortening velocity is related to load, but in heart muscle it is necessary to consider also muscle length and time, so that we are faced with the need to consider the instantaneous relationship between velocity and length and force, all in the context of time during each contraction. As a first step in this seemingly complex analysis, the time course of shortening length and that of shortening velocity are related to each other, so that velocity is displayed, not against time, but against length, thus giving the continuous instantaneous relationship of velocity to length during the shortening phase of contraction (the relaxation phase is not relevant here). Initial muscle length is held at l_{max} with the appropriate preload so that shortening occurs over the physiological range and shortening velocity is not limited by critically short instantaneous length. A series of such phase-plane analyses relating velocity to length is then obtained at a series of different total loads. Loads greater that the preload are obtained, not by applying these loads at rest for this would overstretch the muscle, but by imposing an increment of force (afterload). The muscle is prevented from feeling this at rest by the presence of a stop against which the muscle has to build up force during contraction before it can shorten, which it then does at a constant total force equal to the sum of the preload and the afterload. In order to obtain velocity-length data at loads less than the preload, the applied resting force is electronically reduced to a lower force, again not during rest when it would simply result in short muscle lengths before contraction started and subsequent limitation of velocity on account of short instantaneous length, but immediately after the latent period; thus data may be obtained at minimal loads approximating to zero but at physiological lengths. In this way a series of velocity-length phase-planes are obtained at different forces, ranging from the force of an isometric contraction at one end (where the phase-plane contracts to a point) to near zero force at the other extreme end. These phase-planes may be regarded as a series of slices, cut along the third axis representing force, through a solid 3-dimensional structure whose surface defines the force-velocity-length relations of that muscle in that state (see Fig. 1).* It has been shown that the major portion of this surface is unique for the given contractile state, being independent of time and also independent of initial muscle length unless this is decreased below l_{max} sufficiently far for the surface to be reached at unphysiologically short length (less than about 85 per cent l_{max}).[8 9] Accordingly this time-independent portion of the force-velocity-length relationship has been used to define the contractile state of the muscle. Such a definition clearly has practical limitations for use outside this preparation. However the time independent portion of the surface contains all peak velocity points, and if it has been obtained also at physiological lengths as in the present study, then these peak velocity points can be used to construct a valid force-velocity curve, ranging between isometric (P_0) and zero force. The use of relatively high preloads corresponding to l_{max} has in the past generally been avoided in an attempt to avoid consideration of which muscle model

* *Editor's footnote*: Further illustrations of this can be found in Brutsaert, D. L., Sonnenblick, E. H. (1969). *Circulation Res.* **24:** 137 and Brutsaert, D. L., Claes, V. A., Sonnenblick, E. H. (1971). *Circulation Res.* **29:** 63.

to employ and to minimize the otherwise long and uncertain extrapolation to the theoretical maximum velocity at zero force (V_{max}). These problems do not arise when the velocity values at very low forces can be measured directly by unloading and load clamp techniques.

Anoxia is shown to depress V_{max} to 77 per cent of control value, P_o to 36 per cent of control value, and also the whole intervening surface of the force-velocity-length relationship in the middle of

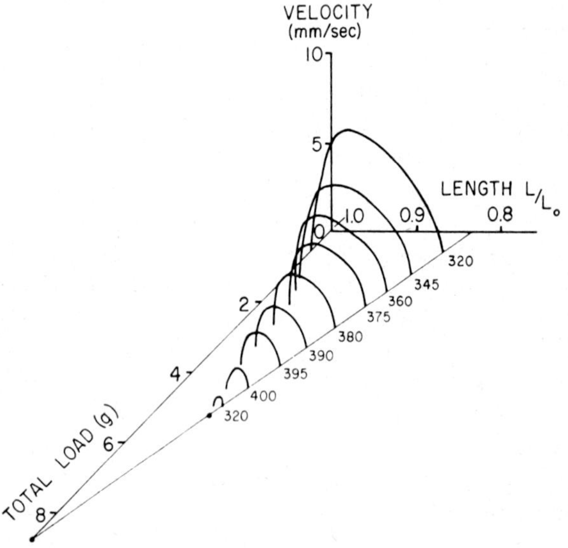

FIG. 17, 1. An example of a three-dimensional construction of the relations between force, velocity and length of the contractile elements corrected for internal shortening due to stretching of the series elastic component (Adapted from Brutsaert and Sonnenblick, 1969[7]: permission of Editors of *Circulation Research*. Ed.).

which lies the physiological range. It was confirmed experimentally that the peak velocity values during anoxia still lay within the unique, time-independent portion of the surface. To exclude the possibility that the observed decrease in velocity at low loads might be attributable solely to a reduction in the number of cross-bridges activated, force-velocity relations were replotted after normalization for the number of cross-bridges activated, as reflected in force, by expressing force as a fraction of isometric force in each curve (P/P_o). Velocities at low relative loads remained lower during anoxia than in control conditions, indicating that the difference in the V_{max} end of the curve could not be removed by correction for the difference in the number of cross-bridges activated in the two states. However the difference between the two normalized curves is represented by only a small difference in force at such low loads, and it might still plausibly be argued that such a small difference could be due to an unrecognized internal load. Further experimental evidence shows that this is unlikely, since maximum unloaded shortening velocity measured under control and anoxic conditions after the muscle had developed the same given amount of force, reflecting activation of the same number of cross-bridges, was not the same. Rather, the maximum unloaded shortening velocity was the same in each condition, whether it was measured before or after the muscle had developed force, and remained clearly lower in anoxia than in control conditions however it was measured. These findings indicate that V_{max} is truly depressed in anoxia and that this cannot be attributed just to a decrease in the number of cross-bridges activated but implies also a decrease in the maximum turnover rate per cross-bridge. Furthermore, a study of the time course of the changes induced by anoxia shows that this decrease in V_{max} is reversible on reoxygenation.

Fig. 17, 2 illustrates also the remarkable changes in the time to peak isometric force (TPF) and in the relaxation time from peak to half developed isometric force (RT 1/2), especially during early reoxygenation.[14 16] The implications of such changes in the aetiology of asynchronous contraction of the ischaemic ventricle have been appreciated.[17] The decrease in V_{max} is notably less than the decrease in P_0. Moreover the changes in V_{max} during the induction of anoxia and subsequent reoxygenation are notably dissociated from the changes in the time course of contraction as shown by TPF and RT 1/2 of the isometric contraction.

These mechanical changes could offer a most useful approach to the understanding of underlying mechanisms if correlated with electrical and biochemical changes measured in the same species and with careful attention to the time course of events.

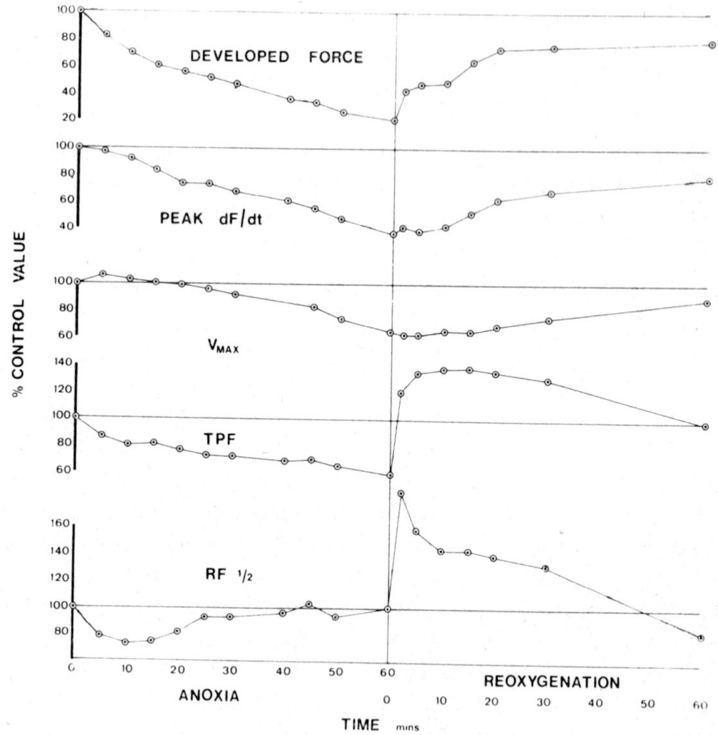

FIG. 17, 2. Time course of changes in mechanical performance during anoxia and reoxygenation in a representative muscle (length 8·0 mm, mean cross-sectional area 0·9 mm², studied at peak of length-force relationship where preload was 1·0 G. and developed force under control conditions was 6·1 G). All values are expressed as a percentage of their respective control values. Developed force, peak rate of force development (dF/dt), time from end of latent period to peak force (TPF), and half relaxation time from peak to half developed force (RF 1/2) were measured in stable isometric beats. Maximum shortening velocity at zero load (V_{max}) was obtained in stable isotonic conditions from a series of measured peak velocity values in consecutive beats at different forces ranging towards zero and a least squares best fit of these points.

REFERENCES

1 HILL, A. V. (1938). Heat of shortening and dynamic constants of muscle. *Proceedings of the Royal Society of London, Series B* **126,** 136-195.

2 ABBOTT, B. C. & MOMMAERTS, W. F. H. M. (1959). A study of inotropic mechanisms in the papillary muscle preparation. *Journal of General Physiology* **42,** 533-551.

3 SONNENBLICK, E. H. (1962). Force-velocity relations in mammalian heart muscle. *American Journal of Physiology* **202,** 931-939.

4 HEFNER, L. L. & BOWEN, T. E. (1967). Elastic components of cat papillary muscle. *American Journal of Physiology* **212,** 1221-1227.

5 BRADY, A. J. (1968). Active state in cardiac muscle. *Physiological Reviews* **48,** 570-600.
6 KATZ, A. M. (1970). Contractile proteins of the heart. *Physiological Reviews* **50,** 63-158.
7 BRUTSAERT, D. L. & SONNENBLICK, E. H. (1969). Force-velocity-length-time relations of the contractile elements in heart muscle of the cat. *Circulation Research* **24,** 137-149.
8 BRUTSAERT, D. L., CLAES, V. A. & SONNENBLICK, E. H. (1971). Effects of abrupt load alterations on force-velocity-length and time relations during isotonic contractions of heart muscle: load clamping. *Journal of Physiology* **216,** 319-330.
9 BRUTSAERT. D. L., CLAES, V. A. & SONNENBLICK, E. H. (1971). Velocity of shortening of unloaded heart muscle and length-tension relation. *Circulation Research* **29,** 63-75.
10 BRUTSAERT, D. L.. CLAES, V. A. & GOETHALS. M. A. (1972). *Submitted for publication.*
11 HENDERSON, A. H., VAN OCKEN, E. & BRUTSAERT, D. L. (1972). *in preparation.*
12 HENDERSON, A. H. & BRUTSAERT, D. L. (1972). *In preparation.*
13 ROSS, J., SONNENBLICK, E. H., TAYLOR, R. R., SPONITZ, H. M. & COVELL, J. W. (1971). Diastolic geometry and sarcomere lengths in the chronically dilated canine left ventricle. *Circulation Research* **28,** 49-61.
14 HENDERSON, A. H., MOST, A. S., PARMLEY, W. W., GORLIN, R. & SONNENBLICK, E. H. (1970). Depression of myocardial contractility in rats by free fatty acids during hypoxia. *Circulation Research* **26,** 439-449.
15 DWYER, E. M. (1970). Left ventricular pressure-volume alterations and regional disorders of contraction during myocardial ischemia induced by atrial pacing. *Circulation* **42,** 1111-1122.
16 TYBERG, J. V., YEATMAN, L. A., PARMLEY, W. W., URSCHEL, C. W. & SONNENBLICK, E. H. (1970). Effects of hypoxia on mechanics of cardiac contraction. *American Journal of Physiology* **218,** 1780-1788.
17 TYBERG, J. V., PARMLEY, W. W. & SONNENBLICK, E. H. (1969). In vitro studies of myocardial asynchrony and regional hypoxia. *Circulation Research* **25,** 569-579.

DISCUSSION

Donald. How long does this preparation last?

Henderson. It can be continued on the next day although I haven't made any studies then.

Conti. I would like to add data we have obtained in the intact beating human heart. Several years ago we were interested in studying left ventricular pressure and relating it to its rate of rise using catheter tip micromanometers. We were able to show that during pacing this measurement of V_{max} increased as heart rate increased. However, once we produced ischaemia (I define ischaemia as typical chest pain, slight elevation of the left ventricular end-diastolic pressure, slight elevation of the systolic pressure and ST segment abnormalities on the electrocardiogram), we noted a definite fall in V_{max} despite tachycardia. I believe this agrees with your data on the isolated heart muscle preparation.

My questions relate to the recovery time you noted in your preparation following anoxia. Your data showed that V_{max} took approximately 40 min to return to normal after you re-oxygenated the preparation. This may be of some practical importance as many laboratories evaluate ischaemia by pacing the heart prior to ventriculography. Is it better to do ventriculography before or after the production of myocardial ischaemia? How long does it take a ventricle to recover from the ischaemia and how does this affect contractility as seen during ventriculography?

Henderson. I don't want to discuss the validity of measuring V_{max} in the whole heart which is quite a different matter. With regard to your finding of a fall in V_{max} during ischaemia, I wonder if it could be related to some unrecognized asynergy since your methods, insofar as they can be used to provide a valid index, refer to the whole heart with its heterogenous population of fibres. Perhaps I should emphasize the altered time course of the contraction during anoxia and reoxygenation which we observe in our small bundle of fibres. In the whole heart this could probably account for asynergy of contraction adequately without needing to consider possible delayed conduction, as Tyberg *et al.*[17], demonstrated in an ingenious preparation using two isolated papillary muscles in series. I cannot directly answer your practical question about the time taken to recover from ischaemia. Our preparation is of course different from the whole heart in many ways. It depends upon inward diffusion for exchange of oxygen and electrolytes and its oxygen requirements are much lower since it is only contracting 12 times per min at a much lower temperature.

Conti. I really think this is important from the standpoint of trying to evaluate the effect of intervention on ventricular function, for example, saphenous vein by-pass surgery. I would caution investigators to perform ventriculography in a standard fashion preferably before ischaemia is produced by pacing.

Wallace. You have shown a rather remarkable decrease in the time to peak tension during anoxia. That's an unusual feature for negative inotropic influence and I wonder, in view of the catecholamine release that has been reported whether you are looking at hypoxia perhaps but also with catecholamine release.

Henderson. I agree that catecholamines are likely to have been released during anoxia and I have not yet extended the experiments to catecholamine-depleted muscles though these are on the agenda. However, Tyberg and his colleagues[16] showed that catecholamine depletion did not substantially alter the findings with respect to the influence of anoxia on isometric contractions using a similar preparation. Time to peak force decreased during anoxia just the same. Clearly an inotropic intervention cannot be adequately characterized simply by its effect on any single index, such as V_{max}. As I mentioned, contractile state is described and defined only by the whole 3-dimensional surface and this can be altered in different ways by different inotropic interventions.

Noble. Did your muscles show the effect of load dependent changes in contractility demonstrated by Parmley *et al.* (Proceedings of the Society for Experimental Biology and Medicine (1968) **27,** 606-609). They showed that in isolated papillary muscle, switched from isotonic to isometric contraction, isometric tension fell off after the first isometric beat. The reason I'm bringing this up is that one possible interpretation of their results is that the isolated papillary muscle in this sort of system is really not getting as much oxygen as it should and if one switches from isotonic contraction, one is increasing the oxygen consumption of the preparation making it even more short of oxygen so that its performance falls off. This would fit in with the results you showed where the effect of hypoxia was much less on velocity shortening at zero load compared with the effect on isometric tension.

Henderson. This phenomenon has been described as the first and stable beat phenomenon, in which the first isometric beat after a series of isotonic contractions develops more force than subsequent stable beats, whereas the converse happens on changing to isotonic beats. There appears to be a difference in contractile state, associated with a difference in action potential, between isotonic and isometric conditions, and it takes several beats to change from one to the other. All our experimental measurements are obtained under stable isometric conditions—that is, after at least five isometric beats, to standardize for this difference. We have studied the phenomenon a little more fully using the methods described earlier, and comparing the 3-dimensional force-velocity-length surface under stable isometric and stable isotonic conditions. The whole surface is shifted symmetrically, as it is with changes in external calcium solution. While I take your point that an isometric contraction costs more energy so that one might wonder whether the phenomenon were due to inadequate oxygenation, the symmetrical shift of the surface contrasts with the asymmetrical shift seen in anoxia, and the decrease in maximum velocity of shortening occurs more quickly than it does after inducing anoxia. Moreover, the phenomenon is independent of muscle thickness in cat muscles where the constant normalized tension development with increasing thickness up to a mean cross-sectional area of about 1·5 mm^2 argues against oxygen limitation in thinner muscle, such as we use. In rat muscles, where I suspect that there may often be oxygen limitation, the phenomenon is scarcely seen. In other words, all the evidence points away from inadequate oxygenation as the cause for this phenomenon. Rather, is it likely to be due to alterations in calcium movement, and one can speculate that it supports recent views of cross-bridge formation, in so far as there is less sliding of myofilaments during force development so that activating calcium may be less easily freed for sequestration and subsequent release by the sarcoplasmic reticulum.

Donald. With regard to possible oxygen limitation, have you repeated these experiments under moderately hyperbaric conditions? They would have to be brief to avoid enzyme changes.

Henderson. No.

Parratt. I wonder if you can comment on the choice of temperature of 29°C and a frequency of 12 beats per minute in view of the fact that some evidence is accumulating that the sensitivity of myocardial tissue to catecholamine stimulation is reduced at lower temperatures. Some people say that the beta receptors 'vanish' when you get to 29°C.

Henderson. I think the reasons for choosing these experimental conditions were initially related to the increased stability of the preparation, associated partly with decreased oxygen requirements, and of course the convenience of having time to turn the necessary knobs between beats. The accumulation of base-line data in this preparation, as used by many different workers, itself provides a reason for continuing in the same way. It has been usual to check the validity of any observations across the temperature and frequency range, though we have not done that in the present experiments.

Parratt. Since 29°C is not the temperature at which the muscle functions normally, do you think your observations would hold good at 37°C?

Henderson. All previous studies on mechanics in this preparation have been repeated at 37°C and shown to remain true at a higher state of contractility as judged by previously measured force velocity relations. These particular studies on anoxia have not been repeated at a higher temperature. One chooses the lower temperature because the oxygen requirements are less.

Thomas. I need some further help in transposing this sort of thinking to the whole heart. You showed that in anoxia there is a drop in V_{max} of perhaps 15 or 20 per cent and force fell about 20 per cent. It is thought that in the centre of a myocardial infarct the muscle actually lengthens during systole. What do we look at in trying to assess the performance of the intact heart muscle in myocardial ischaemia?

Henderson. I don't really know any valid way at the moment. This way of analysing performance in the isolated muscle is valid, I think, and useful because it provides a physiological basis for what must be happening in the whole heart which is made up of muscle fibres. Further, such studies may help us to find out what we should be measuring in the whole heart, but at the moment I don't know the answer.

Thomas. As you yourself say, V_{max} is probably a circumstance which is never reached in health or disease. Shouldn't we perhaps be more simple and look at force developed rather than try to define the whole profile of muscle performance over a wider range of setting?

Henderson. Peak isometric force development seems to be no more physiologically relevant than maximum shortening velocity at zero load. The relevant area is somewhere in the middle of the surface of that three dimensional construction. Maximum shortening velocity and peak isometric force are, however, useful in a different way in so far as they define the extremes of the capability of the muscle.

Noble. You and I always use glucose as substrate. I think this audience might be interested to know whether using any other fuel alters the changes which you have shown here with hypoxia.

Henderson. As you know, I have looked at this in the isolated rat papillary muscle preparation but not yet in the cat muscle. I would expect the effects of using different substrates to be similar in the two species. Glucose improves mechanical performance during anoxia while free fatty acids impair performance. My findings are in line with those of Dr Mjøs so I will leave him to discuss this whole field more fully.

EFFECT OF SUBSTRATE ALTERATION ON MYOCARDIAL OXYGEN CONSUMPTION

O. D. MJØS

TRADITIONALLY, two mechanical factors, myocardial tension and contractility, are assumed to be the main determinants of myocardial oxygen consumption ($M\dot{V}O_2$), whereas external work has been shown to bear little relation to $M\dot{V}O_2$.[1] Myocardial tension is the variable when aortic blood pressure is raised under conditions of constant inotropic stimulation.[1 2] Contractility is raised by infusion of catecholamines, and may be estimated by the maximal rate of pressure generation (dP/dt) during the isovolumic period and by the velocity of shortening of muscle fibres during ventricular ejection.[1 3 4]

However, studies in isolated, aerobically-perfused, contracting rat hearts[5 6 7] suggested that $M\dot{V}O_2$ may also be influenced by the substrate supply to the heart. Thus, in contrast to carbohydrates, e.g., lactate and glucose, free fatty acids (FFA) in high perfusate concentrations were found to enhance $M\dot{V}O_2$ in the isolated rat heart. Similarly, adrenaline raised $M\dot{V}O_2$ in this preparation, and it was concluded that the common cause of the increase was a metabolic stimulation of unbound FFA intracellularly. Since mechanical parameters were not measured in these studies, it was not clear whether the observed rise in $M\dot{V}O_2$ was due to increased mechanical activity of the heart or to a direct effect of FFA (or of related influences) on myocardial metabolic rate. Experimental evidence is also conflicting: Henderson *et al.*[8] found that high concentrations of FFA actually decreased $M\dot{V}O_2$ in the isolated rat heart perfused at a constant flow and paced at constant rate. As contractile force was also depressed, probably due to oxygen limitation, the interpretation of the relationship between $M\dot{V}O_2$ and FFA is less clear. No previous study seems to have been performed on the effect of high plasma-FFA and myocardial uptake of FFA on myocardial function and oxygen consumption in intact hearts, and the present investigation was therefore undertaken to determine the role of FFA in myocardial metabolism in the intact dog heart under controlled haemodynamic conditions.

The following mechanical parameters were measured: left ventricular pressure, maximal rate of rise of left ventricular pressure (dP/dt), heart rate, cardiac output and aortic blood pressure. Myocardial blood flow was measured by the hydrogen desaturation technique.[9] The dogs were intact and anaesthetized with sodium pentobarbital.

In the first series of experiments, raised plasma concentrations and consequently myocardial uptake of FFA were induced by i.v. infusion of a lipid emulsion, Intralipid 'Vitrum', after heparinization.[10 11] Heparin stimulates plasma lipoprotein-lipase activity, thereby hydrolyzing the fat emulsion and releasing FFA. By this procedure, the arterial concentration of FFA was raised from an average of about 500 to 3100 μEq/l, while myocardial uptake of FFA

Table 18, 1. *Metabolic effects of Intralipid infusion in heparinized dogs. Mean ±SE of seven experiments*

	FFA					
	a	a-cs	u	$M\dot{V}O_2$	O_2-extr.	MF
	μEq/litre	*μEq/litre*	*μEq/min /100 g*	*ml/min /100 g*	%	*ml/min /100 g*
Control	488	109	5·7	8·6	57·6	90
±SE	67	32	1·8	0·6	3·0	7
Intralipid infusion	3105	371	22·0	10·7	69·3	93
±SE	286	80	6·5	0·6	1·7	8
P	<0·001	<0·01	<0·05	<0·001	<0·005	NS
Recovery	584	148	8·9	8·3	58·3	90
±SE	80	45	2·8	0·6	3·9	4

n, number of dogs; a, arterial concentrations; a-cs, arterio-coronary sinus differences; u, myocardial uptake of free fatty acids (FFA); $M\dot{V}O_2$, myocardial oxygen consumption; O_2-extr., myocardial oxygen extraction; MF, myocardial blood flow; the values for *P* are the highest probability that the observed differences are due to chance. NS, not significant ($P>0·05$).

increased four fold (Table 18, 1). $M\dot{V}O_2$ rose by about 20 per cent, although mechanical performance remained unchanged.[11] This was evidenced by unaltered left ventricular systolic- and end-diastolic pressure, dP/dt, heart rate and cardiac output (Table 18, 2).

Table 18, 2. *Haemodynamic effects of Intralipid infusion in heparinized dogs. Mean ±SE of seven experiments*

	LVSP	LVEDP	dP/dt	HR	CO
	mmHg	*mmHg*	*mmHg·10⁻³ / sec*	*beats/min*	*ml/min/kg*
Control	149	3·9	2·44	144	131
±SE	3	0·6	0·27	4	15
Intralipid infusion	149	3·8	2·56	140	131
±SE	3	0·6	0·25	4	15
P	NS	NS	NS	NS	NS
Recovery	134	3·6	2·47	143	133
±SE	4	0·6	0·22	3	14

n, number of dogs; LVSP, left ventricular systolic pressure; LVEDP, left ventricular end-diastolic pressure; dP/dt, first derivative of left ventricular pressure; HR, heart rate; CO, cardiac output; NS, not significant ($P>0{\cdot}005$).

It is known that during increased myocardial uptake of FFA, a significant fraction of the FFA taken up is not immediately oxidized, but is stored in the myocardium as triglycerides. However, when calculated according to Ball,[12] the amount of oxygen required for esterification of the additional amount of FFA taken up when plasma FFA were high was less than 10 per cent of the observed rise in $M\dot{V}O_2$. It therefore seems justifiable to assume that a metabolic stimulating effect of FFA is in operation, probably related to increased unbound intracellular FFA.

Stimulation of β-adrenergic receptors—e.g., by isoprenaline—increases the mechanical performance of the heart and markedly affects $M\dot{V}O_2$. Earlier,[1 13] the rise in $M\dot{V}O_2$ caused by catecholamines has been related to increased mechanical performance. Raised basal $M\dot{V}O_2$ represents only a minor fraction of the total $M\dot{V}O_2$.[13 14] Since i.v. infusion of isoprenaline (or other catecholamines) is associated with augmentation of plasma FFA—and hence myocardial uptake of FFA—a series of experiments was undertaken to see whether part of the large increase in $M\dot{V}O_2$ might be related to increased myocardial uptake of FFA. Isoprenaline i.v. raised arterial concentrations of FFA from an average of 450 to 1100 μEq/1 (Table 18, 3). By inhibiting adipose tissue lipolysis with nicotinic acid, β-pyridyl-carbinol (Ronicol 'Roche') or 10 to 20 per cent

Table 18, 3. *Metabolic effects of isoprenaline infusion (2-3 μg/min) before and after inhibition of lipolysis by nicotinic acid or β-pyridyl carbinol. Mean ± SE of five dogs*

	FFA					
	a	a-cs	u	$M\dot{V}O_2$	O_2-extr.	MF
	μEq/litre	*μEq/litre*	*μEq/min /100 g*	*ml/min /100 g*	%	*ml/min /100 g*
Control	449	145	9·5	9·9	72·1	100
± SE	95	37	2·8	0·8	4·8	8
Isoprenaline	1094	209	21·6	17·6	72·7	163
± SE	160	25	4·3	1·2	4·8	26
P	<0·02	<0·05	<0·05	<0·001	NS	<0·05
Inhibition of lipolysis						
Control	350	143	9·4	9·7	70·2	100
± SE	60	37	2·9	1·0	5·5	8
Isoprenaline	340	62	6·1	14·2	59·0	168
± SE	49	13	1·2	1·2	5·6	23
P	NS	NS	NS	<0·001	NS	<0·025

a, arterial concentrations; a-cs, arteriocoronary sinus differences; u, myocardial uptake of free fatty acids (FFA); $M\dot{V}O_2$, myocardial oxygen consumption; O_2-extr., myocardial oxygen extraction; MF, myocardial blood flow; NS, not significant ($P > 0{\cdot}05$).

glucose solution, i.v., the isoprenaline-induced rise in $M\dot{V}O_2$ was about 30 to 40 per cent less than with intact lipolysis.[15] As mechanical responses to isoprenaline were similar before and after inhibition of lipolysis (Table 18, 4) it was concluded that the additional rise (14·2 to 17·6 ml/min/100 g) in $M\dot{V}O_2$ with intact lipolysis was caused by a metabolic stimulation by FFA, as shown for Intralipid/heparin.

Myocardial mechanical performance and $M\dot{V}O_2$ may be increased by inotropic agents other than catecholamines, e.g., glucagon. Glucagon does not raise plasma FFA in the intact organism.[16] Tests were therefore made to determine whether a similar rise in mechanical performance by i.v. infusion of glucagon would result in a smaller rise in $M\dot{V}O_2$ than that effected by isoprenaline. The agents were compared during the same rise in contractility, measured by maximum rate of rise of left ventricular pressure (dP/dt) (Table 18, 5), and the results showed that the rise in $M\dot{V}O_2$ was signifi-

Table 18, 4. *Haemodynamic effects of isoprenaline infusion (2-3 μg/min) before and after inhibition of lipolysis by nicotinic acid or β-pyridyl carbinol. Mean ±SE of five dogs*

	$\overline{AP}$	LVSP	LVEDP	dP/dt	HR	CO
	mmHg	*mmHg*	*mmHg*	*mmHg*/10⁻³ sec	*beats/min*	*ml/min/kg*
Control	132	144	4·4	2·5	160	131
±SE	6	6	1·3	0·3	14	11
Isoprenaline	121	137	3·2	5·4	185	225
±SE	7	6	1·2	0·5	13	13
P	NS	NS	<0·05	<0·001	<0·02	<0·005
Inhibition of lipolysis						
Control	132	144	4·4	2·5	160	130
±SE	6	6	1·3	0·3	15	11
Isoprenaline	122	138	3·1	5·5	185	226
±SE	4	6	1·2	0·5	13	14
P	<0·05	NS	<0·05	<0·001	<0·02	<0·001

$\overline{AP}$, mean aortic blood pressure; LVSP, left ventricular systolic pressure; LVEDP, left venticular end-diastolic pressure; dP/dt, maximal rate of rise of left ventricular pressure; HR, heart rate; CO, cardiac output; NS, not significant ($P>0·05$).

Table 18, 5. *Haemodynamic effects of glucagon and isoprenaline infusion in intact dogs. Mean ±SE of seven dogs*

	$\overline{AP}$	LVSP	LVEDP	dP/dt	HR	CO
	mmHg	*mmHg*	*mmHg*	*mmHg*/10⁻³ *sec*	*beats/min*	*ml/min/kg*
Control	143	158	6·5	2·56	169	138
±SE	9	7	0·9	0·21	8	12
Glucagon inf.	129	146	4·2	4·74	221	195
±SE	10	10	0·6	0·32	10	17
P	<0·005	<0·025	<0·025	<0·001	<0·01	<0·001
Control	144	156	6·4	2·65	166	136
±SE	10	7	0·8	0·21	9	12
Isoprenaline inf.	130	146	4·2	4·80	193	186
±SE	11	10	0·6	0·37	10	16
P	<0·005	<0·02	<0·025	<0·001	<0·02	<0·001

n, number of experiments; $\overline{AP}$, mean aortic blood pressure; LSVP, left ventricular systolic pressure; LVEDP, left ventricular end-diastolic pressure; dP/dt, maximal rate of rise of left ventricular pressure; HR, heart rate; CO, cardiac output; NS, not significant ($P>0·05$).

Table 18, 6. *Metabolic effects of glucagon and isoprenaline infusion in intact dogs. Mean ±SE of seven dogs*

	FFA					
	a	a-cs	u	$M\dot{V}O_2$	O_2-extr.	MF
	μEq/l	*μEq/l*	*μEq/min /100 g*	*ml/min /100 g*	%	*ml/min /100 g*
Control	416	100	8.1	11·3	61·6	118
±SE	42	30	2·6	4·5	4·7	9
Glucagon inf.	353	58	4·4	15·8	68·3	149
±SE	52	40	2·8	3·0	3·1	16
P	NS	NS	NS	<0·001	NS	<0·02
Control	393	88	7·5	11·2	60·8	124
±SE	29	22	2·2	4·0	4·2	10
Isoproterenol inf.	1211	233	24·1	18·6	71·7	163
±SE	38	40	5·3	2·4	2·4	16
P	<0·001	<0·001	<0·005	<0·001	<0·01	<0·01

n, number of experiments; a, arterial concentrations; a-cs, arterio-coronary sinus differences; u, myocardial uptake of free fatty acids (FFA); $M\dot{V}O_2$, myocardial oxygen consumption; O_2-extr., myocardial oxygen extraction; MF, myocardial blood flow; NS, not significant ($P>0{\cdot}05$).

cantly less with glucagon compared with isoprenaline[17] (Table 18, 6). This supports the conclusion that the additional rise in $M\dot{V}O_2$ with isoprenaline was due to metabolic stimulation of the high FFA concentrations.

It is apparent from the present investigation that high plasma concentrations of FFA, in contrast to lactate, glucose and triglycerides, can raise myocardial oxygen consumption considerably in the intact dog heart without changing myocardial performance. Changes in metabolic rate are thus not only caused by the mechanical activity of the heart, but under certain conditions are also influenced by the nature of substrate supply.

The precise mechanism of the $M\dot{V}O_2$-stimulating effect of FFA (or metabolites) remains to be established. The results of the present work may, however, be compatible with *in vitro* studies demonstrating that long chain fatty acids uncouple respiratory chain oxidative phosphorylation.[18 19 20]

In the last few years, attention has been directed towards variations in plasma-FFA as a factor in the development of ventricular arrhythmias and sudden death after myocardial infarction in man. The present experiments were conducted in anaesthetized dogs, but they may well have some clinical relevance in explaining the possible mechanisms involved in the development of certain types of myocardial disorder; some suggestions follow for prophylaxis and treatment.

1. During the initial phase of acute myocardial infarction, plasma concentrations of FFA are often found in excess of 1000 μEq/1 (within the range of high plasma-FFA in the present investigation).[21 22] Ventricular arrhythmias and sudden death have been shown to be more frequent in cases of acute myocardial infarction with the highest values of plasma-FFA,[21] although others disagree.[23]

Agents which increase oxygen demand of the heart more than oxygen supply, e.g. isoprenaline, have recently been shown to enlarge the size of an experimental myocardial infarction in dogs.[24] If this is the case in man, high concentrations of plasma-FFA following acute myocardial infarction may be deleterious by possibly increasing the extent and magnitude of the infarction. Plasma FFA can be reduced by treatment with antilipolytic agents (β-pyridyl-carbinol or nicotinic acid) or i.v. glucose, resulting in a reduction in infarct size, and possibly, also in arrhythmias, due to the consequently reduced oxygen demand.

2. Recent clinical experience suggests that glucagon may be of value in the treatment of myocardial pump failure,[25 26] although in high doses it has been shown to depress myocardial performance.[27] In contrast to some catecholamines, treatment with glucagon is not associated with premature contractions and arrhythmias.[28] According to the present study, one advantage of glucagon over catecholamines is a reduced demand for oxygen, due to failure of plasma-FFA to increase.

3. The present investigation shows that in the normal, intact dog heart high concentrations of FFA (within the clinical range) did not alter myocardial performance. No toxic effects of FFA were therefore observed. These results are in accordance with Henderson *et al.*[29] in isolated rat papillary muscle. When FFA were elevated, under well-oxygenated conditions, they found unaltered developed force, in contrast to reduced force, during hypoxia.

However, as mentioned, increased arterial concentrations, and consequently myocardial uptake of FFA (induced by Intralipid/heparin), raised $M\dot{V}O_2$ by an average of 20 per cent in the intact dog heart, without altering myocardial performance. The purpose of the last series of experiments to be reported here was therefore to determine whether similar high concentrations of FFA (also induced by Intralipid/heparin) would depress mechanical performance at limited oxygen supply, due to increased oxygen demand. This hypothesis was tested in open-chest dogs by producing graded and controlled myocardial ischaemia. Dr Kjekshus co-operated in the study.[30] The circumflex and descending branches of the left coronary artery were directly cannulated close to their origin and perfused from a carotid artery through extracorporeal PVC tubing. Coronary blood flow was gradually reduced by an adjustable clamp above the flowmeter. Aortic flow and left ventricular pressure were continuously recorded. Arterial and coronary sinus blood were sampled to estimate $M\dot{V}O_2$ and uptake of lactate and FFA. Instantaneous changes in left ventricular dimensions were monitored with pairs of ultrasonic distance gauges implanted in the left ventricular wall. The distance gauges were very sensitive to ischaemia. As coronary flow was stepwise reduced by constriction of the shunt, the ventricle dilated and there was good correlation between dilatation and decrease in $M\dot{V}O_2$. As the shunt was stepwise constricted, a good correlation was also obtained between reduction of myocardial lactate uptake and ventricular dilatation. With accentuated constriction, lactate was produced indicating increased anaerobic metabolism. These preliminary experiments therefore showed good correlation between metabolic and mechanical changes due to coronary ischaemia, and demonstrated the reliability of ventricular dilatation as an index of ischaemic injury.

We next investigated what happened when coronary blood flow was fixed at a constant ischaemic level and oxygen demand of the heart was increased by high concentrations of FFA induced by i.v. infusion of Intralipid/heparin, thus activating plasma lipolysis. The dogs were divided into two groups. In both, the shunt was first constricted so as to produce moderate dilatation; this led to an average reduction in $M\dot{V}O_2$ of 20 per cent in each group. Further dilatation was induced in two ways; in one group constriction of the shunt was increased; this resulted in an additional fall in $M\dot{V}O_2$ of about 20 per cent. In the other group, increased dilatation was induced by raising plasma concentration of FFA by Intralipid/heparin, constriction of the shunt remaining unaltered. $M\dot{V}O_2$ in this group was essentially unchanged, despite the fact that the degree of dilatation was the same in both groups. Increased plasma concentrations of FFA therefore increased the ischaemic injury, as evidenced by further dilatation of the heart. Under ischaemic conditions, with limited oxygen supply, this implies that increased consumption of FFA will lead to oxygen being ' stolen ' from processes that will uphold cardiac contractility.

The present data support the contention that elevated concentrations of FFA, within the clinical range, play a significant role in increasing myocardial oxygen requirements in the dog heart, thereby promoting depression of contractility of the oxygen-limited heart. These findings may be of relevance in man.

REFERENCES

1 SONNENBLICK, E. H., ROSS, J. JR. & BRAUNWALD, E. (1968). Oxygen consumption of the heart. *American Journal of Cardiology* **22,** 328-336.

2 MCDONALD, R. H. JR., TAYLOR, R. R. & CINGOLANI, H. (1966). Measurement of myocardial developed tension and its relation to oxygen consumption. *American Journal of Physiology* **211,** 667-673.

3 SONNENBLICK, E. H., ROSS, J. JR., COVELL, J. W., KAISER, G. A. & BRAUNWALD, E. (1965). Velocity of contraction as a determinant of myocardial oxygen consumption. *American Journal of Physiology* **209,** 919-927.

4 TAYLOR, R. R. (1970). Theoretical analysis of the isovolumic phase of left ventricular contraction in terms of cardiac muscle mechanics. *Cardiovascular Research* **4,** 429-435.

5 CHALLONER, D. R. (1968). Evidence for uncoupled respiration in thyrotoxic and epiphrine-stimulated myocardium. *American Journal of Physiology* **214,** 365-369.

6 CHALLONER, D. R. & STEINBERG, D. (1966). Effect of free fatty acids on the oxygen consumption of perfused rat heart. *American Journal of Physiology* **210,** 280-286.

7 CHALLONER, D. R. & STEINBERG, D. (1966). Oxidative metabolism of myocardium as influenced by fatty acids and epinephrine. *American Journal of Physiology* **211,** 897-902.

8 HENDERSON, A. H., CRAIG, R. J., GORLIN, R. & SONNENBLICK, E. H. (1970). Free fatty acids and myocardial function in perfused rat heart. *Cardiovascular Research* **4,** 466-472.

9 AUKLAND, K. B., BOWER, B. F. & BERLINER, R. W. (1964). Measurement of local blood flow with hydrogen gas. *Circulation Research* **14,** 164-187.

10 MENG, H. C. & EDGREN, B. (1963). Source of plasma free fatty acids in dogs receiving fat emulsion and heparin. *American Journal of Physiology* **204,** 691-695.

11 MJØS, O. D. (1971). Effect of free fatty acids on myocardial function and oxygen consumption in intact dogs. *Journal of Clinical Investigation* **50,** 1386-1389.

12 BALL, E. G. (1965). Some energy relationships in adipose tissue *Annals of the New York Academy of Science* **131,** 225-234.

13 KLOCKE, F. J., KAISER, G. A., ROSS, J. JR. & BRAUNWALD, E. (1965). Mechanism of increase of myocardial oxygen uptake produced by catecholamines. *American Journal of Physiology,* **209,** 913-918.

14 HAOGE, A. & ØYE, I. (1966). The action of adrenaline in cardiac muscle. II *Acta Physiologica Scandinavica* **68,** 295-301.

15 MJØS, O. D. (1971). Effect of inhibition of lipolysis on myocardial oxygen consumption in the presence of isoproterenol. *Journal of Clinical Investigation* **50,** 1869-1873.

16 SOKAL, J. E., AJDIN, A. & KRAUS, G. (1966). Effect of glucagon on plasma free fatty acids of normal and pancreatectomized dogs. *American Journal of Physiology* **211,** 1334-1338.

17 MJØS, O. D. (1971). Effect of iso-proterenol, glucagon and calcium on myocardial oxygen consumption in intact dogs. *Scandinavian Journal of Clinical and Laboratory Investigation* **28,** 127-132.

18 BORST, P., LOOS, J. A., CHRIST, E. J. & SLATER, E. C. (1962). Uncoupling activity of long-chain fatty acids. *Biochimica et Biophysica Acta* **62,** 509-518.

19 HITTLEMAN, K. J. & LINDBERG, O. (1970). In *Brown Adipose Tissue,* p. 245. Edited by: O. Lindberg. New York: American Elsevier Publishing Company.

20 PRESSMAN, B. C. & LARDY, H. A. (1956). Effect of surface active agents on the latent ATPase of mitochondria. *Biochimica et Biophysica Acta* **21,** 458-466.

21 OLIVER, M. F., KURIEN, V. A· & GREENWOOD, T. W. (1968). Relation between serum free-fatty-acids and arrhythmias and death after acute myocardial infarction. *Lancet* **I,** 710-714.

22 GUPTA, D. K., YOUNG, R., JEWITT, D. E., HERZOG, M. & OPIE, L. H. (1969). Increased plasma free-fatty-acid concentration and their significance in patients with acute myocardial infarction. *Lancet* **II,** 1209-1213.

23 OWEN, P., THOMAS, M. & OPIE, L. H. (1969). Relative changes in free-fatty-acid and glucose utilisation by ischaemic myocardium after coronary-artery occlusion. *Lancet* **I,** 1187-1190.

24 MAROKO, P. R., KJEKSHUS, J. K., SOBEL, B. E., WATANABE, T., COVELL, J. W., ROSS., JR. & BRAUNWALD, E. (1971). Factors influencing infarct size following experimental coronary artery occlusion. *Circulation* **43,** 67-82.

25 MANCHESTER, J. H., PARMLEY, W. W., MATHOFF, J. M. & SONNENBLICK, E. H. (1969). Prevalence and distribution of coronary atherosclerosis (CA) in a non-selected population. *Clinical research* **17,** 252.

26 WILLIAMS, J. F., CHILDRESS, R. H., CHIP, J. N. & BORDER, J. F. (1969). Hemodynamic effects of glucagon in patients with heart disease. *Circulation* **39,** 38-47.

27 MAYER, S. E., NAMM, D. H. & RICE, L. (1970). Effect of glucagon on cyclic 3′, 5′-AMP, phosphorylase activity and contractility of heart muscle on the rat. *Circulation Research* **26,** 225-233.

28 EPSTEIN, S. E. (1970). Adenyl cyclase and myocardial contractility. *Annals of Internal Medicine* **72,** 561-578.

29 HENDERSON, A. H.. MOST, A. S., PARMLEY, W. W.. GORLIN, R. & SONNENBLICK, E. H. (1970). Depression of myocardial contractility in rats by free fatty acids during hypoxia. *Circulation Research* **26,** 439-449.

30 KJEKSHUS, J. K. & MJØS, O. D. (1972). Effect of free fatty acids on myocardial infarction and metabolism in the ischemic dog heart. *Journal of Clinical Investigation* **51,** 1767-1777.

Discussion

Opie. You referred to perfused rat heart work showing a small increase in oxygen uptake with increased fatty acids in the medium. We should not lose sight of the fact that this is not a specific fatty acid effect. Willebrands in Amsterdam several years ago showed that, compared with glucose, lactate and other substrates all caused an increased oxygen uptake. His work suggests that glucose appears to produce a lower oxygen uptake compared with the other substrates. Could you comment on any work with high fatty acids and infarct size?

Mjøs. My experience from intact dogs is that high concentrations of glucose, lactate or triglycerides (induced by Intralipid *without* heparinization) do not influence $M\dot{V}O_2$. As to the second point, I referred to the work of Maroko *et al.* (1970) showing that agents which alter the balance between oxygen supply and demand influence the extent and magnitude of an experimental myocardial infarction. Thus, agents which increase oxygen demand more than oxygen supply, e.g., isoprenaline, increased the size of experimental infarction in dogs. As far as I know, there is no published study of the effect of FFA in this context.

Opie. We should be very careful in defining our terms in these experiments and bear in mind that we are studying an increased level of free fatty acids in the presence of lipaemia. Regan (*Circulation* **23,** 55-63, 1961) studied the effect of alimentary lipaemia on oxygen uptake in the dog heart, and claimed that lipaemia decreased oxygen uptake. When he gave heparin and the plasma triglyceride level fell and FFA rose, oxygen uptake was restored to normal.

Mjøs. If you raise plasma concentrations of triglycerides by Intralipid without heparin, $M\dot{V}O_2$ remains unchanged. If you administer heparin to the dog during continuous intravenous infusion of Intralipid, plasma triglycerides fall, while plasma FFA rise to about $3000 \mu Eq/1$ due to enhanced intravascular lipolysis. Now, $M\dot{V}O_2$ increased on average by 20 per cent, while mechanical activity of the heart was unchanged throughout the experiment. Thus, there seems to be no effect of triglycerides (or alimentary lipaemia) on $M\dot{V}O_2$ in the intact dog heart.

In unpublished studies we found that average S-T segment elevation following acute coronary occlusion in the presence of high plasma FFA (induced by Intralipid/heparin) was the same as during control occlusion. However, if the dogs were pretreated with an anti-lipolytic drug (β-pyridyl-carbinol or nicotinic acid), average S-T segment elevation following acute coronary occlusion in the presence of high plasma-FFA (induced by Intralipid/heparin) was significantly increased compared with occlusion during inhibition of lipolysis only.

Carlson. During alimentary lipaemia there is no change whatsoever in the arterial coronary sinus oxygen difference. To put it another way, rising exogenous triglycerides do not affect the arterial-coronary sinus oxygen difference. Our studies were carried out without heparin and the results are thus similar to those of Dr Mjøs but opposite to what Dr Opie believes. Did you use heparin?

Møjs. No.

Carlson. I would like to extrapolate Dr Mjøs' interesting results to intact man. About ten years ago Havel and I (*Metabolism* **13:** 1402-1412, 1964) studied the role of plasma FFA as the calorigenic effect of catecholamines. We infused catecholamines and raised the oxygen consumption by about 30 per cent, but when we pretreated the subjects with nicotinic acid to inhibit fat mobilizing lipolysis and thereby the increase in FFA, oxygen consumption fell by about 25 per cent. In a way they are similar to your findings and extend them to the whole body. It may also be of therapeutic importance during acute myocardial infarction because there is a possibility that we might influence total body oxygen consumption and thus reduce the load on the heart.

Mjøs. Your investigation 10 years ago, showing that part of the increase in total body oxygen consumption induced by catecholamines in humans was related to increased concentrations of FFA, was one of the main studies stimulating my enthusiasm to discover whether this was also the case in the heart.

Oliver. Dr Mjøs, you have not told us about your unpublished work on the relationship between elevation of free fatty acids and an increase in ST elevation in the E.C.G. Maroko *et al.*[24] have shown that the elevated ST segments in acute ischaemia are reduced by giving glucose. Does heparin and Intralipid elevate ST segments? Does nicotinic acid lower elevated ST segments? Finally, have you studied the effect of very long chain fatty acids on ventricular dilatation and compared this with shorter chain fatty acids?

Mjøs. We have so far studied only the 'over-all' effect of high concentrations of FFA (induced by Intralipid/heparin) on MVO_2 and mechanical performance of the heart. We are very keen to study the effect of different types of fatty acids (saturated and unsaturated) on $M\dot{V}O_2$ and contractility both during free coronary flow and under oxygen-limited conditions in our shunt-preparation. With regard to the effect of inhibition of lipolysis in ST segment elevation, we have recently shown (*J. clin. Invest.*, in press) that pretreatment with β-pyridyl-carbinol reduced the extent and magnitude of average ST segment elevation following coronary artery occlusion by about 40 per cent, compared with that resulting from coronary artery occlusion alone. Furthermore, during 24 hours' treatment with β-pyridyl-carbinol the extent of depression of myocardial CPK activity from full wall biopsies was significantly less than anticipated from the magnitude of ST segment elevation produced by coronary artery occlusion alone. Tissue damage was therefore less, after inhibition of lipolysis, compared to that which would have been expected from the ST segment elevation after the control occlusion. Our interpretation of the results is that following coronary artery occlusion there is an adrenergic activation of the ischaemic area, leading to enhanced myocardial lipolysis. The consequent accumulation of FFA intracellularly will lead to increased oxygen requirement. β-pyridyl-carbinol presumably acts by inhibiting lipolysis and thus reduces the oxygen demand leading to reduced infarct size. It may be argued that β-pyridyl-carbinol acted by favouring blood flow to the ischaemic area. However, as the doses used in the present experiments had no discernible effect on blood pressure, and as coronary resistance was unchanged by the drug before and during coronary occlusion, any beneficial effect on infarct size through an improvement in coronary collateral circulation is unlikely, although the possibility of redistribution of blood flow cannot be completely ruled out.

The effect of high concentrations of FFA on average ST segment elevation after coronary artery occlusion were mentioned earlier. I would like to add that in other experiments plasma-concentration of FFA was raised by isoproterenol i.v. to an average of 1500 μEq/l.

It was shown that isoproterenol given prior to a repeated coronary artery occlusion increased the severity and extent of the ischaemic injury. On the other hand, the effect of isoproterenol on the occlusion-induced ST segment elevation was markedly reduced when the lipolytic effect of the drug was inhibited by β-pyridyl-carbinol, probably because of the reduced oxygen demand.

Oliver. Did you say that in spite of the reduction of ST elevation by 30 or 40 per cent, there is still the same increase in plasma creatine phosphokinase?

Mjøs. There is an inverse relationship between ST segment elevation and CPK-activity in the heart. In other words, reduction of ST segment elevation by inhibition of lipolysis was followed by a higher level of CPK-activity in the heart than anticipated from the magnitude of ST segment elevation produced by coronary occlusion alone (i.e., without any treatment).

Kurien. It seems likely that there is a redistribution of blood flow in favour of the non-ischaemic myocardium; a 'coronary steal'. It will be very interesting to know if Dr Maseri were able to show in an ischaemic preparation whether the distribution of substrates affects the distribution of coronary flow.

Parratt. I would like to come back to this very interesting finding of the elevation of myocardial oxygen consumption by FFA without a change in myocardial contractility. One of the most pronounced effects of catecholamines on the myocardium is to increase heat production and this can be shown both *in vivo* and *in vitro*. Gibbs has shown *in vitro* that this is partially dependent upon the change in the length of the muscle but there is also a length independent component in heat production. I wonder whether it is this component that is increased by FFA? We must remember that about 70 per cent of the energy of the heart is lost as heat and if FFA are increasing this particular contribution to heat loss, then this would account for the raised oxygen consumption without a change in external work or in contractility.

Mjøs. Since energy provided by myocardial oxygen consumption is transformed into metabolic heat within the myocardium and to external work and, since myocardial performance is not influenced by the uptake of FFA, it follows that metabolic heat production must rise during enhanced uptake of FFA in the myocardium. In other experiments, metabolic heat production in the left ventricular wall in open-chest dogs was estimated from the rate of heat accumulation during acute coronary artery occlusion by recording the initial rise in temperature. The results showed that raised plasma FFA by Intralipid/heparin or isoproterenol i.v. induced a rise in local metabolic rate of the same order of magnitude as that measured as $M\dot{V}O_2$. A metabolic stimulation by FFA was thus confirmed.

Wallace. Before we can interpret any data in relation to nicotinic acid, it is necessary to determine its effect on total and regional coronary blood flow. We cannot at present assume that coronary flow remains unaltered. Secondly, there are a number of potential problems with the ST segment mapping technique. For instance, there is an evolution of the ST segment after coronary occlusion and, therefore, to interpret ST segment changes one has to be meticulous about the time relationship. Finally, you appeared to show that the heart dilated with no increase in oxygen consumption, yet you claim that fatty acids increase oxygen consumption.

Mjøs. High concentrations of FFA (within the clinical range) raised $M\dot{V}O_2$ when there was free coronary blood flow due to increased myocardial oxygen extraction, while mechanical activity of the heart was unchanged. In the experiment you mentioned the heart was 'oxygen-limited' as a result of reducing coronary blood flow by about 20 per cent before raising plasma FFA. Without further increased coronary flow, $M\dot{V}O_2$ could not rise, since oxygen extraction was already maximal and coronary blood flow was kept constant. However, due to the increased oxygen demand by FFA, oxygen was 'stolen' from processes that would uphold cardiac contractility, resulting in further dilatation of the heart and depressed contractility.

Secondly, I agree that it will be of interest to study distribution flow in the heart during these conditions, instead of measuring only total left coronary blood flow.

Thirdly, we have carefully standardized our ST segment mapping after coronary artery occlusion. It is evident that ST segment elevations may be obtained independent of ischaemia. It is therefore of importance to correlate ST segment elevations with other indices of ischaemia, such as loss of CPK-activity in the heart muscle.

Julian. First, may I ask why you used Ronicol? I thought this had quite general vascular effects which would affect heart work irrespective of any effect it might have on FFA. Secondly, you say that FFA are increasing oxygen demand and that is having a deleterious effect on the ischaemic myocardium. If that is the immediate mechanism should not a better supply of oxygen remedy this and does it do so?

Mjøs. First, Ronicol (β-pyridyl-carbinol, the alcohol corresponding to nicotinic acid) is known to be oxidized to nicotinic acid in the liver and to act through nicotinic acid. We frequently used β-pyridyl-carbinol instead of nicotinic acid, since β-pyridyl-carbinol is reported to induce fewer vascular changes in man, while the anti-lipolytic properties are about equal. We found no effect of nicotinic acid or β-pyridyl-carbinol on myocardial haemodynamic parameters in dogs.

Secondly, an improved supply of oxygen should be beneficial, but we have not tested it in the way you suggest.

Opie. In our baboon preparation, the measures to change ST segment have been extremely disappointing. Glucose-potassium-insulin appeared to have little or no effect on ST segment changes although it is possible to achieve minor modifications in cellular metabolism. On the whole it seemed that an infarct was an infarct. If any of the proposed metabolic manipulations are to have an effect, they must reach and involve the ischaemic myocardium. I would support Dr Wallace most strongly that more knowledge is urgently needed concerning the ischaemic myocardium.

Riemersma. Did you measure FFA in the tissue and, secondly, should you measure heat evolved in the myocardium during ischaemia? You suggested that there was a direct uncoupling effect by FFA on the myocardial metabolism. Did you really mean to say that? If so, it is surely necessary to measure FFA concentrations in the tissue to determine whether this is possible or not?

Mjøs. Measurements of intracellular concentrations or turnover of FFA are reported to be very difficult, but are of major importance. A reliable method for measurements of intracellular FFA (or glycerol) would be of great value to workers in this field.

RELATIONSHIP OF ISCHAEMIA TO LOCAL MYOCARDIAL OXYGEN REQUIREMENTS

M. I. M. Noble

Introduction

The layers of left ventricular muscle lying near the cavity, the subendocardium, are more susceptible to ischaemia than the superficial layers, the subepicardium. When there is critical narrowing of all the vessels supplying the left ventricle, the electrocardiographic signs of subendocardial ischaemia develop.[1] In the human it is not possible to prove that subendocardial ischaemia accompanies these ECG signs. However, a few cases progress to subendocardial infarction which can be verified at necropsy.[2] A more usual outcome is full thickness infarction.[1] The phenomenon of subendocardial ischaemia can be studied in experimental animals.[3]

Possible factors contributing to increased susceptibility to ischaemia of the subendocardium

1. *Are the oxygen requirements of the subendocardium greater than those of the subepicardium?*

In order to answer this question directly, it would be necessary to measure the oxygen consumption of subepicardium and subendocardial muscle separately. This would entail collecting coronary venous blood from each layer separately, a technique which has not been achieved to my knowledge. It is therefore necessary to come to an opinion on this question from indirect evidence. Much has been written on the mechanical contractile determinants of oxygen consumption. There is little doubt that active force (tension) development is the major determinant[4] and this is the only factor, which, in any given circumstances, could be different in the subendocardial and subepicardial parts of the ventricular wall. Although total force in the wall of the heart has been measured[5 6 7] no separate measurements of subendocardial and subepicardial wall force have been made to my knowledge. Such an experiment would require a force gauge inside the ventricular cavity coupled to the inner half of the wall while a second gauge on the surface of the ventricle was coupled to the outer half of the wall. Calculations of force (stress) distribution across the wall, based on models, must be dismissed as speculation at the present time because they are not susceptible to experimental verification.

It is therefore necessary to seek even more indirect evidence, namely from estimates of the distribution of myocardial blood flow across the left ventricular wall. The reasoning here is that tissue having a higher oxygen consumption will also have a higher blood flow. Does the subendocardium have a higher blood flow than the subepicardium? According to some authors[8 9 10] it has, others found no difference in blood flow to the two areas,[11 12 13] while a third group found that there was less blood flow to the subendocardium than to the subepicardium.[14 15 16] These different results are due to technical problems on which I will not elaborate here.

Recent studies on regional blood flow have been revolutionized by the introduction of the radioactive microsphere method[17] and its application to the myocardium.[18] The results with this method are critically dependent on microsphere size, the apparent subendocardial: subepicardial blood flow ratio decreasing (from above 1·0) with decreasing microsphere size until, with 8-10 micron diameter, the microspheres are found to distribute uniformly across the ventricular wall.[18 19] The conclusions from these studies, supported by the results of careful measurements using diffusable indicators,[12 13] is that there is no difference in blood flow to the subendocardium and subepicardium under normal circumstances. There is thus no reason to suppose from this evidence that there is any difference in oxygen consumption between the two layers of muscle, although this must remain an uncertain inference in the absence of the A-V difference measurements alluded to at the beginning of this section.

Another approach would be to measure the tissue P_{O_2} of the different layers of the myocardium. Tissue P_{O_2} measurements are fraught with difficulties.[20] However, Lübbers and Schuchhardt[21] reported no difference in tissue P_{O_2} between the inner and outer layers of the myocardium. If this finding is correct, it might be reasonable to infer similar P_{O_2} (and O_2 content) in the venous blood draining the two areas. This evidence, together with the equality of blood flow to the subendocardium and subepicardium, would support the view that the oxygen consumption of the two layers is similar. In section 3 below, changes in subendocardial oxygen demand are assumed to parallel changes in total oxygen consumption.

2. *Is the subendocardium more difficult to perfuse?*

It is well established that blood flow decreases during systole due to occlusion of intramyocardial vessels during contraction.[22] Are subendocardial vessels compressed more than subepicardial vessels? An answer to this question can be obtained from studies of intramyocardial pressure. There has been considerable disagreement about the advantages and disadvantages of the various methods of making this measurement. These arguments are discussed by Van der Meer *et al.*[23] who measured the pressure required to produce flow through a venous segment implanted in the ventricular wall. In the deep layers, some authors found pressures very much higher than left ventricular pressure, e.g. Kirk and Honig,[24] some found lower pressures still in excess of left ventricular pressure,[23] while others found similar values to left ventricular pressure (e.g. Brandi and McGregor[25]). However, all studies on this subject are agreed about the fact that intramural pressure is a function of relative myocardial depth. This means that the subendocardial vessels are subject to a surrounding pressure during systole which is greater than coronary perfusion pressure, and flow in them must therefore stop during this period. The subendocardium is therefore totally dependent on diastolic perfusion. This is not the case in the subepicardium where intramural pressure during systole is less than coronary perfusion pressure. Another fact that emerges from these studies is that subendocardial intramyocardial pressure is a function of left ventricular pressure in both systole and diastole. Since there is no subendocardial flow during systole, subendocardial perfusion depends on the difference between coronary perfusion pressure and left ventricular pressure in diastole. Thus, subendocardial ischaemia develops in the dog with perfused coronary arteries when the coronary artery pressure is reduced below 70 mmHg and the left ventricular diastolic pressure is raised above 25 mmHg.[3] This pressure gradient is not the only factor which affects the volume of oxygenated blood delivered to the subendocardium because this will also depend on the duration of diastole in relation to the total duration of the cardiac cycle. This ratio (diastolic time/total time) decreases with increasing heart rate and extreme tachycardia can result in subendocardial ischaemia.[19] These factors are illustrated in Figure 19, 1 where aortic (coronary perfusion) pressure, left ventricular pressure and phasic left coronary artery blood flow are displayed against time. The volume of blood delivered to

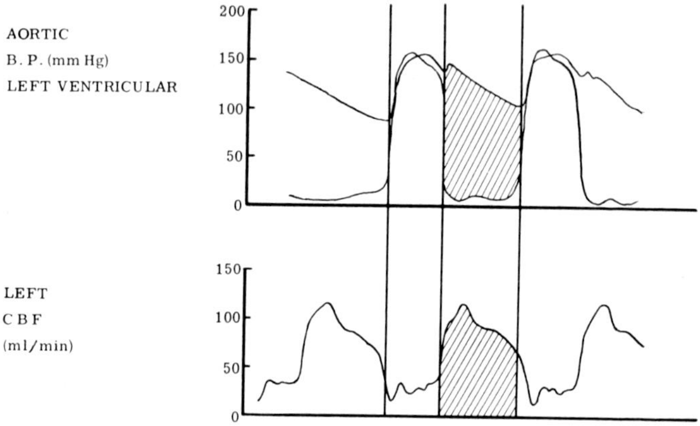

FIG. 19, 1. Aortic (coronary perfusion) pressure, left ventricular pressure and left anterior descending coronary artery flow (left CBF) displayed against time. Subendocardial oxygen supply is dependent on the difference between coronary perfusion pressure and left ventricular pressure during diastole and the duration of the diastole (the cross hatched area, DPTI). Myocardial oxygen demand is mainly determined by the area under the left ventricular (or aortic) pressure curve during systole (TTI) (between first two vertical lines) and left ventricular size.

the subendocardium (and therefore the oxygen supply) depends on the shaded area between the two pressures in diastole. Hoffman's group call this the diastolic pressure time index (DPTI) (using left atrial pressure as an approximation to left ventricular diastolic pressure).

3. *Relationship between subendocardial oxygen supply and demand*
If the DPTI is adequate to maintain subendocardial perfusion under certain control conditions, it may become inadequate if the oxygen demand of the muscle increases. As was mentioned previously, the predominant factor determining oxygen consumption

is force development. An index of oxygen demand could therefore be obtained by integrating wall force over the duration of systole. Wall force is a function of both ventricular pressure and cavity size.[5] In spite of this, Sarnoff[26] suggested using left ventricular or aortic pressure integrated over the duration of systole (called the tension time index or TTI) * This index was also adopted by Hoffman's group in their study, the balance between perfusion and oxygen demand being assessed by the ratio DPTI/TTI. This concept of balance between perfusion and oxygen demand proved useful in predicting the circumstances under which subendocardial ischaemia develops experimentally and provides a rational basis for similar predictions in man. For instance, it might be predicted that the defence reaction accompanied by great tachycardia and hypertension would produce subendocardial ischaemia particularly if the effective perfusion pressure of the myocardium was reduced by the presence of a coronary artery stenosis.

In what other ways can the adequacy of the oxygen supply to the subendocardium be assessed? One useful method is to measure the reactive hyperaemia that follows a period of coronary artery occlusion. Normally coronary blood flow increases so that the time integrated flow 'lost' during the period of occlusion is overpaid during the period of hyperaemia. When the ratio of blood flow in the subendocardium to blood flow in the subepicardium is reduced below 1·0, the reactive hyperaemic response is impaired.[19] The reactive hyperaemic response can therefore be used as an indication of the adequacy of myocardial perfusion. A practical example of this was the recent study of Reneman and Spencer[27] who measured the reactive hyperaemic response after coronary saphenous vein by-pass surgery. A poor response indicated poor anastomosis or further coronary stenosis peripheral to the site of bypass and the likelihood that the operation would be of no benefit to the patient.

* TTI probably underestimates the oxygen demand following manoeuvres (designed to test the validity of the index DPTI/TTI) such as supravalvular and distal aortic occlusion.[19] These not only raise ventricular systolic pressure but also dilate the ventricle so that the rise in wall force is greater than the increase in pressure.

SUMMARY

In an attempt to understand the greater susceptibility to ischaemia of the subendocardium compared with the subepicardium, indirect evidence is presented to suggest that the oxygen demand of the subendocardium is not in excess of that of the subepicardium. The major factor contributing to the subendocardial ischaemia susceptibility appears to be the total dependence of the subendocardial microcirculation on diastolic perfusion due to the distribution of compressive forces within the left ventricular wall. Ischaemia of the subendocardium in the presence of normal coronary arteries depends on the balance between (a) myocardial oxygen consumption and (b) perfusion factors, namely (i) the difference between coronary perfusion pressure and ventricular diastolic pressure and (ii) the ratio of the duration of diastole to the duration of the cardiac cycle.

REFERENCES

1 Master, A. M., Jaffe, H. L., Field, L. E., Donoso, E. (1956). Acute coronary insufficiency: its differential diagnosis and treatment. *Annals of Internal Medicine* **45,** 561-581.

2 Levine, H. D. & Ford, R. V. (1950). Subendocardial infarction: report of 6 cases and critical survey of literature. *Circulation* **1,** 246-263.

3 Salisbury, P. F., Cross, C. E. & Rieben, P. A. (1963). Acute ischemia of inner layers of ventricular wall. *American Heart Journal* **66,** 650-656.

4 McDonald, R. H. Jr. (1966). Developed tension: a major determinant of myocardial oxygen consumption. *American Journal of Physiology* **210,** 351-356.

5 Hefner, L. L., Sheffield, L. T., Cobbs, G. C. & Klip, W. (1962). Relation between mural force and pressure in the left ventricular of the dog. *Circulation Research* **11,** 654-663.

6 Feigl, E. O., Simon, G. E. & Fry, D. L. (1967). Auxotonic and isometric cardiac force transducers. *Journal of Applied Physiology* **23,** 597-600.

7 Lewartowski, B., Sedek, G. & Okalaka, A. (1972). Direct measurement of the tension within left ventricular wall of the dog heart. *Cardiovascular Research* **6,** 28-35.

8 Lowe, W. D. & Tyler, M. D. (1965). Effect of hypoxemia and hyper capnia on regional distribution of myocardial blood flow. *American Journal of Physiology* **208,** 1211-1216.

9 Griggs, D. M. & Nakamura, Y. (1968). Effect of coronary constriction on myocardial distribution of iodoantipyrine ^{131}I. *American Journal of Physiology* **215,** 1081-1086.

10 Fortuin, N. J., Pitt, B. & Kaihara, S. (1968). The distribution of regional myocardial blood flow in the dog. *Circulation* **38,** Suppl. VI, 77.

11 Palmer, W. H., Fam, W. M. & McGregor, M. (1966). The effect of coronary vasodilation (dipyridamole-induced) on the myocardial distribution of tritiated water. *Canadian Journal of Physiology and Pharmacology* **44,** 777-782.

12 Moir, T. W. & De Bra, D. W. (1967). Effect of left ventricular hypertension ischemia and vasoactive drugs on the myocardial distribution of coronary flow. *Circulation Research* **21,** 65-74.

13 COTARELLI, R. & LEVY, M. N. (1963). Intraventricular pressure and the distribution of coronary blood flow. *Circulation Research* **12,** 322-327.
14 MOIR, T. W. & DE BRA, D. W. (1965). Measurement of the endocardial distribution of left ventricular coronary blood flow by Rb-86 chloride. *American Heart Journal* **69,** 795-800.
15 BRANDI, G., FAM, W. M. & MCGREGOR, M. (1968). Measurement of coronary blood flow in local areas of myocardium using Xenon 133. *Journal of Applied Physiology* **24,** 446-450.
16 KIRK, E. S. & HONIG, C. R. (1964). Non uniform distribution of blood flow and gradients of oxygen tension within the heart. *American Journal of Physiology* **207,** 661-668.
17 RUDOLPH, A. M. & HEYMANN, M. A. (1967). The circulation of the fetus in utero. *Circulation Research* **21,** 163-184.
18 DOMENECH, R. J., HOFFMAN, J. I. E., NOBLE, M. I. M., SAUNDERS, K. B., HENSON, J. R. & SUBIJANTO, S. (1969). Total regional coronary blood flow measured by radioactive microspheres in conscious and anesthetized dogs. *Circulation Research* **25,** 581-596.
19 BUCKBERG, G. D., FIXLER, D. E., ARCHIE, J. P. & HOFFMAN, J. I. E. (1972). Experimental subendocardial ischemia in dogs with normal coronary arteries. *Circulation Research* **30,** 67-81.
20 CATER, D. B. (1964). In *Oxygen in the Animal Organism,* p. 230. Edited by: F. Dickens, and E. Neil. London: Pergamon Press.
21 LÜBBERS, D. W. & SCHUCHHARDT, S. (1971). *Proceedings of the International Union of Physiological Science* **8,** 129.
22 GREGG, D. E., FISCHER, L. C. (1963). In *Handbook of Physiology: Circulation* p. 1517. Edited by: W. F. Hamilton and P. Dow. Washington: American Physiological Society.
23 VAN DER MEER, J. J., RENEMAN, R. S., SCHNEIDER, H. & WIEBERDINK, J. (1970). A technique for estimation of intramyocardial pressure in acute and chronic experiments. *Cardiovascular Research* **4,** 132-140.
24 KIRK, E. S. & HONIG, C. R. (1964). An experimental and theoretical analysis of myocardial tissue pressure. *American Journal of Physiology* **207,** 361-367.
25 BRANDIE, G. & MCGREGOR, M. (1969). Intramural pressure in the left ventricle of the dog. *Cardiovascular Research* **3,** 472-475.
26. SARNOFF, S. J., BRAUNWALD, E., WELCH, G. H. JR., CASE, R. B., STAINSBY, W. N., & MACRUZ, R. (1958). Hemodynamic determinants of oxygen consumption of the heart with special reference to the tension-time index. *American Journal of Physiology* **192,** 148-156.
27 RENEMAN, R. S. & SPENCER, M. P. (1972). The use of diastolic reactive hyperemia to evaluate the coronary vascular system. *The Annals of Thoracic Surgery* **13,** 477-487.

DISCUSSION

Parratt. I would like to comment on the problem of increasing oxygenation and blood flow in the subendocardial layers during acute myocardial ischaemia. These results (Fig. 19, 2) were obtained with Dr Ledingham and Mr Marshall at the Western Infirmary in Glasgow. The model, which was the one I described previously, enables blood flow to be measured simultaneously in the normal myocardium and in the ischaemic region and also allows for blood sampling from the normal myocardium and from the infarct. We can thus calculate myocardial oxygen consumption or uptake. We have looked at the effect of a number of drugs, including glucagon, isoprenaline, propanolol and the three very different drugs illustrated in Figure 19, 2. Carbochromen, which is a very active coronary vasodilator drug, increases flow in the normal myocardium, but does not change flow in the ischaemic region: presumably this

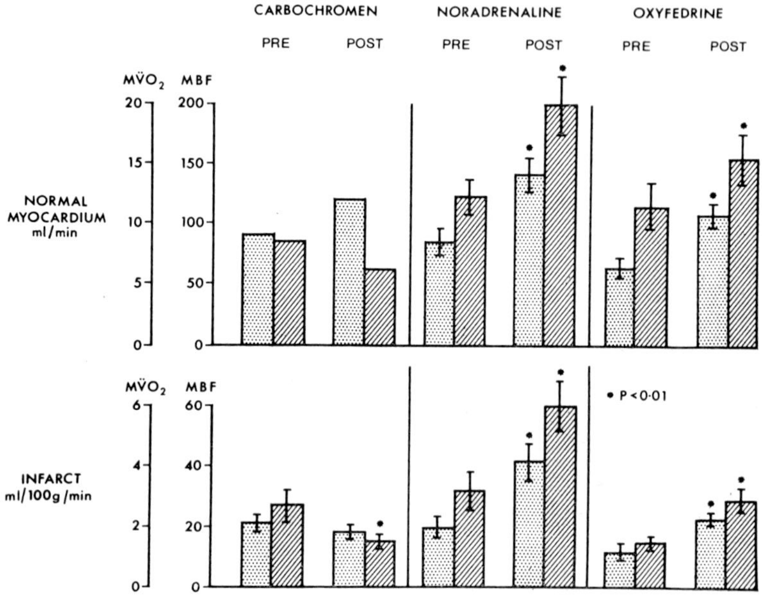

FIG. 19, 2. Top half: changes in the infarct area. Bottom half: changes in the normal myocardium.
First stippled block in each pair represents flow. The second block represents oxygen consumption.

is because the arterioles are already fully dilated in this situation. In some dogs you can get actual 'stealing' of blood from the infarct to the normal myocardium. Noradrenaline, which increases perfusion pressure, will also increase flow and oxygen consumption both in the normal myocardium and in the ischaemic region 2 to 3 hours after ligation. Oxyfedrine is a partial agonist of β-receptors which means it will stimulate β-receptors and then eventually block them. This drug increases blood flow through the infarct. This particular study with oxyfedrine was done four to five hours after ligation when flow was about 12 ml/100 g/min. After oxyfedrine, flow in the infarct was doubled and there was also an increase in flow and in oxygen consumption in the normal myocardium. Two conclusions can be made about changing flow in the ischaemic myocardium: first, you can't do anything to the vasculature if the vessels are fully dilated; and, second, vasodilator drugs will then fail to increase flow. You can only improve flow in two ways: either by increasing the perfusion pressure (which is what happens with noradrenaline) or by decreasing end-diastolic volume and the size of the heart by giving a drug like oxyfedrine.

Muir. I am interested in the vein-graft preparation implanted into the myocardium. First, there is the problem of recording the true intramyocardial pressure, because of fibrosis. Secondly, you did not mention the possible effects of venous pressure changes.

Noble. I didn't detail all the different ways of measuring intramyocardial pressure. The objection you raise to this preparation is a valid one but the other methods available are even worse. I think it is justifiable to ignore myocardial venous pressure because the intramyocardial pressure around the vessels is so much greater. It is rather like a lung in which the alveolar pressure is much in excess of pulmonary venous pressure, when the influence of pulmonary venous pressure is virtually negligible.

Maseri. To comment on this last point, I think that the 'waterfall' phenomenon you mentioned in relation to the lung can probably be applied to the myocardium in that the driving pressure of flow through the heart at various layers from the endo to epicardium depends simply on the difference between coronary arterial pressure and the tissue or venous pressure whichever is higher. This phenomenon assumes greater importance when an elevated left ventricular end-diastolic pressure results in a higher intramyocardial pressure during diastole.

The second point is that the ratio DPTI/TTI was developed earlier in 1968 by Griggs and Nakamura (*Amer. J. Physiol.* (1968) **215:**1081-1086) and should be acknowledged.

Thirdly you may not get reactive hyperaemia after occlusion of the main supply because of adequate collateral arterial blood supply, but still you could have a reduced coronary reserve.

Noble. I agree with your first two statements, but I disagree with your third. Reneman and Spencer[27] showed that an impaired reactive hyperaemia response occurred when the anastomosis wasn't done correctly or when there was distal disease or when the area supplied was already well supplied by collateral flow, in which case it was not necessary to do a by-pass graft. I don't really understand what 'coronary reserve' means and I would like you to explain it to me.

Maseri. The concept and term 'coronary reserve' was introduced by Gregg. When one occludes a coronary vessel for 5 to 20 sec a flowmeter implanted on it will, on reopening the vessel, record a flow 3 to 6 times larger than the preocclusive level. If the lumen of this vessel is chronically restricted following occlusion, the flow through it will increase by only 1 or 2 times, even if basal flow is unchanged. Furthermore, if the stenosis is critical, flow may not increase at all after occlusion. This indicates that there can be no further increase in flow through the vessel even under the maximum vasodilatation produced by complete occlusion. The 'coronary reserve' of such a vessel is said to be zero. This is related to the concept that flow is controlled by two resistances in series, namely R.1 (large vessels: usually negligible) and R.2 (arterioles and resistance vessels: normally very high). R.2 determines 'coronary reserve' as there is a point below which R.2 cannot be decreased after obstruction of a large vessel. Reactive hyperaemia may not be evident on transient occlusion of a stenosed vessel if there is good distal perfusion by a collateral circulation. This is because the myocardium beyond the obstruction is perfused by the collateral circulation and is not exposed to ischaemia. The coronary reserve of that territory may be reduced but to test the extent of the reduction it would be necessary to occlude temporarily the collateral circulation too.

Noble. What you are saying is that if you have constant coronary flow and the distal perfusion pressure is reduced, then clearly there is coronary vasodilatation. I would suggest that it could be considered that this vasodilatation is due to ischaemic metabolites being released; the consequent change in the reactive hyperaemia response can be considered an area of dispute if thought of in this way. It just depends how you define what is happening.

Jennings. There is an alternative hypothesis as to why subendocardial infarction is common; this is that subendocardial myocardial cells are more susceptible to injury because they are structurally or metabolically more sensitive than subepicardial myocardial cells. We have examined this question in some detail in the dog and so far there are no significant structural, chemical or metabolic data that such a difference exists. I therefore think your hypothesis and observations relative to the blood flow are probably correct.

THE EFFECT OF ISCHAEMIA ON MYOCARDIAL FUNCTION

JOHN O. PARKER

WHEN myocardial ischaemia occurs, the oxygen supply may fail to meet myocardial oxygen requirements. Manifestations of ischaemia include pain, electrocardiographic abnormalities, metabolic derangements, liberation of vasoactive substances and dysfunction of the left ventricle.

In man, important alterations of ventricular function develop during myocardial ischaemia. The first observations in man were made by Müller and Rørvik in 1958.[1] These investigators studied patients with coronary artery disease without cardiomegaly or cardiac failure and found elevation of pulmonary arterial and wedge pressure during exertional angina. Johnson and co-workers[2] reported observations in one patient who developed acute coronary insufficiency pain during right heart catheterization, which was accompanied by marked pulmonary hypertension. This was abolished when pain was relieved by sublingual nitroglycerin. Ross and associates[3] reported the development of increased left ventricular end-diastolic pressure (LVEDP) in two patients who developed angina pectoris during selective coronary arteriography. Dimond and Benchimol[4] studied patients with coronary artery disease during exertional angina and were the first to demonstrate elevated LVEDP in this situation. Cohen and associates,[5] however, reported quite different results and showed in their series of patients studied during exertional angina that the maximal increase in LVEDP was 3 mmHg.

In 1965 we first reported our experience in patients studied during supine leg exercise on a bicycle ergometer. In this and later studies, we have found that during angina pectoris precipitated by exercise, the LVEDP was consistently elevated.[6-10] Figure 20, 1 shows LVEDP at rest and during exertional angina in 55 patients without cardiomegaly or signs of cardiac failure (Table 20, 1). The average LVEDP rose from 10 mmHg at rest to 33 mmHg during exertional angina. This elevation of LVEDP usually developed before the onset of pain. In 25 normal patients the average LVEDP rose from 8 mmHg at rest to 10 mmHg during exercise while in 40 patients with coronary artery disease who did not experience angina during this period of exercise, the LVEDP rose from 10 to 17 mmHg. The

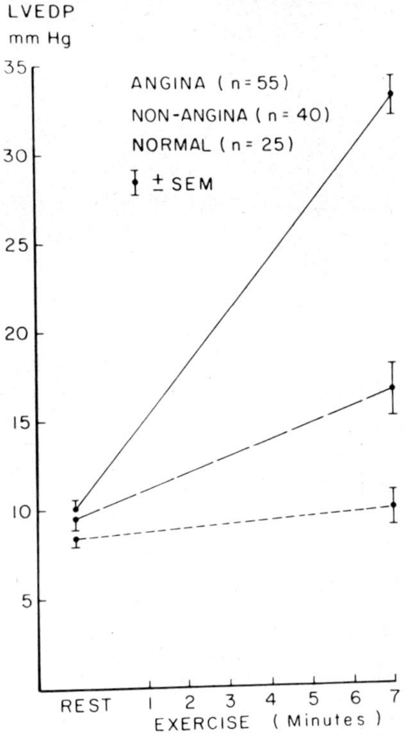

FIG. 20, 1. Left ventricular end-diastolic pressure (LVEDP) at rest and during exercise in three groups of patients.

pattern in this group was variable, ranging from a normal response to one indistinguishable from patients who experienced angina pectoris. Elevation of LVEDP during exertional angina was accompanied by pulmonary hypertension, the average pulmonary arterial mean pressure increasing from 14 to 38 mmHg during exertional angina. In the non-angina group, the pulmonary arterial mean pres-

Table 20, 1 *Summary of haemodynamic data at rest and during exercise*

	BAm (mmHg)	LVEDP (mmHg)	PAm (mmHg)	HR (beats/min)	CI (L/min/m²)	LVSWI (g-m/m²)	SERI ml/sec/m²	TTI mmHg/min × 10⁻¹
Angina Group (n=55)								
Rest	102±14·4	10±3·8	14±3·0	78±13·7	3·92± ·52	49±10·6	118±16·3	1168±301
Exercise	120±17·2	33±7·4	38±7·5	122±18·2	4·58± ·90	45±13·5	122±21·1	2131±517
Non-Angina Group (n=40)								
Rest	96±10·8	10±4·1	14±3·3	76±11	3·10±0·67	48±12·7	128±32·1	1081±241
Exercise	114±11·9	17±9·1	26±7·0	123±19	5·77±1·19	63±17·2	151±33·3	1877±337
Normal Group (n=25)								
Rest	91± 9·3	8±2·0	13±2·7	76±11	3·34±0·59	49± 9·1	137±28·9	965±160
Exercise	106±11·5	10±5·0	22±5·4	123±16	6·29±1·16	66±13·2	170±43·7	1949±352

Data shown are mean ± Standard Deviation.

BAm = mean brachial artery pressure.
LVEDP = left ventricular end-diastolic pressure.
PAm = mean pulmonary artery pressure.
HR = heart rate.
CI = cardiac index.
LVSWI = left ventricular stroke work index.
SERI = systolic ejection rate index.
TTI = tension time index.

sure was 26 mmHg while in the normal subjects this averaged 22 mmHg during exercise.

The elevation of left ventricular filling pressures during exertional angina was accompanied by a subnormal increase in cardiac index and by an abnormal response of left ventricular stroke work index (LVSWI). The average LVSWI fell from 49 to 45 g-m/m^2 in

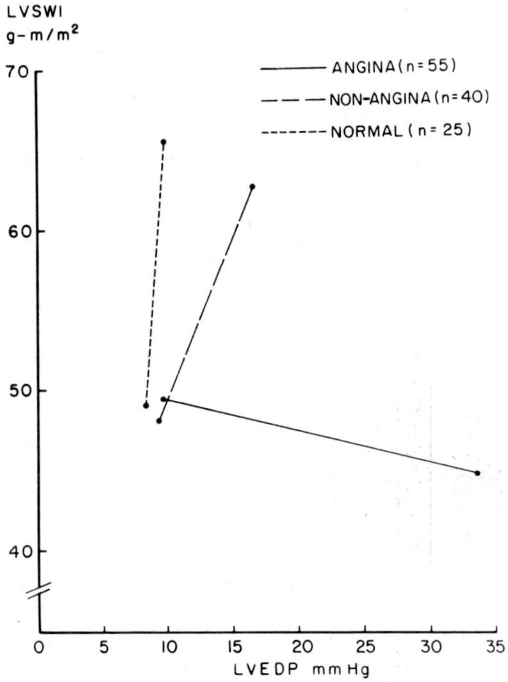

FIG. 20, 2. Relationship between LVSWI and LVEDP showing depressed left ventricular function in the ischaemic group during exertional angina.

contrast to the normal subjects where LVSWI increased from 49 to 66 g-m/m^2 during exercise. In the non-angina group the LVSWI increased from 48 to 63 g-m/m^2 with exercise. In relating left ventricular filling pressure to stroke work, it is apparent that during myocardial ischaemia induced by exercise there is depression of left ventricular function (Fig. 20, 2). Subsequent studies have confirmed these observations.[11 12]

Table 20, 2 *Summary of haemodynamic data before and during pacing*

	BAm (mmHg)	LVEDP (mmHg)	PAm (mmHg)	HR (beats/min)	CI (L/min/m²)	LVSWI (g-m/m²)	TTI mmHg/min × 10⁻¹	dp/dt mmHg/sec
Angina Group (n=56)								
Control	103 ± 14·8	10 ± 3·7	13 ± 3·0	80 ± 13·6	2·94 ± ·56	46 ± 9·3	1139 ± 297	1352 ± 465
Pacing	117 ± 20·9	9 ± 7·0	21 ± 7·7	145 ± 10·8	3·02 ± ·79	31 ± 10·3	2153 ± 406	1738 ± 601
Post-Pacing		22 ± 7·0						
Non-Angina Group (n=20)								
Control	99 ± 11·6	10 ± 2·9	14 ± 2·9	79 ± 15·7	3·15 ± ·47	50 ± 13·4	1081 ± 241	1529 ± 590
Pacing	106 ± 12·2	4 ± 2·3	16 ± 4·0	138 ± 12·7	3·37 ± ·68	33 ± 8·5	1877 ± 337	2029 ± 890
Post-Pacing		12 ± 3·4						
Normal Group (n=23)								
Control	91 ± 11·4	8 ± 2·6	12 ± 2·6	74 ± 11·1	2·94 ± ·36	45 ± 8·4	1067 ± 232	1267 ± 425
Pacing	95 ± 12·3	3 ± 2·4	14 ± 2·3	138 ± 9·2	3·10 ± ·55	28 ± 6·1	1709 ± 235	1765 ± 773
Post-Pacing		10 ± 3·0						

Data shown are mean ± Standard Deviation.

BAm = mean brachial artery pressure.
LVEDP = left ventricular end-diastolic pressure.
PAm = mean pulmonary artery pressure.
HR = heart rate.
CI = cardiac index.
LVSWI = left ventricular stroke work index.
SERI = systolic ejection rate index.
TTI = tension time index.

Atrial pacing has been employed as a stress to induce angina[13-15] and as well to assess haemodynamic[16-19] and metabolic function in patients with coronary artery disease.[16-18] Atrial pacing has been suggested as a superior stress for evaluating patients with coronary artery disease as it is not associated with many of the metabolic and haemodynamic alterations that occur during exercise. This technique may also be more useful in assessing the results of surgical procedures in coronary artery disease as it is more precise and probably less hazardous than exercise. The striking changes in left

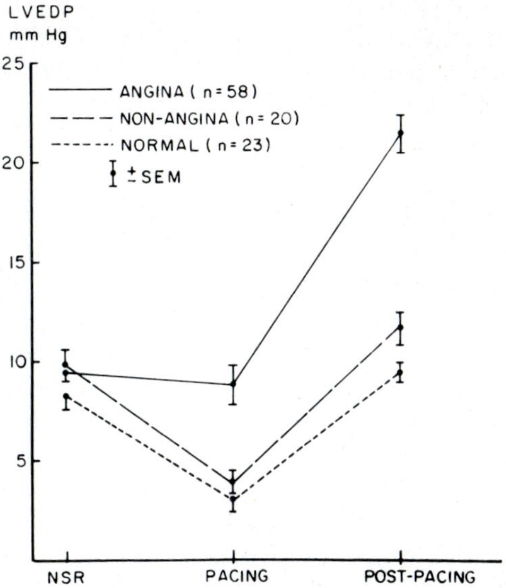

FIG. 20, 3. LVEDP fell during pacing in the normal subjects and in the non-angina group and increased abruptly to control levels in the post-pacing period. The angina group showed no decline during pacing and there was an abnormal increase in LVEDP in the post-pacing period.

ventricular filling pressures seen during exertional angina do not commonly occur during ischaemia precipitated by atrial pacing although haemodynamic alterations indicative of depression of left ventricular function are readily demonstrated.[18] Atrial pacing was carried out at rates of approximately 140/min in 21 normal patients and 78 patients with coronary artery disease. Fifty-eight patients developed angina during pacing while 20 patients had no chest pain. Cardiac index was not altered by atrial pacing at these rates, even in the presence of ischaemia, and thus the stroke index decreased (Table 20, 2). Pacing induced minor changes in brachial artery pressure and thus there was a fall in left ventricular stroke work index (LVSWI) during atrial pacing. Through the Starling relationship this decrease in LVSWI should have been accompanied by a decrease in left ventricular filling pressures and in normal subjects there was a regular decline in LVEDP (Fig. 20, 3). On cessation of atrial pacing and return to sinus rhythm, the stroke index and stroke work rose abruptly to normal and LVEDP returned to control levels. A similar response was seen in patients with coronary artery disease who did not show clinical or biochemical evidence of ischaemia during tachycardia. By relating these changes in stroke work to simultaneous changes in LVEDP, one can construct ventricular function curves (Fig. 20, 4). In patients with coronary artery disease who developed ischaemia during atrial pacing, there was a similar decline in LVSWI but the average LVEDP did not show the expected decline. Some patients showed a decrease in LVEDP and a few rose to very abnormal levels but the majority showed no significant change. The most consistent abnormality seen during angina precipitated by atrial pacing was abrupt elevation of LVEDP when pacing was temporarily interrupted and during the immediate post-pacing period. This post-pacing LVEDP averaged 22 mmHg in contrast to 12 mmHg in the non-angina group and 10 mmHg in normal subjects (Fig. 20, 3). If the changes in stroke work are plotted against LVEDP, it is apparent that left ventricular function is depressed in ischaemia (Fig. 20, 4).

This type of analysis can be extended by measuring stroke work or stroke index and LVEDP at multiple heart rates during atrial pacing and thus obtain a pacing ventricular function curve. Figure 20, 5 shows such a study in one patient where different pacing rates were employed to construct such a curve in the absence of ischaemia. With a longer period of atrial pacing, angina developed and data were obtained at multiple heart rates while angina was present. This was made possible by pacing at rapid rates to maintain ischaemia between observations at lower heart rates. During ischaemia it was apparent from the shift of the ventricular function curve downwards and to the right that ventricular function is depressed in the ischaemic state.[19]

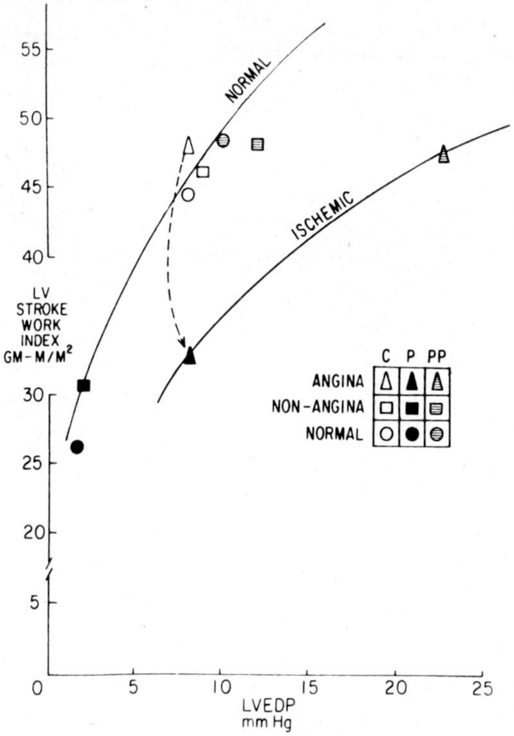

FIG. 20, 4. Ventricular function curves were drawn plotting LVEDP and LVSWI. During sinus rhythm (C), pacing (P) and in the post-pacing (PP) period, the normal and non-angina groups were on a normal ventricular function curve. During angina the patient moved to a depressed ventricular function curve.

We have considered the abnormal LVEDP during exercise and pacing to be a reflection of an increase in left ventricular volume and an indication that there is left ventricular failure during myocardial ischaemia. It must be considered, however, that the changes in filling pressure may reflect alterations in left ventricular diastolic compliance, in that the ischaemic ventricle is less compliant. Dwyer[20] recorded left ventriculograms during pacing-induced ischaemia and showed that left ventricular volume decreased less than in the normal subjects during pacing but only one patient showed an increase in volume during pacing-induced angina. He concluded that both a change in compliance and a volume change may be responsible for the elevated filling pressures during ischaemia.[20]

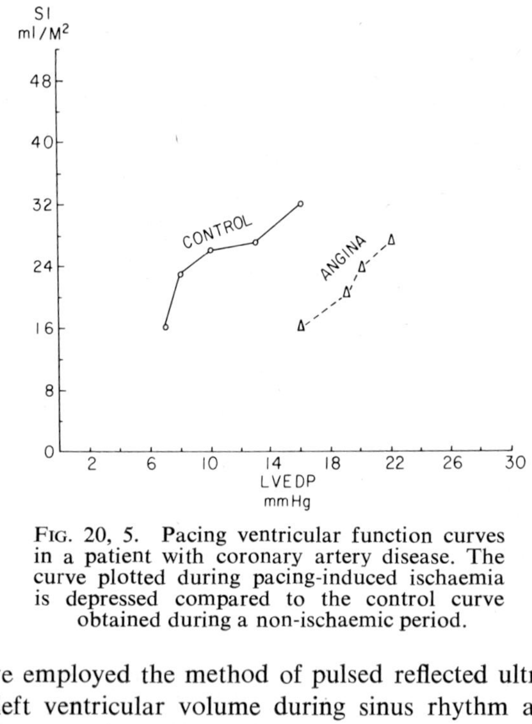

FIG. 20, 5. Pacing ventricular function curves in a patient with coronary artery disease. The curve plotted during pacing-induced ischaemia is depressed compared to the control curve obtained during a non-ischaemic period.

We have employed the method of pulsed reflected ultrasound to estimate left ventricular volume during sinus rhythm and during pacing-induced tachycardia. Left ventricular volume is normally calculated using a formula considering the heart to be a prolate ellipse.[21] This requires knowledge of the long axis and two short axes at right angles. The two short axes are equal and this permits the measurement of left ventricular volume by single plane ventriculography. In both systole and diastole the short axis is approximately one-half of the long axis and thus it is possible to obtain measurements of ventricular volume by knowing only one minor axis. With ultrasound, one can obtain a dimension which approximates the short axis of the left ventricle and studies have demonstrated a close correlation between left ventricular volumes recorded angiographically and by ultrasound.[22 23]

We have measured left ventricular diastolic volume (LVDV) during sinus rhythm, during atrial pacing and at points of interruption of pacing. In normal subjects LVDV decreased abruptly with tachycardia and remained low during atrial pacing. With an increase in heart rate from 84 to 150 beats/min, LVDV decreased from 84 to 60 ml. At points of interruption, LVDV returned to control values.

In patients with coronary artery disease, the LVDV also decreased during the early portion of the pacing period, falling from 136 to 95 ml with an increase in heart rate from 76 to 145 beats/min. During this early pacing period when ischaemia had not developed, the LVDV returned to values only slightly exceeding control at points of interruption, the average value being 143 ml. During the later period of pacing when ischaemia had developed, LVDV increased to 110 ml ($P<0{\cdot}005$) and at this time when pacing was interrupted the volume increased to 178 ml, a volume significantly greater than control ($P<0{\cdot}001$).

In an attempt to assess the left ventricular diastolic compliance, the proportion of LVDV contributed to by atrial systole was calculated for the angina group during the control period of sinus rhythm, during interruption of pacing when not ischaemic and during interruption of pacing during ischaemia. The percentage of LVDV due to atrial systole was 25 per cent, 22 per cent, and 23 per cent during these 3 periods. The change in diastolic pressure related to atrial systole at these periods was 7, 8 and 11 mmHg. It would be tempting to consider these greater changes in pressure as a manifestation of decreased ventricular compliance but assessment of left ventricular compliance in man is complicated because of the curvilinear relationship between pressure and volume and the different LVDV during these three phases of the study. In relating LVEDP to LVDV in the angina group, the pressure-volume relationships during ischaemia did not appear different from those obtained during the non-ischaemic phase.

Nitroglycerin is the oldest and most effective drug in the treatment of angina pectoris although its exact mode of action is still in doubt. The effects of nitroglycerin on the response to exercise in

Table 20, 3 *Summary of haemodynamic data at rest and during exercise before and after nitroglycerin*

	BAm (mmHg)	LVEDP (mmHg)	PAm (mmHg)	HR (beats/min)	CI (L/min/m²)	LVSWI (g-m/m²)	TTI mmHg/min × 10⁻¹
Angina Group (n=20)							
Rest	98 ± 11·8	10 ± 3·2	14 ± 3·4	77 ± 14·7	3·07 ± ·55	49 ± 13·0	1113 ± 276
Exercise	113 ± 14·5	33 ± 6·3	36 ± 7·0	116 ± 15·8	4·75 ± 1·1	45 ± 16·6	1919 ± 396
Recovery	96 ± 11·0	8 ± 3·4	14 ± 2·7	81 ± 12·5	2·80 ± ·47	41 ± 9·6	1105 ± 204
Rest NG	87 ± 13·1	3 ± 3·0	9 ± 2·6	91 ± 14·2	2·75 ± ·54	36 ± 9·8	1137 ± 294
Exercise NG	106 ± 16·3	12 ± 10·7	22 ± 8·7	118 ± 14·4	5·17 ± 1·0	56 ± 20·0	1940 ± 465
Non-Angina Group (n=18)							
Rest	92 ± 8·5	11 ± 3·6	14 ± 3·3	74 ± 10·9	3·11 ± ·77	47 ± 14·7	947 ± 179
Exercise	107 ± 22·9	20 ± 9·8	28 ± 7·6	118 ± 18·4	5·47 ± 1·02	57 ± 15·6	1886 ± 386
Recovery	90 ± 10·4	9 ± 5·0	13 ± 3·9	79 ± 13·2	3·03 ± ·82	48 ± 17·2	976 ± 166
Rest NG	83 ± 8·1	4 ± 3·5	8 ± 2·9	87 ± 13·3	2·97 ± ·81	38 ± 11·2	975 ± 180
Exercise NG	101 ± 9·3	9 ± 7·6	19 ± 4·8	120 ± 18·1	6·02 ± 1·01	64 ± 16·0	1801 ± 352
Normal Group (n=7)							
Rest	90 ± 9·4	9 ± 1·7	12 ± 2·4	72 ± 10·9	3·42 ± ·33	55 ± 7·4	890 ± 170
Exercise	108 ± 9·3	15 ± 3·9	18 ± 6·0	111 ± 12·7	6·85 ± 1·18	78 ± 10·4	1732 ± 244
Recovery	94 ± 6·3	9 ± 2·5	12 ± 2·6	75 ± 8·1	—	—	968 ± 178
Rest NG	81 ± 11·9	3 ± 2·1	8 ± 1·5	87 ± 7·9	3·38 ± ·77	41·1 ± 10·2	927 ± 178
Exercise NG	101 ± 8·9	7 ± 3·4	14 ± 1·9	115 ± 11·8	6·25 ± ·88	67 ± 10·0	1694 ± 550

Data are mean ± Standard Deviation.

patients with coronary heart disease and normal subjects were studied in our laboratory[7 8] (Table 20, 3). Twenty patients who had experienced angina during exercise carried out the same exercise period after administration of a chewable form of nitroglycerin and only three had chest pain during this second exercise period. The haemodynamic alterations were compared with those seen in normal subjects and in patients with coronary artery disease

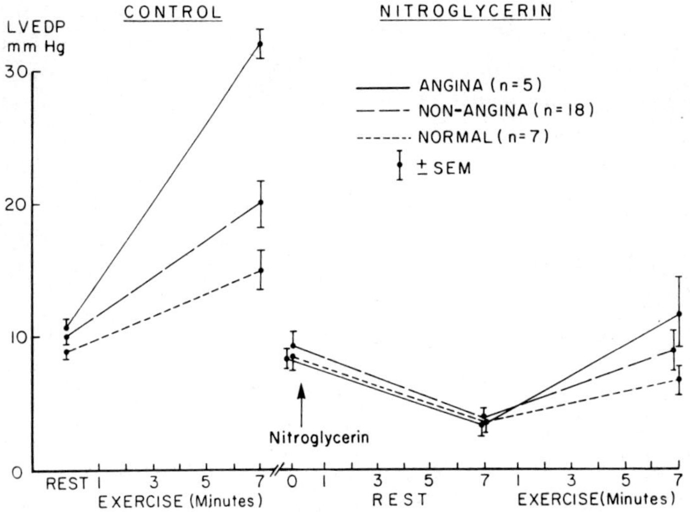

FIG. 20, 6. LVEDP at rest and during exercise in the three groups of patients during the initial exercise period and following nitroglycerin administration. There was a uniform decline in resting LVEDP following nitroglycerin administration. The LVEDP remained normal during exercise in each of the three groups.

who did not develop angina during exercise. Resting LVEDP decreased after nitroglycerin administration in every patient studied. In those patients where angina was prevented, there was a normal increase in LVEDP during exercise (Fig. 20, 6). The average LVEDP during exertional angina was 33 mmHg but only 12 mmHg in this group during exercise after nitroglycerin. The LVEDP during exercise was also lower in the normal group and in the non-angina group. In relating changes in stroke work to changes in LVEDP, improvement in ventricular function was apparent during exercise following nitroglycerin in patients where angina was prevented by administration of the drug. The administration of nitroglycerin was also effective in preventing the development of angina during atrial pacing.[18] Following nitroglycerin, the LVEDP during sinus rhythm decreased and this pressure fell again during pacing, similar to the pattern seen in normal subjects. When pacing was interrupted in the immediate post-pacing period, the LVEDP returned to control levels. This haemodynamic response was similar to that seen in normal subjects. In relating these changes in LVEDP to simultaneous changes in LVSWI, it appears that when angina is prevented by the prior administration of nitroglycerin that the depression of myocardial function seen during myocardial ischaemia does not occur.

The mechanism of action of nitroglycerin is uncertain. It has been considered to be a coronary dilator. Although one can demonstrate angiographically that the nitrates induce coronary dilatation, there is as yet no clear evidence in man that the drug effects total coronary flow or its distribution. Studies in which coronary blood flow was measured with Krypton^{85} at rest and exercise before and after nitroglycerin administration showed no increase in coronary blood flow either at rest and exercise following drug administration.[24] There is at present considerable evidence that nitroglycerin acts through a reduction in myocardial oxygen requirements rather than an increase in oxygen delivery to the myocardium. The determinants of myocardial oxygen consumption are heart rate, myocardial contractility and ventricular wall tension which is related to left ventricular pressure and volume. In our studies during exercise the heart rate, brachial artery mean pressure and tension time index and systolic ejection rate were similar during exercise before and after nitroglycerin administration (Table 20, 3). Thus the major haemodynamic alteration that could have prevented the occurrence of angina during the second period of exercise was the decline in wall tension brought about by a decrease in left ventricular volume. The regular decrease in LVEDP, both at rest and during exercise following nitroglycerin administration, suggests a decrease in volume and such a change has been shown using radiographic techniques. We have found a similar reduction in volume employing the technique of echocardiography. This decrease in left ventricular volume appears to be related to a reduction in venous return as the afterload was not significantly affected and the contractility not reduced. During the atrial pacing studies the situation is less clear. As with nitroglycerin administration the systemic pressure, tension time index and LVEDP were all significantly lower. Thus changes in several variables could have led to a decrease in left ventricular oxygen requirements.

The decrease in left ventricular volume induced by nitroglycerin would reduce left ventricular wall tension through the LaPlace relationship and thus lower left ventricular oxygen requirements. Two studies demonstrate the importance of changes in left ventricular volume on myocardial oxygen consumption. Firstly, the effect of blood volume expansion with low molecular weight dextran on the anginal threshold was determined by the pacing stress test.[25] Thirteen patients with coronary artery disease underwent atrial pacing to determine the anginal threshold. This period of pacing was repeated following the administration of low molecular weight dextran in a volume adequate to increase LVEDP to approximately double the control values. Four patients did not develop angina during either pacing period. Five patients developed angina during both pacing periods, the time of onset of angina from the initiation of pacing averaged 5 minutes before dextran infusion and 1·8 minutes following volume expansion. Two of these patients developed chest pain during the infusion period before the onset of the second period of atrial pacing. Of the four patients who remained free of pain during the first pacing period, one developed angina during the infusion period before the onset of the second period of atrial pacing, and all developed angina during pacing after blood volume expansion. The average time of onset of angina in these four patients was two minutes. It is unlikely that dextran would have any deleterious effect on coronary flow and in all probability through its reduction in viscosity, coronary flow might be augmented. There were only minor changes in arterial haematocrit and thus there would be no significant reduction in the arterial oxygen transport.

In assessing the haemodynamic alterations during the two pacing periods that could have significantly lowered the anginal threshold, there was no significant change in the systemic pressure, heart rate, LV dP/dt or tension time index during the two pacing periods (Fig. 20, 7). The major change was the marked increase in LVEDP following dextran infusion. This suggested that the increase in left ventricular volume induced by blood volume expansion significantly increased ventricular oxygen consumption and thus decreased the anginal threshold.

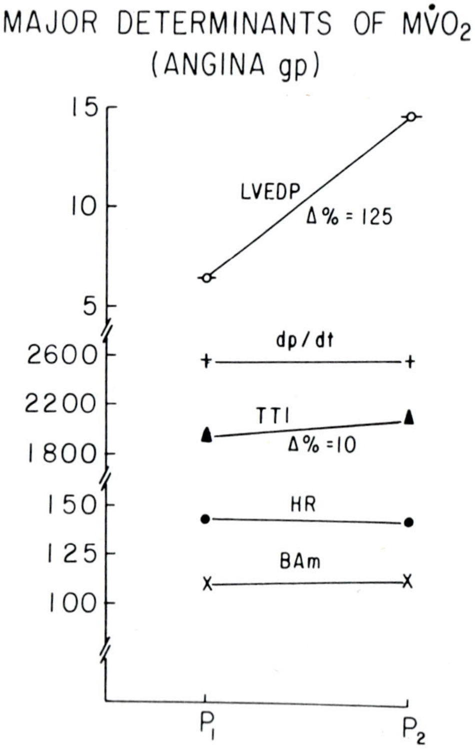

FIG. 20, 7. Alterations in haemodynamic parameters during pacing before and after dextran administration. The only change of significance was the increase in LVEDP following dextran administration. This suggests an increase in left ventricular volume which may have been responsible for the more ready precipitation of angina by atrial pacing.

The consistent decrease in LVEDP following nitroglycerin administration is related to the decrease in afterload, tachycardia and a decrease in venous return—changes which would reduce left ventricular volume. The reduced filling pressures, however, persist after systemic pressure has returned to normal. It thus appears that venous dilatation and decreased venous return are the most important mode of action of nitroglycerin. In an attempt to reproduce

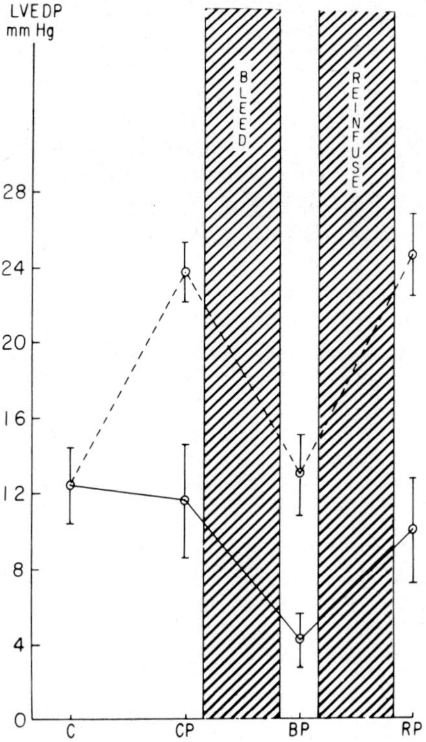

FIG. 20, 8. LVEDP during control pacing, phlebotomy and reinfusion. The LVEDP fell during phlebotomy with relief of pacing-induced angina and returned to near control levels with reinfusion and a return of angina.

this venous pooling effect of nitroglycerin, we studied the effect of phlebotomy on the clinical and haemodynamic response to atrial pacing in patients with angina pectoris.[26] A group of eight patients with coronary artery disease were studied during atrial pacing.

When angina had been established and while pacing continued, venous blood was withdrawn through a cannula at an everage rate of 68 ml/min until pain was relieved for a total of 400 ml removed. In seven of the eight patients, angina was relieved during phlebotomy after an average volume of 275 ml had been removed. Pacing was continued and blood was reinfused at a rate of 30 ml/min and in all but one patient angina recurred during or immediately following blood infusion. Phlebotomy did not significantly alter cardiac output, systemic pressure, left ventricular stroke work, LV dP/dt or TTI and the heart rate was constant. The only alterations during the relief of angina by phlebotomy was a reduction in LVEDP (Fig. 20, 8). This pressure increased with blood infusion and the reappearance of angina. These data support the concept that nitroglycerin may exert its major beneficial effects through peripheral pooling, a reduction in LVEDP and ventricular volume.

REFERENCES

1 MÜLLER, O. & RØRVIK, K. (1958). Haemodynamic consequences of coronary heart disease. *British Heart Journal* **20,** 302-310.
2 JOHNSON, J. B., FAIRLEY, A. & CARTER, C. (1959). Effect of sublingual nitroglycerin on pulmonary arterial pressure in patients with left ventricular failure. *Annals of Internal Medicine* **50,** 34-42.
3 ROSS, R. S., SCHWARTZ, N., GAERTNER, R. A. & FRIESINGER, G. C. (1962). Electrocardiographic and hemodynamic observations during selective coronary cineangiocardiography. *Journal of Clinical Investigation* **41,** 1395.
4 DIMOND, E. G. & BENCHIMOL, A. (1963). Correlation of intra cardiac pressure and praecordial movement in ischaemic heart disease. *British Heart Journal* **25,** 389-392.
5 COHEN, L. S., ELLIOTT, W. C., ROLETT, E. L. & GORLIN, R. (1965). Hemodynamic studies during angina pectoris. *Circulation* **31,** 409-416.
6 PARKER, J. O., DI GIORGI, S. & WEST, R. O. In *Proceedings of International Symposium on Cardiovascular and Respiratory Effects of Hypoxia,* p. 360. Kingston.
7 PARKER, J. O., DI GIORGI, S. & WEST, R. O. (1966). A hemodynamic study of acute coronary insufficiency precipitated by exercise. *American Journal of Cardiology* **17,** 470-483.
8 PARKER, J. O., DI GIORGI, S. & WEST, R. O. (1967). The hemodynamic response to exercise in patients with healed myocardial infarction without angina. *Circulation* **36,** 734-752.
9 PARKER, J. O., DI GIORGI, S. & WEST, R. O. (1968). Hemodynamic effects of propranolol in coronary heart disease. *American Journal of Cardiology* **21,** 11-19.
10 PARKER, J. O., WEST, R. O., CASE, R. B. & CHIONG, M. A. (1969). Temporal relationship of myocardial lactate metabolism, left ventricular function, and S-T segment depression during angina precipitated by exercise. *Circulation* **40,** 97-111.
11 MCCALLISTER, B. D., YIPINTSOI, T., HALLERMAN, F. J., WALLACE, R. B. & FRYE, R. L. (1968). Left ventricular performance during mild supine leg exercise in coronary artery disease. *Circulation* **37,** 922-931.

12 WIENER, L., DWYER, E. M. JR., & COX, J. W. (1968). Left ventricular hemodynamics in exercise-induced angina pectoris. *Circulation* **38,** 240-249.
13 SOWTON, G. E., BALCON, R., CROSS, D. & FRICK, M. H. (1967). Measurement of the angina threshold using atrial pacing. *Cardiovascular Research* **1,** 301-307.
14 BALCON, R., MALLY, W. C. & SOWTON, E. (1968). Clinical use of atrial pacing test in angina pectoris. *British Medical Journal* **3,** 91-92.
15 PITT, B., FORTUIN, N., DAGENAIS, G., FRIESINGER, G. C. & HODGE, M. (1968). The pacing stress test in the evaluation of patients with angina pectoris. *Circulation* **38,** Suppl. VI, 157.
16 FRICK, M. H., BALCON, R., CROSS, D. & SOWTON, E. (1968). Hemodynamic effects of nitroglycerin in patients with angina pectoris studied by an atrial pacing method. *Circulation* **37,** 160-168.
17 FRIESINGER, G. C., CONTI, C. R. & PITT, B. (1967). Observations on left ventricular pressure during angina pectoris. *Circulation* **36,** *Suppl. II,* 115.
18 PARKER, J. O., LEDWICH, J. R., WEST, R. O. & CASE, R. B. (1969). Reversible cardiac failure during angina pectoris. *Circulation* **39,** 745-757.
19 PARKER, J. O., KHAJA, F. & CASE, R. B. (1971). Analysis of left ventricular function by atrial pacing. *Circulation* **3,** 241-252.
20 DWYER, E. M. (1970). Left ventricular pressure-volume alterations and regional disorders of contraction during myocardial ischaemia induced by arterial pacing. *Circulation* **42,** 1111-1122.
21 DODGE, H. T., SANDLER, H., BALLEW, D. W. & LORD, J. D. (1960). Cardiovascular effects of isoproterenol in normal subjects and subjects with congestive heart failure. *American Heart Journal* **60,** 94-105.
22 POPP, R. L. & HARRISON, D. C. (1970). Ultrasonic cardiac echography for determining stroke volume and valvular regurgitation. *Circulation* **41,** 493-502.
23 POMBO, J. F., TROY, B. L. & RUSSELL, T. O. (1971). Left ventricular volumes and ejection fraction by echocardiography. *Circulation* **43,** 480-490.
24 PARKER, J. O., WEST, R. O., DI GIORGI, S. (1971). The effect of nitroglycerine on coronary blood flow and the hemodynamic response to exercise in coronary artery disease. *American Journal of Cardiology* **27,** 59-65.
25 KHAJA, F., SANGHVI, V., MARK, A. & PARKER, J. O. (1971). Effect of volume expansion on the anginal threshold. *Circulation* **43,** 624-635.
26 PARKER, J. O., CASE, R. B., KHAJA, F., LEDWICH, J. R. & ARMSTRONG, P. W. (1970). The influence of changes in blood flow on angina pectoris. *Circulation* **41,** 593.

DISCUSSION

Donald. Did you try the effects of bleeding in patients with angina during exercise?

Parker. No.

Donald. Did you investigate how long the effect of nitroglycerin lasted as judged by the improved haemodynamic findings?

Parker. We were studying its effects 15 to 20 minutes after drug administration. The effect is much longer than generally thought.

Donald. Did you find out how long it is?

Parker. No, but we have reason to believe that the effects are certainly present 30 minutes after the final study.

Henderson. With reference to the diastolic compliance, I stated earlier that in the cat papillary muscle there was no change in the resting diastolic compliance in anoxia, whereas previous work in the rat showed that there was a reversible increase in stiffness. This seemed to be related to severity of anoxia and possibly to the increased fatty acid content. May I have other people's comments on a change in the diastolic volume force relationship?

Parker. Dwyer reported this but it has not been published. He looked at left ventriculograms during pacing in patients with coronary disease and found that during pacing-induced angina the reduction in volume was not quite as great as observed in normal subjects, only in one subject did he actually show an increase in ventricular volume. He concluded from the study that in some patients there is a change in compliance but in others the findings can be entirely explained by an increase in left ventricular volume. Remember he was doing two left ventriculograms in each case. We don't really know the effect of this on ventricular function, or whether some effects are transient or longer lasting.

Noble. Regarding this particular point, I would have thought it would be very difficult to come to any conclusion about changes in diastolic compliance in view of the great difficulty in measuring volume with any of the current methods and also in view of the fact that one has to compare two pressure volume curves which are alinear. I was dubious about the fact that you plotted, on a single ventricular performance curve, points obtained at completely different heart rates.

Parker. I agree that increasing heart rate is a positive inotropic factor and that your objection is valid. I think, however, that when one plots the data in a single patient the effect of heart rate is the same on both of these curves and they are clearly different. This certainly supports the fact that we have depressed left ventricular function.

Conti. What is your success rate in trying to measure the minor axis using ultrasonography in patients with ischaemic heart disease?

Parker. Roughly 50 per cent. We bring all these patients to the laboratory the day before. In many patients, particularly in the late middle aged group who have chronic chest disease, it is difficult if not impossible to get clear septal and posterior wall patterns.

Conti. That has been our experience too. We get reasonable measurements in 40 to 45 per cent. There may be an alternative method of studying ventricular volume during an intervention such as pacing. This involves measurement of stroke volume by a catheter tip velocity transducer and ejection fraction by thermal dilution and then deriving ventricular volume. However, there are still a number of problems.

Maseri. There is a rapid progressive increase in the wedge pressure and pulmonary arterial pressure closely related to the rate of pacing. We have had considerable trouble measuring the filling pressure of the left ventricle and consequently use pulmonary wedge or pulmonary artery pressure. Some recordings are rather difficult to interpret in this regard.

Parker. It is necessary to record at a high sensitivity. We relate the end-diastolic pressure to the R waves. I am not sure that you can use wedge pressures as an indication of end-diastolic pressure. In several patients we have found, during simultaneous measurements, that pulmonary artery, pulmonary wedge or left atrial pressure diverge from left ventricular end-diastolic pressure.

Maseri. Which is more meaningful—indirect left atrial or direct left ventricular end-diastolic pressure?

Parker. Left ventricular fibre length is the important physiological factor. From angiocardiographic data left ventricular pressure appears a good index of left ventricular volume and, therefore, of fibre length.

Jennings. It seems to me that, in the presence of angina and elevated end-diastolic pressure, there is decreased subendocardial blood flow. Consequently there is accumulation of metabolites of the ischaemic process (e.g. lactic acid) perhaps causing the pain of angina. Then the nitroglycerine effect is quite a simple one, it lowers the end-diastolic pressure, increases subendocardial flow, washes out the metabolites and the pain disappears.

Parker. I don't know which is cause and which is effect. I imagine that the high filling pressures certainly interfere with subendocardial flow but the improvement with nitroglycerine could be related to either the washing out of metabolites or due to reduced ventricular compression. I would favour the latter hypothesis. I don't think lactic acid produces the pain because during exercise one can sample from the coronary sinus and one has much higher lactate levels than one does during pacing-induced angina.

Parratt. Have you seen the development of exercise-induced anginal pain without an increase in diastolic pressure? In other words, is there any evidence of some form of coronary vasospasm in any group of angina patients?

Parker. In answer to your first question, we had one or two patients who had had pain and electrocardiographic changes without a marked rise in end-diastolic pressure but I don't think that your next statement about vasospasm necessarily follows. One could, under these circumstances, have pain by some mechanism which was not associated with enough derangement of left ventricular function to produce the usual haemodynamic abnormalities. I don't think that one has to make any hypothesis to describe the occasional angina without haemodynamic abnormalities.

Donald. One point concerning the compliance of the hypoxic myocardium is that in severe respiratory failure you may have a high normal cardiac output maintained at very low levels of blood oxygenation often without raised filling pressure, so there must be normal diastolic myocardial compliance under these conditions.

REGULATION OF THE MOBILIZATION OF FREE FATTY ACIDS FROM ADIPOSE TISSUE

L. A. CARLSON

Plasma FFA and myocardial metabolism

It is well known that the albumin-bound free fatty acids (FFA) in plasma play a major role in caloric homeostasis in man. One hundred to two hundred grams of fatty acids may be mobilized daily from adipose tissue and transported as FFA to other tissues. The heart is one of many tissues which utilize FFA as a major source of energy. As we have heard in this meeting, about half of the heart's energy requirement in fasting man may be covered by the uptake of FFA. FFA are taken up by the heart in amounts proportional to the plasma levels of FFA. This indicates that the rate of mobilization of FFA from adipose tissue is one determinant for the uptake of FFA by the heart. Fatty acids derived from exogenous plasma triglycerides may also be quite an important source of energy in the fed state for the human myocardium.

In addition to being a major fuel contributor to the heart, FFA may also exert certain regulatory functions. FFA may regulate the uptake of carbohydrate substrates, not only glucose—the so-called Randle fatty acid-glucose cycle[1]—but also lactate and pyruvate.[2] Furthermore, FFA may stimulate whole body as well as myocardial oxygen consumption.[3 4 5] Finally, the work of Dr Oliver and co-workers suggests that high plasma levels of FFA may be arrhythmogenic.[6 7]

Against this background it is natural that cardiologists should be interested in the regulation of mobilization of FFA from adipose tissue. Normally about 90 per cent of plasma FFA are derived from adipose tissue. The artificial situation with infusion of Intralipid[R] and heparin so much discussed at this symposium is, of course, quite different. Here the majority of circulating FFA are derived from hydrolysis of the highly unsaturated Intralipid[R] triglycerides.

Mobilization of FFA, a balance between fat-mobilizing lipolysis and fatty acid re-esterification

The two major processes which determine the availability of free fatty acids inside the adipocyte are *lipolysis* (hydrolysis) of the triglycerides and *re-esterification* of the fatty acids. It is very likely that the rate of mobilization of fatty acids out of the cell into blood is proportional to the intracellular concentration of the free fatty acid pool depicted schematically in Figure 21, 1.

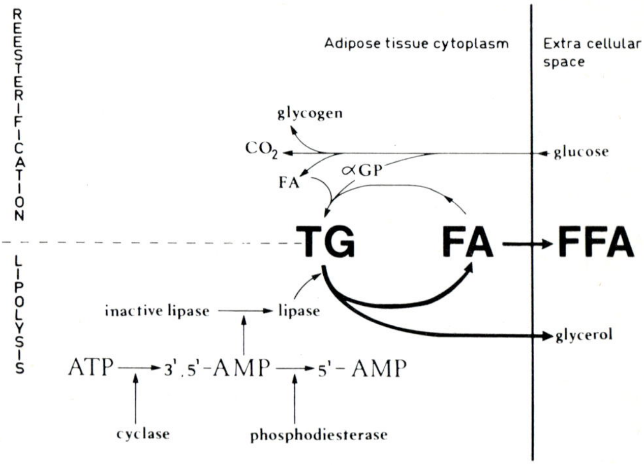

FIG. 21, 1. Schematic diagram of the mobilization of free fatty acids (FFA) from adipose tissue. Lipolysis and re-esterification are the two main processes regulating FFA mobilization, αGP=α-glycerophosphate.

One major regulator of the lipolytic process is cyclic-AMP. The role of cyclic-AMP in this process has been reviewed recently.[8] Cyclic-AMP activates an inactive form of the triglyceride lipase to an active form probably in the usual way by stimulating a protein kinase to phosphorylate the inactive enzyme. The phosphorylated form is the active form of the lipase. As yet no phosphatase which dephosphorylates the active lipase has been described.

Two enzyme systems regulate the intracellular concentration of cyclic-AMP. The membrane bound adenyl cyclase system forms cyclic-AMP from ATP while the cytoplasmic phosphodiesterase system breaks down cyclic-AMP to inactive 5-AMP. The level of cyclic-AMP is of course a balance between these two processes of synthesis and breakdown as indicated in Figure 21, 1.

One major regulator of the re-esterification process is the availability of α-glycerophosphate. Adipose tissue appears to lack glycerokinase and thus cannot synthesize α-glycerophosphate from glycerol. The major part of the α-glycerophosphate is derived from glycolysis, although at least under *in vitro* conditions α-glycerophosphate may be synthesized from pyruvate. The rate of glycolysis and the availability of NADH are two important factors determining the rate of formation of α-glycerophosphate.

Factors of importance for the mobilization of FFA

In the context of this meeting the factors influencing FFA mobilization will be considered from the clinical point of view. Table 21, 1 lists factors which may be of importance for regulating the rate of mobilization of FFA.

Table 21, 1 *Principle factors influencing the rate of mobilization of FFA from adipose tissue*

BLOOD FLOW
HORMONES
Circulating
Local
SUBSTRATES
Circulating
Local
ELECTROLYTES AND pH
Circulating
Local
PHARMACOLOGICAL AGENTS

Blood flow. It is self-evident that major changes in blood flow through adipose tissue could markedly influence the rate of mobilization of FFA. Relatively little is known about blood flow in human adipose tissue in clinical conditions such as myocardial infarction and shock. In canine subcutaneous adipose tissue, nerve stimulation and noradrenaline infusion causes constriction of arterioles and veins while prostaglandin E_1 (PGE_1) was found to be a most pronounced vasodilator.[9] While noradrenaline stimulates and PGE_1 inhibits lipolysis in adipose tissue, the above mentioned effects of these compounds appear to exercise an opposite effect on the mobilization of FFA. However, in man increased lipolysis such as seen during fasting and after glucagon may be associated with increased blood flow through adipose tissue.[10] It is clear that we need much more information in this area of control of FFA mobilization.

Hormones. A number of hormones are known to influence the rate of mobilization of FFA. They may either act on the lipolytic machinery or on re-esterification or both, such as is the case with insulin. The interplay is indeed still more complex in the intact organism where hormones not only interact on the adipocyte at different biochemical sites but also directly interact with each other's secretion. An example of this, which may be of interest in connection with myocardial infarctions, is the inhibitory effect adrenaline exerts on insulin secretion.

Table 21, 2 lists the effect of several hormones on the mobilization of FFA. It is important to realize that there is a considerable species difference for the actions of hormones on adipose tissue, especially with regard to lipolysis. ACTH, for instance, is a very potent stimulator of lipolysis in rat fat but devoid of activity in this regard in man. Also catecholamines are the most important fast-acting stimulants of lipolysis in man but without such effect on, for example, bird adipose tissue. The so-called α- and β-adrenergic receptors appear to have opposite effects on the lipolytic process in human adipose tissue, β-receptors stimulating and α-receptors inhibiting lipolysis.[11] In fact, a β-stimulating compound such as isoprenaline causes the cyclic-AMP level of human fat to increase about 100 times more than an equivalent amount of an α, β-stimulating compound such as noradrenaline.[12]

As some hormones may act inside the cell, intracellular hormone concentrations may be of importance. A special role is played here by the prostaglandins, in particular PGE_1, which is a most active inhibitor of fat mobilizing lipolysis and of accumulation of cyclic-AMP.[8] The prostaglandins are probably synthesized locally in cells and not transported to cells in the blood.

Substrates. Glucose is one of the most important circulating substrates. It exerts a major and inhibitory regulatory role on FFA mobilization. During *in vitro* conditions, a major part of its inhibitory effect is by increasing re-esterification. *In vivo* the action is more complex and the effects of glucose on various hormones, which in turn may act on adipose tissue, must be considered in addition to the stimulation of glucose uptake and metabolism in adipose tissue.

Table 21, 2 *Substances influencing the rate of mobilization of FFA from adipose tissue*

STIMULATION	INHIBITION
Cyclic-AMP	Insulin
Catecholamines (FA)	Prostaglandin E_1
ACTH (FA)	β-adrenergic blockers
Glucagon (FA)	Glucose
Growth hormone (FA)	Lactate
Secretin (FA)	Na^+
TSH (FA, SA)	Acidosis
Thyroxin	
Corticosteroids (SA)	
Methylxanthines (FA)	
α-adrenergic blockers	
Pyruvate?	
K^+, Ca^{++}	
Alkalosis	

FA=fast acting stimulation. This is in general induced by raising the tissue concentration of cyclic-AMP.
SA=slow acting stimulation. This is not caused by direct effects on the tissue level of cyclic-AMP.

Also other circulating substrates have important effects on FFA mobilization. Furthermore, local substrate levels such as glycogen concentration in the adipocyte may be of importance for regulating FFA mobilization, as may also the NADH/NAD ratio. A high concentration or a high ratio may stimulate the formation of α-glycerophosphate and thus diminish FFA mobilization by enhancement of re-esterification.

Electrolytes. Ions such as potassium and calcium are of importance *in vitro* for the mobilization process and lack of them leads to considerable depression of lipolysis. On the other hand sodium ions may inhibit lipolysis and hypernatraemia *in vivo* is associated with a reduced FFA mobilization. It is not unlikely that local shifts in the ionic milieu inside and around the adipocyte may be quite important for the lipolytic process.

Pharmacologic agents. A number of compounds have been found to inhibit mobilization of FFA from adipose tissue (for review see[13 14]). Salicylates were the first group of pharmacologic compounds shown to lower plasma FFA levels.[15] Certain heterocyclic acids have been found to be most effective inhibitors of fat mobilizing lipolysis and at the same time they prevent the accumulating of cyclic-AMP in adipose tissue. Nicotinic acid is a very potent inhibitor of FFA mobilization[16] and has been used in a number of clinical and experimental conditions as a pharmacological tool for reducing FFA levels in blood.[17 18] However, the clinical usefulness of nicotinic acid as an inhibitor of FFA mobilization is at least in certain situations limited because its well known vascular effects (flush). The development of nicotinic acid derivatives with more potent antilipolytic effects and less vascular effects is therefore highly desirable. 5-fluoronicotinic acid is an example of such a derivative which we have found to be about 5 times as antilipolytic as nicotinic acid[19] and to have less vascular effect. Such a compound might be useful to try in acute myocardial infarction to evaluate the arrhythmogenic effect of high plasma levels of FFA.

REFERENCES

1 RANDLE, P. J., GARLAND, P. B., HALES, C. N. & NEWSHOLME, E. A. (1963). The glucose fatty-acid cycle. *Lancet* **I,** 785-789.

2 LASSERS, B. W., KAIJSER, L. & CARLSON, L. A. (1972, in press). *European Journal of Clinical Investigation.*

3 HAVEL, R. J., CARLSON, L. A., EKELUND, L. G. & HOLMGREN, A. (1964). Studies on the relation between mobilization of free fatty acids and energy metabolism in man: effects of nor-epinephrine and nicotinic acid. *Metabolism* **13,** 1402-1412.

4 WAHLQVIST, M. L., LASSERS, B. W., KAIJSER, L. & CARLSON, L. A. (1972, in press). *Acta Medica Scandinavica.*

5 MJØS, O. D. *This symposium.*

6 OLIVER, M. F., KURIEN, V. A. & GREENWOOD, T. (1968). Relation between serum free-fatty acids and arrhythmias and death after acute myocardial infarction. *Lancet* **1,** 710-714.

7 KURIEN, V. A., YATES, P. A. & OLIVER, M. F. (1971). The role of free fatty acids in the production of ventricular arrhythmias after acute coronary artery occlusion. *European Journal of Clinical Investigation* **1,** 225-241.

8 BUTCHER, R. W. (1970). In *Adipose Tissue,* p. 5. Edited by B. Jeanrenaud and D Hepp. New York: Academic Press.

9 FREDHOLM, B. B., ÖBERG, B. & ROSELL, S. (1970). Effects of vasoactive drugs on circulation in canine subcutaneous adipose tissue. *Acta Physiologia Scandinavica* **79,** 564-574.

10 NIELSEN, S. L. et al. (1968). Blood flow through human adipose tissue through lipolysis. *Scandinavian Journal of Clinical Investigation* **22,** 124-130.
11 ÖSTMAN, J. & EFFENDIC, S. (1970). Catecholamines and metabolism of human adipose tissue. *Acta Medica Scandinavica* **187,** 471-474.
12 CARLSON, L. A. & BUTCHER, R. W. (1972, in press). In *Advances in cyclic nucleotide research*. Edited by P. Greengard and G. A. Robinson. New York: Raven Press.
13 CARLSON, L. A. (1970). In *Atherosclerosis: 2nd International Symposium,* p. 516. Edited by R. Jones. Springer Verlag.
14 KUPIECHI, F. P. (1971). In *Progress in Biochemical Pharmacology,* p. 274. Edited by R. Jones. Springer Verlag.
15 CARLSON, L. A. & ÖSTMAN, J. (1961). Effect of salicylates on plasma free fatty acid in normal and diabetic subjects. *Metabolism* **10,** 781-787.
16 CARLSON, L. A. & ORÖ, L. (1962). The effect of nicotinic acid on the plasma free fatty acid. *Acta Medica Scandinavica* **172,** 641-654.
17 CARLSON, L. A. (1969). Antilipolysis as a tool in the study of clinical and experimental diabetes. *Diabetologia* **5,** 361-365.
18 CARLSON, L. A. (1971). In *Metabolic Effects of Nicotinic Acid and its Derivatives,* p. 157. Edited by K. F. Gey and L. A. Carlson. Bern: Hans Huber Publishers.
19 CARLSON, L. A., HEDBOM, CH., HELGSTRAND, E., SJÖBERG, B. & STJERNSTRÖM, N. E. (1969). In *Drugs Affecting Lipid Metabolism. Advances in Experimental Medicine and Biology,* p. 85. Edited by W. L. Holmes, L. A. Carlson and R. Paoletti. New York: Plenum Press.

PROSTAGLANDIN E_1 IN CARDIAC ARRHYTHMIA DUE TO ACUTE LOCAL ISCHAEMIA IN A DOG

A. J. VERGROESEN. IN COLLABORATION WITH W. G. ZIJLSTRA, J. R. BRUNSTING AND F. TEN HOOR

ELEVATED serum-levels of free fatty acids (FFA) after acute myocardial infarction might cause cardiac arrhythmia[1] by increasing myocardial oxygen consumption due to the utilization of FFA as the major energy substrate. Opie (1970)[2] postulated that the accumulation of intracellular FFA is toxic to heart function and can result in decreased contractility and rhythm disturbances. In isolated rat hearts, perfused with 1 mM palmitic acid, prostaglandin E_1 (PGE_1) will increase the oxidation of this fatty acid but not in hearts perfused with glucose + palmitic acid.[3] In our experiments[4] and in other still unpublished results with isolated hypo-dynamic rat and frog hearts, some of the results suggested an anti-arrhythmic action of PGE_1. The following observation applying to the normalization of heart rhythm and the restoration of arterial blood pressure in a dog with myocardial ischaemia caused by ligation of the circumflex branch of the left coronary artery is of interest.

The figure 21, 2 shows the ECG and the arterial and right atrial blood pressure recordings immediately before ligation (A), 41 min after ligation during the injection of 50 μg PGE_1 through a cardiac catheter into the right atrium (B), and 15 sec and 100 min after the injection of PGE_1 (C and D) demonstrating a lasting improvement of the ECG and the arterial and venous blood pressure.

In a recent publication,[5] the relationship between prostaglandins and cardiac rate and rhythm has been discussed. The available

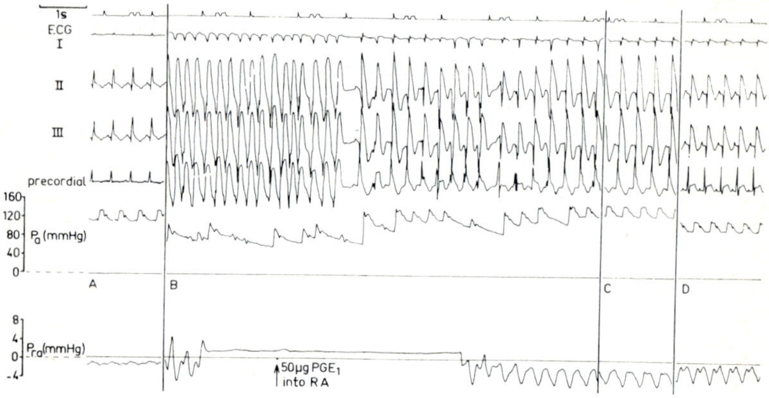

FIG. 21, 2. In a male dog (25 kg) serious arrhythmia developed after ligation of the circumflex branch of the left coronary artery resulting in local myocardial ischaemia.

A: ECG, arterial blood pressure (P_a) and right atrial pressure (P_{ra}) before ligation: heart rate (f_c)=140 min^{-1}.

B: Ventricular tachycardia 40 min after ligation, f_c=280 min^{-1}; injection of 50 μg PGE_1 through the catheter in the right atrium. There is a rapid rise of P_a and a decrease of P_{ra}.

C: Record obtained 15 s after injection of PGE_1 : f_c=160 min^{-1}.

D: Record obtained 100 min after injection of PGE_1: f_c=180 min^{-1}; ECG is still clearly improved.

Intermittent positive pressure breathing (N_2O/O_2) using a Bird respirator. Arterial blood gases and acid-base status were frequently checked. Immediately before the injection of PGE_1 the oxygen saturation was 97·5 per cent, pH 7·30, plasma bicarbonate 16·8 mEq l^{-1} and P_{co2} 33·8 mmHg.

evidence suggests that PGE_1 is involved in the mechanism controlling the equilibrium between sympathetic and parasympathetic influences on the heart. This could explain reported discrepancies as to the effects of PGE_1 on heart rate, cardiac output and myocardial contractility, the direction of the effects being dependent on the experimental conditions existing before the PGE_1 administration.

One of the most promising hypotheses on the origin of cardiac arrhythmias is the theory of re-entry[6]. A prerequisite for the re-entry phenomenon is the presence of a delay in conduction of the stimulus. PGE_1 might suppress cardiac arrhythmias through its moderating influence on the sympathetic-parasympathetic balance, which influences impulse conduction in the heart. Another possible cause of the anti-arrhythmic action of PGE_1 could be its repolarizing effect as suggested by the results in the K^+-arrested frog and rat heart.[4] As a delay in stimulus conduction may be the result of local depolarization of the conduction system, a repolarizing effect of PGE_1 could restore or partly restore normal conduction, thus abolishing a prerequisite for re-entry.

Oliver *et al.* (1968) concluded that the high level of FFA is the main arrhythmic factor in myocardial ischaema. However, they could not rule out the possible harmful effects of a high sympathetic tone. The observed anti-arrhythmic effect of PGE_1 suggests that a locally increased catecholamine concentration might be the more important factor in respect to the induction of arrhythmia. The possibility that an anti-arrhythmic effect of PGE_1 proceeds via a stimulation of myocardial FFA metabolism resulting in lower intracellular FFA concentration seems to be another but less probable explanation.

REFERENCES

1 Oliver, M. F., Kurien, V. A. & Greenwood, T. W. (1968). Relation between serum-free-fatty-acids and arrhythmias and death after acute myocardial infarction. *Lancet* **1,** 710-714.

2 Opie, L. H. (1970). Effect of fatty acids on contractility and rhythm of the heart. *Nature* **227,** 1055-1056.

3 Willebrands, A. F. & Tasseron, S. J. A. (1968). Effect of hormones on substrate preference in isolated rat heart. *American Journal of Physiology* **215,** 1089-1095.

4 Vergroesen, A. J. & de Boer, J. (1968). Effects of prostaglandins E1 and F1-alpha on isolated frog and rat hearts in relation to the potassium-calcium ratio of the perfusion fluid. *European Journal of Pharmacology* **3,** 171-176.

5 Zijlstra, W. G., Brunsting, J. R., ten Hoor, F. & Vergroesen, A. J. (1972, accepted for publication). *European Journal of Pharmacology.*

6 Cranefield, P. F. & Hoffman, B. F. (1971). Re-entry: slower conduction, summation and inhibition. *Circulation* **44,** 309-311.

Discussion

Barrett. How many cups of coffee would a patient with recent infarction and high circulating noradrenaline need to take before there are grossly elevated free fatty acid levels?

Carlson. I am sure you do not expect an answer. Nevertheless the synergistic effect of caffeine and catecholamines may be important.

Mjøs. A group in Oslo gave glucagon to patients with heart disease, but found no change in plasma FFA concentrations. A group from Vienna found a decrease in FFA concentration after glucagon and another report has indicated that in intact dogs glucagon has no effect on plasma FFA, but it has a strong lipolytic effect on adipose tissue.

Carlson. In birds, glucagon is the main fat mobilizing factor and yet bird adipose tissue does not respond at all to catecholamines. Now in man, glucagon has several effects: it raises blood sugar and stimulates insulin production and both these effects might initiate fat mobilization. Time influences the effects of glucagon. In man, there is an increase in glycerol output during the first few minutes after injection of glucagon, but later there may be no stimulation of fat mobilization or even a decrease in plasma glycerol concentration due to other metabolic changes produced by glucagon.

Mjøs. Did you say that noradrenaline decreased blood flow in adipose tissue?

Carlson. Yes, but not in human adipose tissue. I referred to isolated dog adipose tissue.

Mjøs. I think a group in Denmark gave noradrenaline intravenously and showed a rise in human adipose tissue blood flow. We have given it intravenously in dogs and measured flow in perfused *in vivo* inguinal adipose tissue preparations. When arterial blood pressure rose to 150 mmHg, there was an initial slight fall in blood flow. This increase was also seen after treatment with nicotinic acid. So there are some indications that noradrenaline given intravenously both to humans and to the dog inguinal adipose tissue preparation increases blood flow. The Stockholm group stimulated adipose tissue sympathetic nerves and this definitely reduced blood flow in adipose tissue.

Carlson. If noradrenaline increases blood flow in human adipose tissue, it simplifies life as noradrenaline stimulates lipolysis and at the same time increases blood flow. On the other hand, you say that nerve stimulation has the opposite effect on flow. What conclusion do you draw from that? In adipose tissue the nerve supply only goes to the blood vessels. This suggests that nerve stimulation would have a similar effect to noradrenaline.

Mjøs. Well, there is a discrepancy here. It is not clear whether nerve endings in adipose tissue go only to the blood vessels. It is possible that fat cells may be supplied by nerve endings.

Carlson. I am quite sure the histochemists in Hillarp's group in Stockholm were unable to demonstrate any nerve supply to fat cells.

Mjøs. Can ketone bodies be formed in the heart when there are high concentrations of free fatty acids?

Opie. Yes, ketone bodies are formed in the myocardium.

Oliver. Do you think that there is any evidence that there is a differential rate of release of fatty acids? Might some fatty acids, particularly long chain fatty acids, be released at a greater or slower speed? This might be of interest if long chain fatty acids have greater toxicity. If the composition of omental fat is different from that of peripheral adipose tissue and the rate of lipolysis in omental fat is greater than that of adipose tissue, one could envisage the situation where the intake of certain dietary fats might be associated with preferential mobilization of long chain acids.

Carlson. The composition of the free fatty acids is a very important aspect of the problem. One thing which makes me unhappy about Intralipid and heparin is that the plasma FFA you create by that method are very different from those which are mobilized from adipose tissue. Intralipid has a very high content of linoleic and linolenic acid. The composition of plasma free fatty acids is similar to that of adipose tissue and by long term dietary manipulation we could change adipose tissue composition and alter the composition of plasma free fatty acids.

Kurien. Is there any evidence to show that nicotinic acid interferes with mobilization of intracellular triglyceride in cardiac muscle?

Carlson. This is a very interesting question. Before this meeting my feeling was that nicotinic acid did not affect lipolysis in the myocardium. The major reason for this view was that when we injected nicotinic acid into the intact rat and reduced adipose tissue lipolysis and plasma FFA levels, there was also a very rapid fall in the content of triglyceride in the myocardium suggesting that there was active lipolysis (*Acta med. Scand.* **180,** 571 (1966)). Now Dr Mjøs has suggested that nicotinic acid might inhibit lipolysis in the myocardium.

Mjøs. A temporary occlusion of the whole descending branch of the coronary artery results in an increased release of glycerol from the heart. It is possible that a lipase is activated resulting in increased glycerol release from the heart. We are investigating the possibility that nicotinic acid could block this release of glycerol found with infarction. Glycerol may be blocked after an arterial occlusion but this observation requires confirmation.

Carlson. Dr Lassers reported the same finding during exercise in man (pp. 200 to 211). There is quite a considerable release of glycerol but after administration of nicotinic acid there is no such release. We feel it is unwise to draw the conclusion that this means inhibition of lipolysis in the myocardium because the myocardium, in contrast to adipose tissue, has an active glycerokinase and could metabolize its own glycerol.

Barrett. The difference in stimulation of cyclic-AMP which you showed between noradrenaline and isoprenaline is very interesting. I wonder if you could state what the relative concentrations were of these two substances to produce these effects.

Carlson. It was supra-maximal stimulation. Maximal stimulation of lipolysis occurs in human fat with concentrations of about 1 mg/ml and we used 10 mg/ml for both compounds.

Oliver. Do you know if there is any evidence that the administration of nicotinic acid is associated with reduction of plasma cyclic-AMP levels?

Carlson. No.

Barrett. I thought cyclic-AMP was a cell bound compound.

Oliver. It is also present in plasma and there is evidence that noradrenaline increases plasma cyclic-AMP. It has a half life of about 30 minutes.

THE ROLE OF BETA-ADRENERGIC BLOCKADE IN ACUTE MYOCARDIAL ISCHAEMIA

J. D. FITZGERALD

Introduction

BETA-adrenergic blocking drugs are highly specific competitive antagonists of adrenergic agonists at their beta receptor sites.[1] Therefore, any discussion of their clinical role is intimately connected with the actions of adrenaline and noradrenaline in the organism. In the absence of catecholamine activity, beta-adrenergic blocking drugs have no significant pharmacological actions in the doses used in man. The results of administration of a beta blocking drug to man are determined not only by the degree of autonomic activity prior to its application, but also by the beneficial or harmful effects of that activity. In order to delineate the role of beta blocking drugs in the management of myocardial ischaemia, it is therefore necessary to consider first the actions of these catecholamines in this situation.

Catecholamines and myocardial ischaemia

Myocardial ischaemia implies a diminution in the supply of oxygenated blood to part of the myocardium. Its occurrence and severity are determined by: (a) Myocardial blood flow and distribution (b) Oxygen content of the arterial blood (c) Myocardial work.

The primary results of myocardial ischaemia range from impaired cellular metabolism to cell death. The consequences can be loss of contractile activity and serious cardiac dysrhythmias leading frequently to sudden death. In such a situation, the overall effect of catecholamines is the result of a complex series of interactions (Fig. 22, 1). The view is commonly held that the effects of catecholamines in myocardial ischaemia are detrimental to the heart and that the prevention of these effects should be beneficial. This view has been most closely argued by Raab.[2] It is based on the fact that catecholamines increase myocardial oxygen consumption and would therefore be expected to increase any myocardial hypoxia resulting from ischaemia. There is now convincing evidence that myocardial ischaemia, whether reversible or irreversible, is accompanied by the release of catecholamines locally within the myocardium,[3] and by increased circulating and urinary catecholamine levels.[4] Irreversible myocardial ischaemia accompanied by infarction and the cardiac shock syndrome is associated with the highest elevation of circulating and urinary catecholamines (Fig. 22, 2).[5 6] The effects of increased catecholamine activity in myocardial ischaemia can be classified into haemodynamic, electrophysiological, metabolic and ionic.

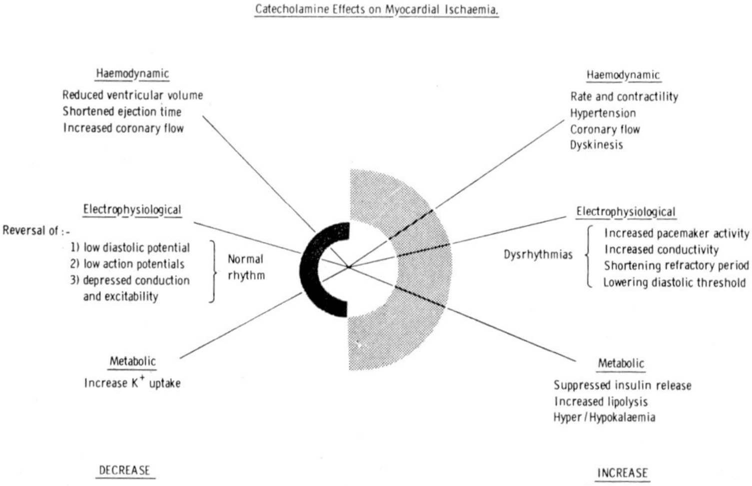

FIG. 22, 1. Diagrammatic representation of the possible ways in which catecholamines may increase or decrease the area of myocardial ischaemia.

Haemodynamic effects of catecholamines

Cardiac. Catecholamines increase myocardial oxygen consumption by increasing heart rate and the velocity of contraction. It now seems unlikely that they alter significantly the basal metabolic rate or that they uncouple oxidative phosphorylation in the myocardium.[7] Their effect on myocardial wall tension depends on the initial size of the ventricle. If the ventricle is dilated, catecholamines will reduce ventricular volume and wall tension, thereby reducing myocardial oxygen consumption. Though ejection time is shortened by catecholamines, the increased velocity of contraction will offset the possible oxygen sparing effect.

Vascular. The peripheral vasoconstrictor actions of noradrenaline, and to a lesser extent of adrenaline, may increase the 'afterload' on the left ventricle which in turn will increase myocardial oxygen demand. The action of catecholamines on coronary flow is complex. According to Berne,[8] their primary effect on coronary

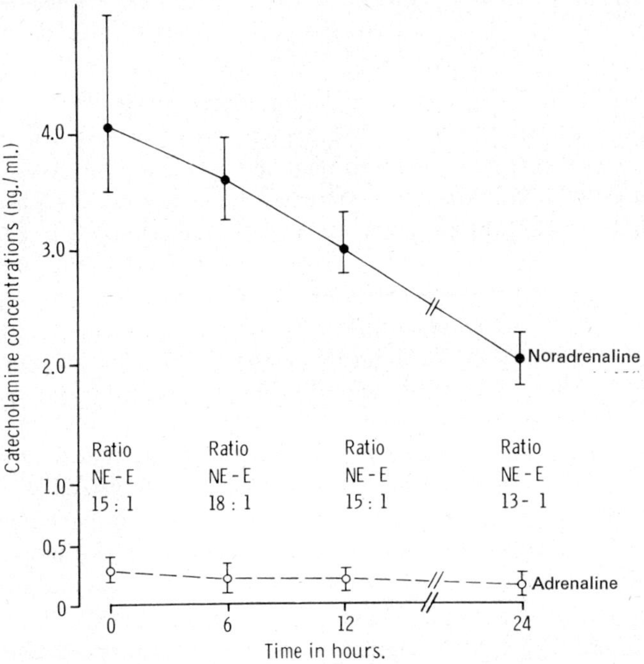

FIG. 22, 2. Circulating levels of noradrenaline and adrenaline over the first 24 hours. Mean results in 9 patients in clinical shock. (From Griffiths and Leung 1971[6] by kind permission of the Editors of the *American Heart Journal.*)

vessels is vasoconstriction. They also elevate blood pressure, increase extravascular compression of the coronary circulation, alter the relationship between systole and diasystole, and enhance myocardial metabolic activity by increasing cardiac work. The observed effect of catecholamines on coronary flow in man will be the resultant of all these interactions and will vary according to which factor is dominant.

Electrophysiological effects of catecholamines

Pacemaker cells undergo slow depolarization during diastole. When depolarization reaches a threshold level, the cell depolarizes completely resulting in a propagated action potential. This process can be observed in the sinus node, the bundle of His and its branches, as well as in the Purkinje tissue of the ventricle. Diastolic depolarization is not normally observed in the ventricle unless the normal cardiac impulse fails to reach the ventricle. The slope of the depolarization and the excitability of Purkinje tissue is increased by catecholamines.[9] Adrenaline and noradrenaline therefore cause an increase in heart rate and in the conduction velocity in the auricle and ventricle and particularly through the AV node.[10]

Catecholamines may also increase the temporal dispersion of recovery of excitability in the Purkinje tissue. Han[11] has observed that there is a greater asynchrony of recovery of the ventricle when catecholamines are liberated locally than when adrenaline is given systemically. Adrenaline infusion increased the temporal dispersion of refractory periods and decreased the fibrillation threshold. As the infusion continued, temporal dispersion decreased and the fibrillation threshold increased.

The appearance of re-entrant pathways and the development of serious dysrhythmias in myocardial ischaemia is favoured by the catecholamine-induced reduction in the slope of diastolic depolarization, the induction of focal ectopic activity and the increase in temporal dispersion of the recovery phase.[12] There are nevertheless situations in which catecholamines can reduce ectopic formation rate in myocardial ischaemia by increasing ventricular rate and shortening the refractory period. Damaged myocardial fibres may have a low diastolic potential, depressed action potentials with slow conduction and varying degrees of block. When catecholamines are added to such a preparation, the reduced excitability and conduction are improved and the diastolic potential may become normal. Regan *et al.*[13] have demonstrated reversal of ventricular arrhythmias, due to myocardial ischaemia in dogs, by infusions of low doses of noradrenaline (0·05 μg/kg/min).

It may be concluded that whilst catecholamines may favour dysrhythmia formation in myocardial ischaemia, they can in certain situations exert a favourable effect.

Metabolic effects of catecholamines

Adrenaline and noradrenaline increase triglyceride breakdown in adipose tissue, resulting in an elevation of circulating levels of free fatty acids (FFA), glycerol and ketone bodies. Continuing adrenergic stimulation can lead to increased esterification of FFA, and accumulation of lipid in the liver. These changes are mediated by activation of adenyl cyclase. Stimulation of the sympathetic nervous system also causes a rise in FFA and glycerol. Adrenergic mediated lipolysis is strongly inhibited by insulin.

The effects of adrenaline and noradrenaline on carbohydrate metabolism are complex.[14] Glucose, lactate and pyruvate levels are elevated but part of this elevation may be due to an indirect effect of the simultaneous elevation of glucose and FFA. Thus it has been observed that infusion of glucose in the presence of high FFA levels increases the concentration of lactate and pyruvate. In the heart, adrenaline decreases ATP levels and increases ADP, AMP and phosphate concentrations.[15] There is an increase in glycolysis, glucose or glycogen being used as substrate according to the intensity of the adrenergic stimulus. Catecholamines, particularly adrenaline, can cause a rise in circulating potassium levels followed by hypokalaemia.[15] Noradrenaline has less effect in this respect and in very low concentrations may, in fact, promote potassium uptake in ischaemic tissue.[13]

The complexity of the possible interactions of catecholamines during myocardial ischaemia indicates that it is not possible simply to conclude that they are either beneficial or harmful. The complexity of the situation is summarized in Figure 22, 1.

Beta-adrenergic blockade

In 1958 Dr J. Black initiated a research programme in the laboratories of ICI Pharmaceuticals Division aimed at discovering a compound which would specifically antagonize the cardiac actions of catecholamines. He has written 'We hoped that beta-adrenergic blockade would reduce the consumption of oxygen by the ischaemic myocardium and thus have the same net effect as increasing its oxygen supply. The possibility that the treatment of patients with myocardial ischaemia, with or without an actual infarction with adrenergic beta receptor antagonists might prolong their lives was part of our speculations about the therapeutic use of these drugs'.[17]

Evidence proving that there is an increased local and systemic release of catecholamines in acute myocardial ischaemia has been obtained only in the last ten years.[5 6]

The original findings of Gazes *et al.*[4] are given in Table 22, 1 and show that both angina and infarction in man are accompanied by increased circulating levels of catecholamines, particularly noradrenaline. Initially, it was easier to appreciate the potentially harmful

Table 22, 1 *Plasma catecholamine levels (μg/L) in normal subjects and anginal subjects at rest and after exercise; catecholamine levels 36 and 72 hours after myocardial infarction*

	NUMBER	NORADRENALINE	ADRENALINE
Non-cardiac pain	6	1·85	0·40
Myocardial infarction	13 a)	5·28	0·78
	b)	2·01	0·48
Normal subjects	7 c)	2·43	0·22
	d)	2·53	0·24
Anginal subjects	12 c)	2·53	0·68
	d)	5·55	1·09

Modified from Gazes *et al.* 1959.[4]
a) 36 hours after infarct.
b) 72 hours after infarct.
c) Resting levels.
d) Post exercise levels.

effects of catecholamines than their possible beneficial effects in this situation. At that time the detailed knowledge which we now have concerning the haemodynamic, electrophysiological and metabolic effects of catecholamines was not available. Since it is now appreciated that there must be a balance between the potentially beneficial and harmful effects of catecholamines in myocardial ischaemia, the original ideas concerning the effects of antagonism of catecholamines in this situation have had to be modified. The remainder of this paper will be concerned with a consideration of where this balance is thought to lie.

Acute reversible myocardial ischaemia

It has been recognized for the last fifty years that sympathetic activity could precipitate acute reversible myocardial ischaemia in situations where myocardial oxygen demand could not be met. Cardiac sympathectomy was found to be very effective in a limited number of studies.[18 19] Irradiation of the adrenal glands and reduction in thyroid function have been used, based partly or wholly on the rationale of reducing catecholamine activity and hence myocardial work. The introduction of beta-adrenergic blockade into the therapy of acute reversible myocardial ischaemia has proved to be a major therapeutic advance. Reports of 51 double blind trials involving 1150 patients have been published (Table 22, 2).[20 21] Whilst the criteria used to evaluate efficacy are very imprecise, they are the best presently available. If it is agreed the criteria used for evaluation are valid, then it must be concluded that beta-adrenergic blockade can cause a significant symptomatic improvement in many patients with this condition.

Table 22, 2. *Summary of results of trials of beta blocking drugs in angina pectoris*

NUMBER OF CONTROLLED TRIALS	NUMBER OF PATIENTS	NUMBER OF TRIALS: DRUG BETTER THAN PLACEBO*	TRIALS WITH NO BENEFICIAL EFFECT
51	1152	48	3

* Criteria:—
Effort tolerance.
TNT consumption.
Incidence of anginal pain.

Mode of action

Reversible myocardial ischaemia suggests that there has been a temporary imbalance between myocardial oxygen demand and the ability of the coronary vasculature to supply sufficient oxygenated blood to meet it. In man, even at rest, catecholamine activity modulates heart rate and myocardial contractility. The administration of a beta blocking drug, such as propranolol, causes a reduction in heart rate, in speed of myocardial fibre shortening, and possibly in ‘after-load’. All these actions will reduce myocardial oxygen demand and will therefore favour a reversal of the results of ischaemia. Dwyer and colleagues have shown[22] that the greatest beneficial effect from propranolol is observed in those patients in whom it causes a maximal reduction in heart rate and myocardial contractility, as reflected by dP/dt. Furthermore, Sowton and colleagues[23] have shown that propranolol does not reduce the threshold to pain in patients in whom ischaemic pain is produced, at rest, by electrical pacing of the heart. In other words, the failure of propranolol to slow the heart in this situation prevents it having a beneficial effect, suggesting that its major action in angina is to lower heart rate. The additional actions of beta-adrenergic blockade in possibly increasing cardiac size and systolic ejection time, and promoting ventricular dyskinesis, will tend to increase myocardial oxygen consumption and offset the previously described beneficial effects. It is not possible to predict which of these actions will predominate in an individual patient, though clinical experience suggests that a significant number of patients with reversible myocardial ischaemia are benefited by beta-adrenergic blockade. There is still a need to investigate subjects with reversible myocardial ischaemia who fail to respond to beta-adrenergic blockade, so that an insight might be gained into the mechanisms responsible for pain in these cases.

Irreversible myocardial ischaemia

A reduction in myocardial oxygen consumption brought about by reducing the cardiac effects of catecholamine activity should also be beneficial in irreversible myocardial ischaemia. Recent studies from Braunwald's group[24] have provided experimental evidence that beta-adrenergic blockade will reduce the area of myocardial ischaemia in dogs following experimental ligation of the anterior descending coronary artery. The severity of ischaemia was assessed by measuring the height and extent of ST segment elevation during occlusion and the extent of the depletion of creatine phosphokinase (CPK) 24 hours after ligation of the artery. Inotropic intervention with such drugs as isoprenaline and ouabain increased the severity and extent of the ST segment elevation (Fig. 22, 3). Beta-adrenergic blockade by propranolol reduced the area of ischaemia (Fig. 22, 4). Propranolol also lessened the extent of creatine phosphokinase depletion in the myocardium. Similar results have been obtained using the cardio-selective beta blocking drug practolol.[25] Practolol (2·5 mg/kg iv) was given to six open-chest dogs after a control occlusion had been made of the descending coronary artery. The ST segment elevation decreased from an

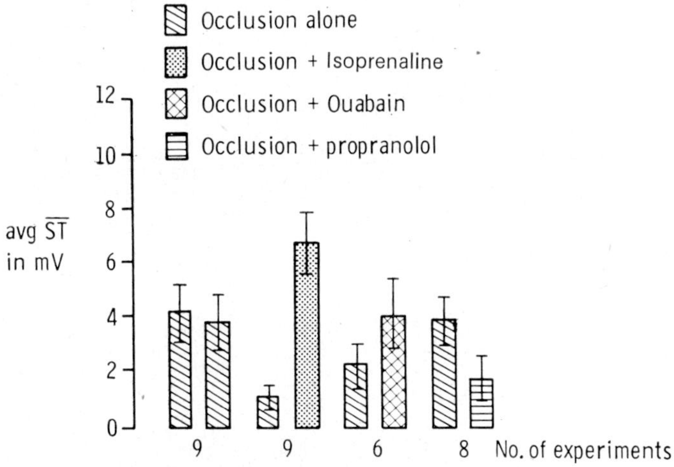

FIG. 22, 3. Influence of repeated occlusions of anterior descending coronary artery of dogs under the influence of isoprenaline, ouabain and propranolol. (From Maroko *et al.* 1971[24] by kind permission of the editors of *Circulation*.)

average of 4·5 ± 0·6 mm before practolol to 2·4 ± 0·4 mm after practolol. Similarly, the number of areas with elevation of the ST segment exceeding 2 mm diminished from 8·30 ± 0·4 to 4·5 ± 0·8. Both these reductions were statistically significant. The only significant change in haemodynamic function during administration of practolol was a reduction in heart rate. There was no change in dP/dt or end-diastolic pressure. Studies have already been carried out in man to determine the effect of beta blockade on the extent of ST segment elevation during myocardial infarction.[26] A multiple electrode 'ECG blanket' technique was used to measure the area of ischaemia as accurately as possible. It was found that propranolol (5 mg iv) caused a clear reversal of ST segment elevation (Fig. 22, 5). Similar results have been reported using practolol.[27] The use of the

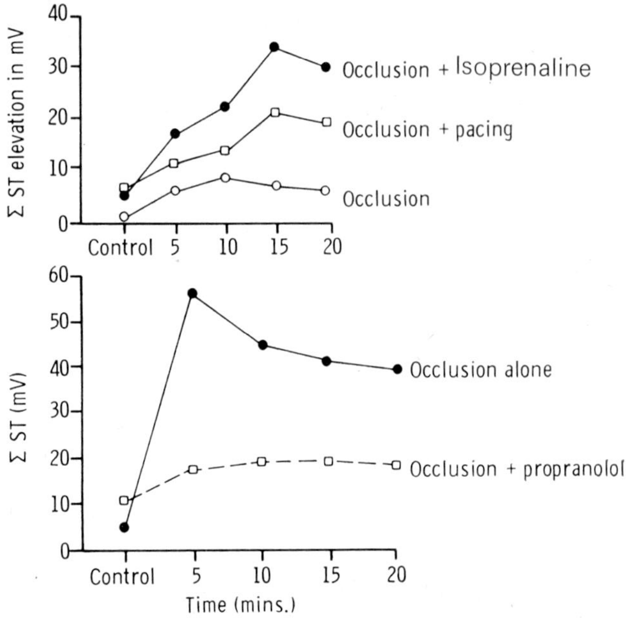

FIG. 22, 4. The effects of tachycardia and isoprenaline (upper graph) and of propranolol (lower graph) on the area of ischaemia as measured by the sum of the ST segment elevations (ST). (From Maroko *et al.* 1971)[24] by kind permission of the Editors of *Circulation.*)

degree and extent of ST segment elevation as a measure of myocardial ischaemia has been questioned,[28] since ST segment elevation indicates transmural injury and does not necessarily signify permanent cell damage. Nevertheless, the good correlation between ECG changes and CPK levels suggests that beta adrenergic blockade can reduce the area of myocardial ischaemia.

Mechanisms of reversing myocardial ischaemia

The mechanism by which this is achieved is not known but the following factors are certainly relevant.

Cardiac work

Left ventricular work is reduced under the influence of beta-adrenergic blockade. Hence myocardial oxygen consumption should

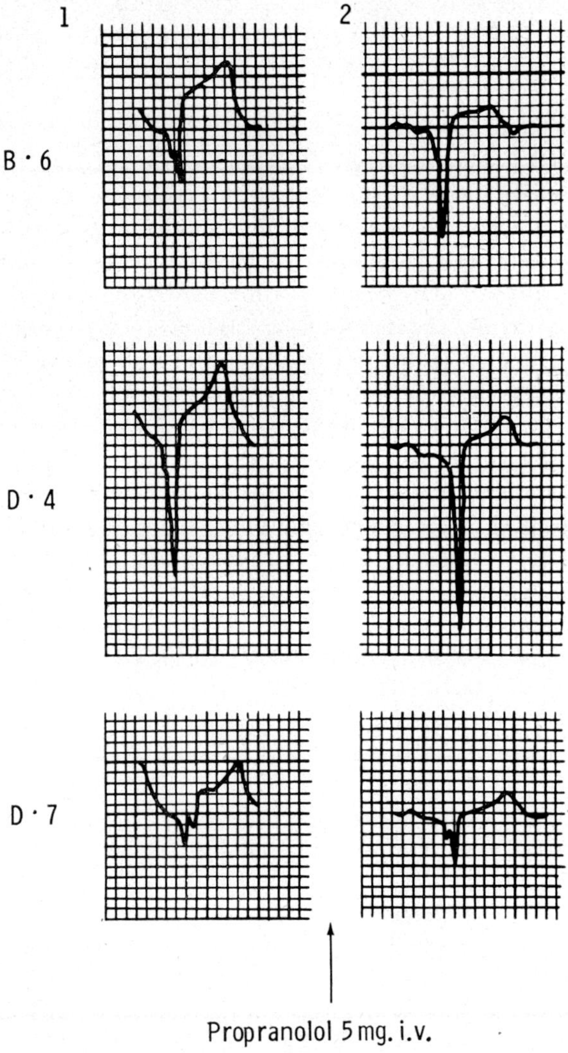

FIG. 22, 5. The influence of propranolol on S-T segment elevation in a 50-year-old man with acute myocardial infarction.
Column 1—immediately before.
Column 2—one hour after propranolol 5 mg i.v.
B.6, D.4, D.7 refer to site of chest leads.
(From Maroko, P. R. *et al.* 1972[26] by kind permission of the Editors of the *American Journal of Cardiology*).

be reduced as well though whether the overall reduction in total myocardial demand or the reduction in the poorly perfused area around the infarct is the important factor is not clear.

Coronary blood flow

The effects of beta-adrenergic blockade on coronary blood flow may also be important. Experimental partial coronary occlusion is followed by a disproportionate fall in endomyocardial blood flow.[29] Studies on canine and guinea pig hearts *in vitro* show that propranolol causes a redistribution of myocardial blood flow from the epicardium to the endocardium.[30 31] Winbury[30] has suggested that this redistribution is due not only to an overall reduction in myocardial metabolism but also to a greater relative resistance in epicardial vessels, due to the higher tissue oxygen tension in this area. It is possible therefore that one of the mechanisms by which beta blockade reduces the area of ischaemia is redistribution of blood flow. The effect of beta blockade on intramyocardial oxygen tension at different myocardial depths before and after coronary artery ligation has not been reported.

Several workers have shown that beta-adrenergic blockade reduces *total* myocardial blood flow. There has been controversy concerning its potentially harmful effects in myocardial ischaemia. The reduction in blood flow is primarily due to the reduction in myocardial work and is evidence of the auto-regulatory control of myocardial blood flow.[32] This view may need some qualifying as a result of the studies reported by Vatner *et al.*[33] who showed that when arterial pressure, myocardial contractility and heart rate were reduced by stimulation of the carotid sinus nerve in the conscious dog, there was a reduction in diastolic coronary resistance. An elevation of resistance would be expected if myocardial metabolism was the sole controlling factor. The reduction in coronary resistance that occurred despite the reduction in myocardial work was thought to be due to a reduction of resting sympathetic vasoconstrictor tone mediated through alpha receptors. It has been suggested that an important element in the reduction of flow following beta-adrenergic blockade is due to an increase in coronary vascular resistance caused by 'unmasking' of alpha receptor activity in coronary vessels.[34] Clinical experience both in patients with angina and myocardial infarction shows that there is an overall increase in myocardial lactate extraction after beta blockade by propranolol.[35 36] This observation suggests that even if unmasking of alpha receptors in the coronary vessels does occur, it is not of crucial importance. The fact that propranolol has little effect on coronary flow in conscious dogs at rest or after atrial pacing (120-210 beats per min) also supports this interpretation.[37 38] In addition, it would be expected that anginal subjects who develop pain during atrial pacing would do so at a lower pacing rate after beta-adrenergic blockade, if significant alpha-adrenergic constriction was exposed by the presence of beta-adrenergic blockade. This has been shown not to occur.[23] Clinical experience supports the experimental findings of Whitsett and Lucchesi that propranolol lowers myocardial blood flow in proportion to the reduction in cardiac work.[39]

The introduction of the cardio-selective beta blocking drug practolol into clinical medicine has reawakened interest in the question of the adrenergic control of coronary vasculature. Practolol antagonizes the chronotropic and inotropic actions of isoprenaline on the heart, without affecting its coronary vasodilator actions in rats,[40] guinea pigs[41] and dogs.[42 43] These various investigators have concluded that the coronary vessels contain predominantly beta receptors related to the peripheral vascular tree and are not blocked by practolol but are blocked by propranolol. These findings are contested by Lucchesi and Hodgeman[44] as well as Somani and Laddu.[45] They find that practolol blocks the coronary vasodilator actions of isoprenaline at doses which also block its inotropic and chronotropic effects. The explanation for the discrepancy in these findings is not clear. Most of the present evidence supports the view that the coronary vessels contain beta receptors which are similar in nature to the peripheral vascular beta receptors. It has also been shown in dogs that practolol potentiates the coronary vasoconstrictor actions of noradrenaline and also of stimulation of the sympathetic nerves to the heart.[42 46] The changes were determined by measuring perfusion pressure in the coronary artery. On the other hand, studies by Somani and Laddu[47] indicate that practolol prevents the reduction by catecholamines of the *nutritional blood* flow in the dog myocardium. It is not possible on present evidence to extrapolate these pharmacological findings to the clinical situation. Evidence is still awaited as to whether practolol has less effect on coronary flow than propranolol in doses which are equally effective in antagonizing the cardiac beta receptors.

In summary, present evidence suggests that the effect of beta adrenergic blockade of coronary blood vessels during myocardial ischaemia is either beneficial or at least certainly not detrimental to the myocardium.

Propranolol and the oxygen dissociation curve

It has recently been shown that propranolol alters the oxygen dissociation curve for haemoglobin in intact human erythrocytes both *in vivo* and *in vitro*.[48] This finding implies that the affinity of haemoglobin for oxygen is reduced at any given partial pressure of oxygen and hence more oxygen is available for utilization by the tissues. This effect has been demonstrated only for propranolol and has been shown not to occur with the other beta blocking drugs, INPEA, KO592, and MJ1999 (sotalol).[49] Propranolol exerts its effects by increasing the concentration of unbound 2,3-diphosphoglycerate (DPG) in the erythrocyte. The concentration of DPG in the human erythrocyte plays a central role in regulating the affinity of haemoglobin for oxygen. An increase in intracellular concentration of DPG reduces the affinity of haemoglobin for oxygen. It is too early to evaluate the relative importance of this action of propranolol in reducing myocardial ischaemia but the importance of abnormal haemoglobin oxygen dissociation in the genesis of angina pectoris has recently been demonstrated.[50,51]

The Anti-arrhythmic Effects of Beta Blocking Drugs in Myocardial Ischaemia

Experimental studies

Cardiac arrhythmias induced by adrenaline or noradrenaline in experimental animals during volatile anaesthesia are prevented or reversed by beta-adrenergic blockade.[52] During experimental myocardial ischaemia, catecholamines have a significant influence on the early occurrence (0-10 min) of ventricular ectopic beats following coronary artery occlusion in dogs.[53] Catecholamines probably are of less importance in the genesis of late onset (greater than eight hours) dysrhythmias.[54] The arrhythmogenic action of catecholamines in myocardial ischaemia has been appreciated but their significance has been disputed.[54] Harris and Bisteni[55] studied the effects of cervical sympathectomy on ventricular ectopics in the early post-coronary occlusion phase in dogs. They showed that sympathectomy reduced the incidence of arrhythmias in this phase and also in the intermediate 4½-8 hours post-occlusion phase. It did not change the time of onset of phase III arrhythmias but may have shortened their duration. According to Maling *et al.*,[54] depletion of cardiac catecholamines by reserpine did not affect early or late arrhythmias induced by coronary ligation in dogs. However, Somers[56] did demonstrate reduction in ventricular fibrillation in reserpinized dogs after 20 minutes transient occlusion of the left coronary artery.

The effect of beta-adrenergic blockade on coronary ligation arrhythmias was first reported by Moran *et al.* in 1962.[57] The action of dichloroisoprenaline (DCI) on adrenaline-induced dysrhythmias in conscious dogs after ligation of the anterior descending coronary artery was studied. DCI (16 mg/kg iv) antagonized the exaggerated ectopic response to intravenous noradrenaline given

Table 22, 3. *The effect of beta blocking drugs on the development of ventricular arrhythmias following experimental infarction in conscious animals*

BETA BLOCKADE IN EXPERIMENTAL INFARCTION ON ARRHYTHMIAS (CONSCIOUS ANIMALS)

Investigator	Ref. No.	Species	Drug	Early	Intermediate	Late	Catecholamine challenge
Lown	58	Dog	Propranolol	+	0	0	0
			Dexpropranolol	+	0	0	0
			Practolol	+	0	0	0
Morris	62	Pigs	Propranolol	+	+	0	0
Harris	59	Dogs	Propranolol	+	+	−	+*
Kaplan	60	Dogs	Bunalolol	0	0	−	+
Shanks	61	Dogs	Propranolol	0	0	−	+
	72	Dogs	Practolol				
Duce	63	Dogs	Alprenolol	0	0	+	0
			Dexalprenolol			+	0

* sympathetic stimulation

on the fourth day after ligation. DCI did not affect the spontaneous ectopic activity at this time. Many studies of the effect of beta blockade on arrhythmias in experimental infarction have appeared since that time (Tables 22, 3 and 22, 4). The experimental protocols

Table 22, 4. *The effect of beta blocking drugs on the development of ventricular arrhythmias following experimental infarction in anaesthetized animals*

BETA BLOCKADE IN EXPERIMENTAL INFARCTION (ANAESTHETIZED ANIMALS)

Investigator	Ref. No.	Species	Drug	Early	Late	Catecholamine challenge
Pentecost	65	Dog	Propranolol	+	0	0
Fearon	66	Dog	Propranolol	+	0	0
Grayson	67	Dog	Propranolol	+	0	0
Nami	73	Dog	Propranolol	—	0	0
Ceremuzynski	3	Dog	Practolol Propranolol	+	0	+
Kaumann	68	Dog	Sotalol	+	0	0
		Depleted Dog	Sotalol	+	0	0
Moran	57	Dog	D.C.I.	0	—	+

— = no effect
\+ = positive effect
0 = not done

used in the various studies differ but they may be considered under two headings: (a) acute studies in anaesthetized animals; (b) acute and chronic studies in conscious animals. In each group the effect of the beta blocking drug on the phase I and phase III (Harris) dysrhythmias are considered separately.*

Phase I arrhythmias

There is a general agreement that blockade of cardiac beta receptors by several different types of beta blocking drug will reduce the

* Editor's footnote. *Phase I* lasts 5 to 20 minutes and is characterized by single ectopic beats and bigeminy; it frequently terminates in ventricular fibrillation. *Phase II* is a period of relative quiescence lasting up to 4 hours in survivors of phase I. *Phase III* lasts up to 36 hours during which there are runs of consecutive beats and bigeminy.

incidence of dysrhythmias in the first 30 minutes following acute myocardial ischaemia in either conscious[72 58 59] or anaesthetized[3 65 66] dogs. It is particularly interesting to note that stimulation of the cardiac sympathetic nerves induce dysrhythmias following coronary artery ligation in dogs and that this is prevented by propranolol.[59] Kaumann and Aramendia[68] observed that sotalol (10 mg/kg iv) was effective in preventing ventricular fibrillation in anaesthetized ligated dogs, both normal and catecholamine depleted. It is difficult to explain this latter finding unless a small residual amount of catecholamine activity was still present. Lown[58] has shown that practolol and propranolol will significantly reduce or prevent ventricular fibrillation in conscious dogs either during occlusion of the coronary artery or after release of the occlusion. Curiously the dextroisomer of propranolol, which has minimal beta blocking activity but important membrane stabilizing properties,[58] completely protected these dogs against ventricular fibrillation after release of temporary occlusion.

The mechanism of the anti-arrhythmic action of beta blockers in phase I infarction arrhythmias is not known. Recent experimental studies indicate that the fibrillation threshold is reduced within two minutes of occlusion and reaches a nadir within five minutes. It returns to normal 30 minutes after occlusion.[69] Han[12] has shown that the fibrillation threshold is reduced in the non-ischaemic part of the myocardium as well as in the ischaemic part. Propranolol (0·2, 1·0, 5·0 mg/kg cumulatively) has no effect on the ventricular fibrillation threshold in normal anaesthetized dogs.[70] Since beta-adrenergic blocking drugs in low doses are specific in that they block only beta receptors, it is reasonable to conclude on present evidence that the anti-arrhythmic effects observed are due to blockade of catecholamine activity. This interpretation is supported by the finding that coronary artery ligation in dogs is accompanied by an increase in catecholamine levels in coronary sinus blood and that both practolol and propranolol will prevent the associated arrhythmia without reduction in the catecholamine levels[3 71] (Fig. 22, 6).

Phase III arrhythmias

Blockade of cardiac beta receptors does not influence the incidence of phase III dysrhythmias in dogs.[60 61 72] All the blocking drugs studied (Table 22, 3 and 22, 4) reduce or prevent catecholamine induced arrhythmias during phase III. Duce *et al.*[63] have shown that large doses of the laevo (7·5 mg) and dextro (15 mg/kg) isomers of alprenalol as well as racemic alprenalol (3·5 mg/kg) reduce the incidence of arrhythmias in phase III. Since the doses of drug used are at least 100 times higher than those needed for beta-adrenergic blockade, it seems likely that the anti-arrhythmic action is due to the membrane stabilizing action of this drug. In contrast, Shanks and Dunlop[61] did not observe any change in the incidence

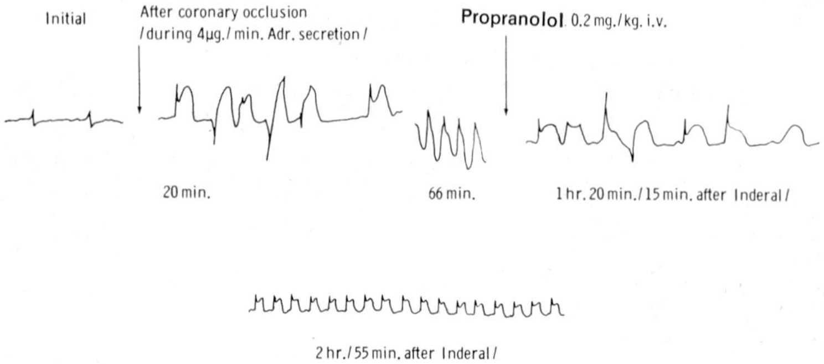

FIG. 22, 6. Lead I ECG recordings in anaesthetized dog (chloralose) before and after ligation of anterior descending coronary artery. After occlusion the arterial level of adrenaline rose to 4 µg/min and was followed by ventricular tachycardia. Propranolol suppressed the tachycardia and sinus rhythm returned. (From Ceremuzynski *et al.* 1969)[3] by kind permission of the Editors of *Cardiovascular Research.*

of phase III ectopic arrhythmias after dexpropranolol (3·0 mg/kg). The failure of beta blocking drugs to control arrhythmias in phase III suggests that catecholamine activity is less important in the maintenance of this class of arrhythmia. This may explain why beta blockade has failed in preventing the development of dysrhythmias in patients with myocardial infarction because all these are occurring in the ' late ' phase III stage. Alternatively, these experimental arrhythmias may not resemble those found in man. No studies of the prophylactic administration of beta blocking drugs in man prior to the onset of myocardial infarction have been reported.

Mortality studies

Morris *et al.*[62] observed that propranolol (0·2 mg/kg per 6 hours) prolonged survival time from the control of 28 hours to 49 hours in pigs in which infarction was produced by means of an ameroid constrictor.[67] Grayson also reported prolonged survival in dogs following acute ligation of the anterior descending coronary artery.[67] In contrast, Nami and Proger[73] were unable to show a significant improvement in mortality in anaesthetized dogs after ligation of the anterior descending coronary artery. There is insufficient experimental evidence to form any opinion as to the effect of beta blockade on survival in acute experimental myocardial infarction.

Clinical studies

The use of beta adrenergic blocking drugs during myocardial infarction has been reviewed.[74,75] Two types of study have been carried out. Firstly, those in which the drugs have been used to treat dysrhythmias as they arise in patients with myocardial infarction. Secondly, studies in which patients with myocardial infarction have been given beta blocking drugs as soon as the diagnosis has been made in an attempt to reduce mortality and the incidence of dysrhythmias.

A. Therapeutic studies

There are relatively few reports relating specifically to the use of beta blocking drugs in post-infarction arrhythmias in man. It is clear from these sporadic reports that propranolol, alprenolol, oxprenolol and practolol have successfully controlled supraventricular and ventricular dysrhythmias. The largest series reported so far is that of Lemberg *et al.*[76] who used propranolol to control 43 episodes of tachyarrhythmias and Jewitt *et al.*[77] who studied practolol in 75 patients with infarction.

Supraventricular arrhythmias

In Lemberg's series the arrhythmias included atrial fibrillation, atrial flutter and supraventricular tachycardia. In all but one of these patients sinus rhythm returned and the ventricular rates slowed to 80 beats per min after 0·5 to 0·75 mg of propranolol intravenously. All the patients initially had ventricular rates in excess of 140 beats per min.

In the series reported by Jewitt *et al,* there were 35 patients with supraventricular arrhythmias and a majority of these also had ventricular rates above 140 beats per min. Of 18 patients with atrial fibrillation, 14 responded with a reduction of ventricular rate to below 100 beats per min and in 5 sinus rhythm returned. Of 13 patients with atrial flutter or tachycardia, in which the ventricular rates were above 140 beats per min, 12 had a reduction in the ventricular rates associated with clinical benefit. Eight of these 12 patients reverted to sinus rhythm and in the others the slowing of the ventricular rate was due to increased atrio-ventricular block, the rate of atrial flutter being unchanged.

Ventricular arrhythmias

Ventricular ectopic beats were suppressed in 14 of 17 patients with myocardial infarction receiving propranolol (9 cases) or alprenolol (8 cases).[74] In 13 of 24 patients with ventricular ectopics, practolol 5 to 25 mg i.v. suppressed the ventricular ectopics.[77] All these patients were resistant to lidocaine (2 mg/kg i.v.) given previously. Lemberg[76] has reported control of ventricular tachycardia in 8 patients resistant to lidocaine or quinidine. Forty patients with myocardial infarction who developed ventricular tachycardia have been treated with either propranolol (20 cases)[74,76] or practolol (20 cases).[77,78] In the propranolol treated cases, fourteen reverted to sinus rhythm, whilst in the practolol treated group ten returned to sinus rhythm.

Beta-adrenergic blockade has been used in an attempt to maintain sinus rhythm after DC counter shock in forty-five patients. Sinus rhythm was restored by propranolol in 23 of 38 such patients. Six patients in whom ventricular fibrillation developed after acute infarction and who failed to respond to DC shock, did so after practolol (5 to 15 mg i.v.).

These clinical findings suggest that beta-adrenergic blockade will control a significant number of supraventricular and ventricular dysrhythmias in acute myocardial infarction. There is no evidence to indicate the true proportion of responsive subjects with myocardial infarction or how to select the likely responders.

B. Prophylactic (mortality) studies

The first report of studies of the effect of beta-adrenergic blockade on mortality in myocardial infarction was published by Snow in 1965.[79] Propranolol (20 mg orally 8 hourly) was given to every second patient admitted with myocardial infarction. The mortality of the treated group was 16 per cent as opposed to 35 per cent in the control group. This trial was extended until a total of 52 treated patients and 55 control patients had been studied. The mortality in the treated group was 13 per cent and in the control was 25 per cent. The differences were significant at the 5 per cent level.[80] Since then there have been ten studies of the effect of beta blockade, given prophylactically, on the mortality and morbidity in myocardial infarction which failed to reproduce these results. Eight of these concerned propranolol, one of them has concerned oxprenolol and one has concerned alprenolol.[81 82] There is now no doubt that beta blocking drugs given prophylactically in patients presenting with symptoms of myocardial infarction will effect neither the incidence of cardiac arrhythmias nor the overall death rate in these cases. The reasons for this failure are probably many. The most important may be that the drugs were given after the patient had presented with symptoms and were therefore presumably in a clinical phase equivalent to phase III of experimental infarction. It may well be that catecholamines do not play such an important part in the genesis of arrhythmias at this phase. However, it is known that the majority of patients who die, die within an hour of the onset of the infarct and they may die an arrhythmic death which would be equivalent to the Harris phase I experimental arrhythmia. It would therefore be unjustifiable to conclude that beta-adrenergic blocking drugs have no part to play in the prevention of arrhythmias due to myocardial infarction. The fault may lie in not being able to administer the drug at a time when its pharmacological action is most appropriate.

Disadvantages of beta blockade in irreversible myocardial ischaemia

The evidence presented suggests that beta-adrenergic blockade may reduce the size of the ischaemic area and control established dysrhythmias associated with irreversible myocardial ischaemia. What is the price paid for these actions? The paradox concerning the use of beta blocking drugs in ischaemia is that they must reduce cardiac function if they are to achieve the reduction in ischaemia. But clearly there is an optimal degree of cardiac function and the effect of beta-adrenergic blockade depends where that optimum lies. On the positive side, subjects with high ventricular rates, even with heart failure, are improved by beta-adrenergic blockade.[76 77] This improvement is brought about probably by reducing the high ventricular rate which permits better ventricular filling and improved coronary flow and reduced myocardial oxygen consumption. This may explain why Lemberg[76] observed such favourable results with propranolol since all his myocardial infarction patients had ventricular rates in excess of 140 bts/min.

On the other hand, patients who have modest ventricular rates which fall rapidly after propranolol may deteriorate clinically. Stannard *et al.*[83] have shown that the simultaneous administration of atropine (1 to 2 mg i.v.) together with propranolol (0·1 mg/kg) will prevent the reduction in cardiac output in patients with myocardial infarction. It is possible that a considerable element of the unwanted reduction in haemodynamic function in patients with myocardial infarction after beta-adrenergic blockade is due to unopposed vagal activity.

A further disadvantage of beta-adrenergic blockade may be that it can cause or enhance ventricular dyskinesis as demonstrated by Gorlin's group in Boston.[84] Thus by reducing myocardial contractility, there is an increased stretching of the myocardial tissue in the ischaemic area which further impairs cardiac output. Stretching in this area may also act as a trigger for dysrhythmias.[12] In addition non-selective beta-adrenergic blocking drugs may increase 'afterload' by a reflex rise in peripheral resistance due to a fall in cardiac output. This response may not only embarrass the heart but potentiate catecholamine arrhythmias by increasing ventricular wall tension. It has been suggested that the absence of unwanted haemodynamic sequelae following the use of practolol in myocardial infarction is due to its cardioselectivity,[85] because by not blocking peripheral vascular beta receptors, alpha adrenergic activity should not be unmasked. Non-selective beta blockade could increase 'afterload' as well as diminish venous return by enhancing the alpha stimulating action of adrenaline. There is no firm evidence to support this theory at present.

Another aspect of the problem concerns the possible effects of non-selective beta-adrenergic drugs on pulmonary function. Though beta blockade does not cause significant reduction in pulmonary function in normal subjects,[86] a small increase in airways resistance in patients with myocardial infarction may aggravate hypoxia by disturbing ventilation/perfusion relationships. The importance of this factor has not been evaluated. The prior administration of atropine should prevent this as well as an unwanted bradycardia. The favourable and unfavourable effects of beta-adrenergic blockade in myocardial ischaemia are shown in Figure 22, 7 where the disadvantages already discussed are shown on the right hand side. Against these disadvantages must be set the undoubted antidysrhythmic actions of beta blocking drugs in acute myocardial

Beta Blockers in Myocardial Ischaemia.

Positive	Negative
Reduce heart rate	Bradycardia
Reduce contractility	Negative inotropic effect
Redistribute regional blood flow	Potentiate α effects (coronary / peripheral) vessels
Antagonize catechol. dysrhythmias	Reduce ventilators function
? Reduce lipolysis	Increase myocardial dyskinesis
? Oxygen dissociation curve (2,3 D.P.G.)	Increase bradyarrythmias
	Increase size of ventricle

FIG. 22, 7. Summary of the unwanted (negative) and desirable (positive) pharmacological effects of nonselective beta blocking drugs in myocardial ischaemia.

ischaemia, as well as the possible favourable action in re-distributing myocardial blood flow. The possible advantages of the non-cardiac effects of beta blocking drugs is less certain but may merit further study. The unwanted actions of high circulating levels of free fatty acids in the setting of acute myocardial ischaemia have been recently reviewed[87] and it is possible that beta blockade may reduce the enhanced lipolysis occurring in this situation. It is also possible that the recently described effects of propranolol on the oxygen dissociation curve may be of relevance.[48]

What may be needed, perhaps, is a drug with all the beneficial actions listed in Figure 22, 7 and none of the unwanted ones. The cardio-selective beta blocking drug practolol may go some way toward meeting this requirement. The haemodynamic effects of practolol in subjects suffering from myocardial infarction differ markedly from those of propranolol (Fig. 22, 8). Cardiac output does not change after practolol (5 mg i.v.) though there is a small fall after 25 mg intravenously. Thus in patients reported by Jewitt and Croxson there was a fall in cardiac output from 4·9 to 4·5 litres per min ten min after administration of 25 mg of practolol (i.v.).[89]

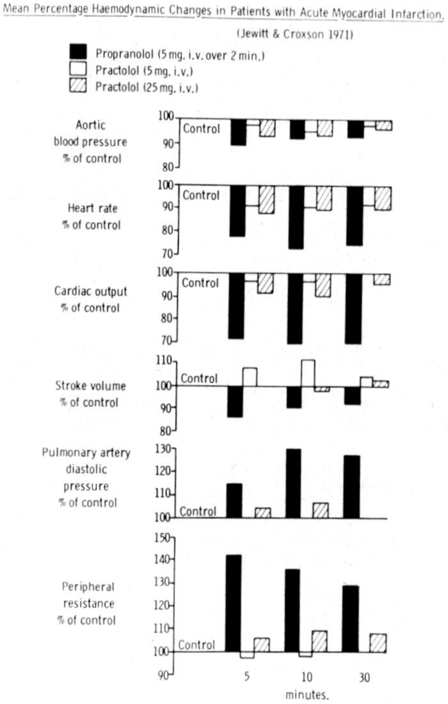

FIG. 22, 8. Haemodynamic changes (expressed as mean percentage change) in patients with acute myocardial infarction who received propranolol 5 mg intravenously over 2 min (5 patients), practolol 5 mg intravenously over 2 min (5 patients) and practolol 25 mg intravenously over 2 min (10 patients). (From Jewitt and Croxson 1971[71] by kind permission of the Editors of the *Postgraduate Medical Journal*).

There was also a very small rise in pulmonary artery pressure, and total peripheral resistance with a small fall on heart rate and diastolic blood pressure. These modest changes are in marked contrast to those observed after propranolol (5 mg) administered in a similar clinical setting.

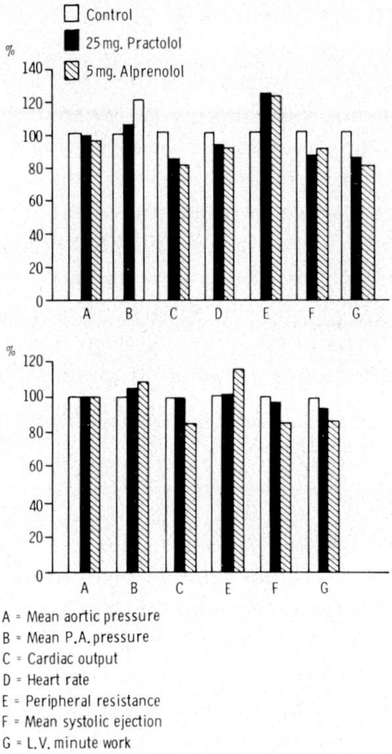

FIG. 22, 9. A comparison of the haemodynamic effects of practolol 25 mg and alprenolol 5 mg intravenously in a patient with myocardial infarction: upper histogram heart rate unpaced. Lower histogram: similar comparison in a patient with sinus bradycardia and myocardial infarction atrially paced at 90 beats min. (Jewitt, D. E. 1971[85].) (By kind permission of the Editors of 'Symposium on Cardiac arrhythmias'.)

It is interesting to speculate on the reasons for these differences. Are they due to the selectivity of action of practolol, or to the partial agonist activity, or to both these differences from propranolol? Jewitt[89] has explored the possible role of partial agonist activity by comparing the haemodynamic effects of alprenolol and practolol, both of which have equivalent partial agonist or intrinsic activity in subjects with myocardial infarction. Both drugs caused a fall in cardiac output when given to a patient with myocardial infarction (Fig. 22, 9). However when the heart rate was held constant by atrial pacing, alprenolol still lowered the cardiac output whilst practolol had no effect. These findings suggest that the cardio-selective action of practolol may be important. It is extremely unlikely that the absence of membrane stabilizing properties in practolol is an important factor in determining its absence of deleterious haemodynamic effects since Bennett *et al.*[90] have shown that dexpropranolol (25 mg i.v.) does not cause significant haemodynamic changes in patients suffering from myocardial infarction. Since dexpropranolol and racemic propranolol have equivalent membrane stabilizing activity[91] it seems extremely unlikely that this pharmacological property is of relevance in the clinical situation.

Conclusion

This paper has set out to show that the original view that catecholamine activity is inimicable in myocardial ischaemia is not necessarily true. Therefore the specific inhibition of the action of catecholamines by beta blocking drugs is not always beneficial. Present evidence indicates that beta blockade is of undoubted value in acute reversible myocardial ischaemia. In irreversible myocardial ischaemia, it can be valuable in controlling supraventricular and ventricular dysrhythmias. The unwanted haemodynamic and respiratory effects can be largely nullified by using practolol with or without atropine. There may yet be an important role for beta adrenergic blocking drugs in the management of myocardial ischaemia if a means is found to administer the correct dose at the correct time. A further advance would be to discover a beta blocking drug without negative inotropic actions and perhaps find one with additional electrophysiological properties. The role of beta-adrenergic blockade in myocardial ischaemia will be clarified further as new types of beta blocking drugs are developed.

REFERENCES

1 BARRATT, A. M. & FITZGERALD, J. D. (1968). What is a β-blocker? *American Heart Journal* **76,** 712-714.

2 RAAB, W. (1962). The sympathogenic biochemical trigger mechanism of angina pectoris. *American Journal of Cardiology* **9,** 576-590.

3 CEREMUZYNSKI, L., STASZEWSKA-BARCZAK, J. & HERBACZYNSKA-CEDRO, K. (1969). Cardiac rhythm disturbances and the release of catecholamines after acute coronary occlusion in dogs. *Cardiovascular Research* **3,** 190-197.

4 GAZES, P. C., RICHARDSON, J. A. & WOODS, E. F. (1959). Plasma catecholamine concentrations in myocardial infarction and angina pectoris, *Circulation* **19,** 657-661.

5 JEQUIER, E. & PERRET, C. (1970). Urinary excretion of catecholamines and their main metabolites after myocardial infarction; relationship of the clinical syndrome. *European Journal of Clinical Investigation* **1,** 77-83.

6 GRIFFITHS, J. & LEUNG, F. (1971). The sequential estimation of plasma catecholamines and whole blood histamine in myocardial infarction. *American Heart Journal* **82,** 171-179.

7 BRAUNWALD, E. (1971). Control of myocardial oxygen consumption. *American Journal of Cardiology* **27,** 416-432.

8 BERNE, R. M. (1966). In *The Myocardial Cell,* p. 355. Edited by S. A. Briller and H. J. Conn. Philadelphia: University of Pennsylvania Press.

9 BROOKS, C. M., HOFFMAN, B. F. & SUCKLING, E. (1955). In *Excitability of the Heart.* New York/London: Grune and Stratton.

10 HOFFMAN, B. F. & SINGER, D. H. (1967). Appraisal of the effect of catecholamines on cardiac electrical activity. *Annals of the New York Academy of Science* **139,** 914-939.

11 HAN, J. (1969). Mechanism of ventricular arrhythmias associated with myocardial infarction. *American Journal of Cardiology* **24,** 800-813.

12 HAN, J., DE JALON, G. & MOE, G. K. (1964). Adrenergic effects on ventricular vulnerability. *Circulation Research* **14,** 516-524.

13 REGAN, T. J., MURKOV, A., OLDEWURTAL, H. H. & BURKE, W. M. (1970). Myocardial metabolism and function during ischaemia: response to l-noradrenaline. *Cardiovascular Research* **4,** 334-342.

14 HIMMS-HAGEN, J. (1967). Sympathetic regulation of metabolism. *Pharmacological Review* **19,** 367-461.

15 WILLIAMSON, J. R. (1966). Kinetic studies of epinephrine effects in the perfused rat heart. *Pharmacological Review* **18,** 205-210.

16 COSTIN, J. C. & SKINNER, N. S. (1971). Effects of systemic hypoxemia and catecholamines on arterial potassium in concentrations before and after β-adrenergic blockade. *European Journal of Pharmacology* **16,** 142-147.

17 BLACK, J. W. (1967). In *Drug Responses in Man,* p. 121. Edited by G. Wolstenholme and R. Porter. London: Churchill.

18 BIRKETT, D. A., ALTHORP, G. H., CHAMBERLAIN, D. A., HAYWARD, G. W. & TUCKWELL, E. G. (1965). Bilateral upper thoracic sympathectomy in angina pectoris: result in 52 cases. *British Medical Journal* **2,** 187-190.

19 LINDGREN, I. (1950). Angina pectoris. A clinical study with special reference to neurosurgical treatment. *Acta Medica Scandinavica* **138,** *Suppl.* **243,** 389-404.

20 ELLIOTT, W. C. & STONE, J. M. (1969). Beta-adrenergic blocking agents for the treatment of angina pectoris. *Progress in Cardiovascular Diseases* **12,** 83-98.

21 FITZGERALD, J. D. (1972). Beta-adrenergic blocking drugs: present position and future development. *Acta Cardiologica Suppl.* **15,** 199-216.

22 DWYER, E. M., WEINER, L. & COX, J. W. (1967). Effect of beta-adrenergic blockade on left ventricular hemodynamics and electrocardiogram during exercise-induced angina pectoris. *Circulation* **36 II,** 99-100.

23 BALCON, R. (1971). Assessment of drugs in angina pectoris: *Postgraduate Medical Journal* **47,** *Suppl.,* 53-58.

24 MAROKO, P. R., KJEKSHUS, J. K., SOBEL, B. E., WATANABE, T., COVELL, J. W., ROSS, J. & BRAUNWALD, E. (1971). Factors influencing infarct size following experimental coronary artery occlusion. *Circulation* **43,** 67-82.

25 LIBBY, P., MAROKO, P. R., COVELL, J. W., MALLOCH, C. I., ROSS, J. & BRAUNWALD, E. (1972). Reduction in infarct size following experimental coronary occlusion by hydrocortisone treatment. *Clinical Research* **20,** 207.

26 MAROKO, P. R., LIBBY, D., COVELL, J. W., SOBELL, B. E., ROSS, J. & BRAUNWALD, E. (1972). Precordial S-T segment elevation mapping. *American Journal of Cardiology* **29,** 223-230.

27 REID, D., PELIDES, L. J., THOMAS, M. & SHILLINGFORD, J. P. (1971). Surface mapping of the RS-T segment in acute myocardial infarction and effect of beta-blockade. *British Heart Journal* **33,** 609.

28 HOOD, W. D. (1971). Salvage of myocardium in acute ischemia. *Circulation* **43,** 11-13.

29 WINBURY, M. M., HOWE, B. P. & WEISS, H. R. (1971). Effect of nitroglycerin and dipyridamole on epicardial and endocardial oxygen tension —further evidence for redistribution of myocardial blood flow. *Journal of Pharmacological and Experimental Therapy* **176,** 184-199.

30 WINBURY, M. M., WEISS, H. R. & HOWE, B. P. (1971). Effects of β-adrenoreceptor blockade and nitroglycerin on myocardial oxygenation. *European Journal of Pharmacology* **16,** 271-277.

31 VIRTANEN, K. & FRICK, N. H. (1971). Effect of beta blockade on myocardial blood content during the cardiac cycle in guinea pigs. *Scandinavian Journal of Clinical & Laboratory Investigation* **27,** *Suppl.* **166,** 22.

32 SHANKS, R. G. (1967). Propranolol in myocardial infarction. *Lancet* **I,** 788-789.

33 VATNER, S. F., FRANKLIN, D., VAN CITTERS, R. L. & BRAUNWALD, E. (1970). Effects of carotid sinus nerve stimulation on the coronary circulation of the conscious dog. *Circulation Research* **27,** 11-21.

34 PARRATT, J. R. & GRAYSON, J. (1966). Myocardial vascular reactivity after beta-adrenergic blockade. *Lancet* **I,** 338-340.

35 WOLFSON, S. & GORLIN, R. (1969). Cardiovascular pharmacology of propranolol in man. *Circulation* **40,** 501-511.

36 MUELLER, H., AYRES, S. M. & GRACE, W. S. (1972). Effects of propranolol and L-norephinephrine in acute myocardial infarction in man. *American Journal of Cardiology* **29,** 282-283.

37 PITT, B. & GREGG, D. E. (1968). Coronary hemodynamic effects of increasing ventricular rate in the unanesthetized dog. *Circulation Research* **22,** 753-761.

38 BERGAMSCHI, M., SHANKS, R. G., CARAVAGGI, A. M. & MANDELLI, V. (1971). A comparison of the cardiovascular actions of four adrenergic β-receptor blocking agents in resting, conscious dogs. *American Heart Journal* **82,** 338-351.

39 WHITSITT, L. S. & LUCCHESI, B. R. (1967). Effects of propranolol and its stereoisomers upon coronary vascular resistance. *Circulation Research* **21,** 305-317.

40 DEPRECZENI, L. & VFENYVEZI, T. (1971). Effect of β-adrenoceptor blocking compounds on isoprenaline induce changes in regional blood flow in the rat. *British Journal of Pharmacology* **41,** 171-176.

41 BROADLEY, K. J. (1970). An analysis of the coronary vascular responses to catecholamines, using a modified Langendorff heart preparation. *British Journal of Pharmacology* **40,** 617-629.

42 ROSS, G. & JORGENSEN, C. R. (1970). Effects of a cardio-selective beta-adrenergic blocking agent on the heart and coronary circulation. *Cardiovascular Research* **4,** 148-153.

43 McRaven, D. R., Mark, A. L., Abboud, F. M. & Mayer, A. H. (1971). Responses of coronary vessels to adrenergic stimuli. *Journal of Clinical Investigation* **50,** 773-778.

44 Lucchesi, D. R. & Hodgeman, R. J. (1971). Effect of 4(2-hydroxy-3-isopropylaminopropoxy) acetamilide (AY 21,011) on the myocardial and coronary vascular response to adrenergic stimulation. *Journal of Pharmacology and Experimental Therapeutics* **176,** 200-211.

45 Somani, P. & Laddu, A. R. (1969). Blockade of cardiac effects of isoproterenol by 4-(2-hydroxy-3-isopropylaminopropoxy)-acetanilide. *Journal of Pharmacology and Experimental Therapeutics* **170,** 72-78.

46 Adam, K. R., Boyles, S. & Scholfield, P. C. (1970). Cardio-selective β-adrenoceptor blockade and the coronary circulation. *British Journal of Pharmacology* **40,** 534-536.

47 Somani, P., Laddu, A. R. & Hardman, H. F. (1970). Nutritional circulation in the heart. *Journal of Pharmacology and Experimental Therapeutics* **175,** 577-592.

48 Oski, F. A., Miller, L. D., Delivoria-Papadoulos, M., Manchester, J. H. & Shelburne, J. C. (1972). Oxygen affinity in red cells: changes induced in vivo by propranolol. *Science* **175,** 1372-1373.

49 Pendleton, R. C., Newman, D. J., Sherman, S. S., Braun, E. C. & Maya, W. E. (1972). The effect of propranolol upon the haemoglobin oxygen dissociation curve. *Journal of Pharmacology and Experimental Therapeutics* **180,** 647-657.

50 Elliot, R. S. & Bratt, G. (1969). The paradox of myocardial ischemia and necrosis in young women with normal coronary arteriograms. *American Journal of Cardiology* **23,** 633-638.

51 Shapell, S. D., Murray, J. A., Nasser, M. O., Wills, H. E., Torrance, J. D. & Lenfant, C. J. M. (1970). Acute change in hemoglobin affinity for oxygen during angina pectoris. *New England Journal of Medicine* **282,** 1219-1224.

52 Black, J. W., Duncan, W. A. & Shank, R. G. (1965). Comparison of some properties of pronethalol and propranolol. *British Journal of Pharmacology* **25,** 577-591.

53 Harris, A. S., Estandia, A. & Tillotson, R. F. (1951). Effects of diphenylhydantion sodium (dilantin sodium) and phenobarbital sodium upon ectopic ventricular tachycardia in acute myocardial infarction. *American Journal of Physiology* **163,** 505-516.

54 Maling, H. M., Cohn, V. H. & Highman, B. (1959). The effect of coronary occlusion in dogs treated with reserpine and in dogs treated with phenoxybenzamine. *Journal of Pharmacology and Experimental Therapeutics* **127,** 229-235.

55 Harris, A. S. & Bisteni, A. (1955). Effects of sympathetic blockade drugs on ventricular tachycardia resulting from myocardial infarction. *American Journal of Physiology* **181,** 559-566.

56 Sommers, H. M. (1966). The effect of reserpine and propranolol on spontaneous ventricular fibrillation and myocardial necrosis following transient coronary artery occlusion. *Federation Proceedings* **25, Part 1,** 666.

57 Moran, N. C., Moore, J. I., Holcomb, A. K. & Mushet, G. (1962). Antagonism of adrenergically induced cardiac arrhythmias by dichloroisoproterenol. *Journal of Pharmacology and Experimental Therapeutics* **136,** 327-335.

58 Lown, B. & Wolf, M. (1971). Approaches to sudden death from coronary heart disease. *Circulation* **44,** 130-142.

59 Harris, A. S., Otero, H. & Bocage, A. J. (1971). The induction of arrhythmias by sympathetic activity before and after occlusion of a coronary artery in the canine heart. *Journal of Electrocardiography* **4,** 34-43.

60 KAPLAN, H. P. & ROBSON, R. D. (1970). Anti-arrhythmic activity of bunolol, a new beta adrenergic blocking agent. *Journal of Pharmacology and Experimental Therapeutics* **175,** 168-177.

61 SHANKS, R. G. & DUNLOP, D. (1967). Effect of propranolol on arrhythmias following coronary artery occlusion in dogs. *Cardiovascular Research* **1,** 34-41.

62 MORRIS, J. J., WOHLGEMUTH, S., JACKSON, D., WHALEN, R. E. & MCINTOSH, H. D. (1967). Quinidine, propranolol and polarizing solution in the treatment of experimental myocardial infarction. *Clinical Research* **15,** 57.

63 DUCE, B. R. & GURBERG, L. (1969). Effect of alprenolol, a new beta-adrenergic receptor isomer, on arrhythmias following coronary artery occlusion in dogs. *Federation Proceedings* **28,** 1230.

64 SOMANI, P. & LUM, B. K. B. (1965). The anti-arrhythmic action of beta-adrenergic blocking agents. *Journal of Pharmacology and Experimental Therapeutics* **147,** 194-204.

65 PENTECOST, B. L. & AUSTEN, W. O. (1966). Beta-adrenergic blockade in experimental myocardial infarction. *American Heart Journal* **72,** 790, 796.

66 FEARON, R. E. (1967). Propranolol in the prevention of ventricular fibrillation due to experimental coronary artery occlusion. *American Journal of Cardiology* **20,** 222-228.

67 GRAYSON, J. (1967). Propranolol in myocardial infarction. *Lancet* **1,** 788-789.

68 KAUMANN, A. J. & ARAMENDIA, P. (1968). Prevention of ventricular fibrillation induced by coronary ligation. *Journal of Pharmacology and Experimental Therapeutics* **164,** 326-332.

69 BURHESS, M. J., ABILDSKOW, J. A., MILLAR, K., GEDDES, J. S. & GREEN, L. S. (1971). Time course of vulnerability to fibrillation after experimental coronary occlusion. *American Journal of Cardiology* **27,** 617-621.

70 ALLAN, J. D., PANTRIDGE, J. F. & SHANKS, R. G. (1971). Effect of lignocaine, propranolol and bretylium on ventricular fibrillation threshold. *American Journal of Cardiology* **28,** 555-562.

71 SERRANO, P. A., CHAVEZ-LARD, B., BISTENI, A. & SODI-PALLARES, D. (1971). Effect of propranolol on catecholamine content of injured cardiac tissue. *Journal of Molecular and Cellular Cardiology* **2,** 91-97

72 SHANKS, R. G. & DUNLOP, D. (1968). Selective blockade of adrenoceptive beta receptors in the heart. *British Journal of Pharmacology* **32,** 201-218.

73 NAMI, S. & PROGER, S. (1966). Propranolol in myocardial infarction. *Lancet* **II,** 1465-1466.

74 GIBSON, D. & SOWTON, E. (1969). The use of beta-adrenergic receptor blocking drugs in dysrhythmias. *Progress in Cardiovascular Diseases* **12,** 16-39.

75 JEWITT, D. & SINGH, B. (1972). In *Textbook of Coronary Care*. Edited by: A. J. Dunning and L. E. Meltzer. In press.

76 LEMBERG, L., CASTELLANOS, A. & ARABAL, A. C. (1970). The use of propranolol in arrhythmias complicating acute myocardial infarction. *American Heart Journal* **80,** 479-487.

77 JEWITT, D. E., MERCER, C. J. & SHILLINGFORD, J. P. (1969). Practolol in the treatment of cardiac dysrhythmias due to acute myocardial infarction. *Lancet* **II,** 227-232.

78 ALLAN, J. D., PANTRIDGE, J. F. & SHANKS, R. G. (1967). Practolol in the treatment of ventricular dysrhythmias in acute myocardial infarction. *Postgraduate Medical Journal* **47,** *Suppl.*, 29-35.

79 SNOW, P. J. D. (1965). Effect of propranolol in myocardial infarction. *Lancet* **II,** 551-553.

80 SNOW, P. J. D (1966). Treatment of acute myocardial infarction with propranolol. *American Journal of Cardiology* **18,** 458-462.

81 Sowton, E. (1968). Beta-adrenergic blockade in cardiac infarction. *Progress in Cardiovascular Diseases* **10,** 561-574.
82 Reynolds, J. L. & Whitlock, R. M. L. (1972). Effects of a beta-adrenergic receptor blocker in myocardial infarction treated for one year from onset. *British Heart Journal* **34,** 252-259.
83 Stannard, M., Sloman, G. & Sangster, L. (1968). The haemodynamic effects of atropine combined with propranolol in acute myocardial infarction. *Medical Journal of Australia* **1,** 333-334.
84 Helfant, R. H., Herman, M. V. & Gorlin, R. (1971). Abnormalities of left ventricular contraction induced by beta-adrenergic blockade. *Circulation* **43,** 641-647.
85 Gibson, D. C. (1971). Haemodynamic effects of practolol. *Postgraduate Medical Journal* **47,** *Suppl.,* 16-21.
86 Richardson, P. S. & Sterling, C. M. (1969). Effect of beta-adrenergic receptor blockade on airway conductance and lung volume in normal and asthmatic subjects. *British Medical Journal* **3,** 143-145.
87 Kurien, V. A., Yates, P. A. & Oliver, M. F. (1971). The role of free fatty acids in the production of ventricular arrhythmias after acute coronary artery occlusion. *European Journal of Clinical Investigation* **1,** 225-241.
88 Jewitt, D. E. & Croxson, R. (1971). Practolol in the management of cardiac dysrhythmias following myocardial infarction and cardiac surgery. *Postgraduate Medical Journal* **47,** *Suppl.,* 25-29.
89 Jewitt, D. E. (1970). In *Symposium on Cardiac Arrhythmias,* p. 517. Edited by E. Sandoe, E. Flensted-Jensen and K. H. Olsen. Södertälje/Sweden: Astra AB.
90 Bennett, S., Balcon, R., Hoy, J. & Sowton, E. (1970). Haemodynamic effects of dextro-propranolol in acute myocardial infarction. *Thorax* **25,** 86-88.
91 Barratt, A. M. & Cullum, V. (1968). The biological properties of the optimal isomers of propranolol and their effects on cardiac arrhythmias. *British Journal of Pharmacology* **34,** 43-55.

Discussion

Thomas. About a year ago we gave practolol to a series of patients after myocardial infarction but without pulmonary oedema and showed that it was feasible to lower the ST segments. Like others, we tried to evaluate the biological value of ST segment inhibition in experimental animals. One approach was to study the metabolic changes in the blood draining from ischaemic segments following coronary artery ligation. We have been hesitating over the results largely because of the regional flow problem. Even though one can confidently measure the changes in concentration of a metabolite in the blood draining from the ischaemic area through the local vein, it seems from our most recent microsphere studies that the blood in these veins is the net effluent from tissues with a wide range of blood flow. Of course, to calculate metabolic balance without knowing regional blood flow is risky. We have therefore equated regional flow with ST segment change. This is possible on a very precise point-to-point basis and it seems quite clear that practolol can lower the ST segment considerably in an area where the blood flow is as little as 1 or 2 ml 100 g/min. If we fractionate the tissue from the ischaemic area, according to the range of blood flow, we find that propranolol lowers the ST segment most markedly in the centre of the lesion and without shifting flow. Between flows of say 30 to 60 per cent of control values, propranolol lowers regional myocardial flow only slightly. Towards the periphery, where the flow is highest, propranolol lowers flow most of all.

Fitzgerald. It is possible that the reversal of abnormal ST segment elevation by propranolol is due chiefly to its effect in reducing loss of potassium from the cell.

Thomas. We know that the ST segment can be shifted by the transmembrane potassium gradient. Regan showed by infusing the ischaemic area with a high potassium concentration that the ST segment increases. One of the problems is to know the potassium concentration just outside the cell membrane.

Wallace. There are problems in ST segment analysis that I would like to illustrate by reference to propranolol. Propranolol reduces the duration of the action potential in Purkinje and muscles cells. Dr Herbaczynska-Cedro showed that current leaked from non-ischaemic depolarized cells to the injured cells which had repolarized prematurely because of their short action potential, thereby leading to ST segment elevation. If, therefore, an agent (*e.g.* propranolol) is given which shortens the duration of action potential, it should result in less leakage of current to the ischaemic cells and thus lower ST segment elevation. In experimental isolated heart preparations, this certainly occurs but similar changes can be achieved by hypothermia in the absence of ischaemia. I find it difficult to interpret ST segment changes alone. I like the concept of limiting the size of a myocardial infarct by a pharmacological agent, if one can get to the patient early enough. The San Diego work[24] on the use of propranolol for this purpose is interesting but I do not think the final answer has come yet.

Fitzgerald. If an agent is developed which will reduce the area of myocardial ischaemia by antagonizing the actions of catecholamines, it is almost certainly going to reduce myocardial function simultaneously. It is likely that the reduction in the area of ischaemia results from the reduction in myocardial function. I would like to draw attention to the problem of the correct dose of beta blocking drug to be used in controlling arrhythmias. The first study of propranolol in angina pectoris was carried out using a dose of 60 mg per day. This dose was chosen because satisfactory control of arrhythmias had been obtained previously with it. Subsequent experience has shown that 400 to 600 mg per day of propranolol is needed to control angina. In the case of arrhythmias, control can be obtained with far lower doses and it is possible that adequate control of arrhythmias might be obtained with a dose that causes minimal haemodynamic changes. This aspect has not been adequately studied.

Opie. Dr Fitzgerald mentioned that catecholamines in very low doses prevented potassium loss from the heart and also phosphate loss. The phosphate probably comes from ATP and phosphocreatine so that catecholamines would be beneficial. In larger doses, there is evidence that these changes are accelerated and in high doses catecholamines cause cardiac necrosis. Is the problem of knowing whether catecholamines are good or bad simply dependent on their concentration? If so, one could decide which patient needed beta-blockers by measuring the levels of circulating catecholamines.

Fitzgerald. The problem of how much catecholamine activity is good for you after irreversible myocardial ischaemia is a difficult one. It is theoretically possible that there is an optimal degree of activity in the three categories I mentioned—namely haemodynamic, electrophysiological and metabolic (including ionic). If these optima differ markedly in a given subject, then it is going to be very difficult to adjust the dose of beta blocking drug to the circulating level of catecholamine activity, as you suggest.

Wallace. Although isoprenaline made the infarct larger, noradrenaline made the infarct smaller because it raised the perfusion pressure. It is important to remember that obstructed arteries need an adequate perfusion pressure.

METABOLIC INTERVENTION

M. F. OLIVER, M. J. ROWE, N. VETTER

HALF of all the deaths which occur during the first four weeks after acute myocardial infarction take place within two hours of the onset of symptoms.[1] The majority of patients seek medical aid after this time[2] and treatment of serious ventricular arrhythmias and of impaired myocardial contractility is seldom initiated soon enough to reduce this early mortality. It is often difficult to decide which patients should be given prophylactic treatment and which should be left untreated. Therefore, an attractive and logical, although at present impractical prophylactic approach, is to try to provide the incipiently ischaemic myocardium with a metabolic milieu adequate for it to withstand the consequences of subsequent ischaemia.

The occurrence of serious ventricular arrhythmias and of impaired ventricular contractility during impending myocardial infarction might theoretically be prevented, or at least the risk reduced, by providing ischaemic myocardial cells with the optimum concentration of substrates, by preventing cation loss, by minimizing the consequences of catecholamine depletion and by improving oxygenation. Each of these aspects have been considered in detail in previous papers. We propose to deal with the first approach.

Plasma substrate changes during infarction

The hypothesis[3] has been put forward that, in the presence of myocardial ischaemia, accumulation of intracellular free fatty acids (FFA) could be deleterious and lead to serious ventricular arrhythmias and impaired contractility. A simple approach, therefore, to the attainment of an optimum metabolic milieu is either to reduce excess arterial FFA levels or to increase the available glucose, or both.

The evidence that elevated levels of plasma FFA may be harmful to the ischaemic myocardium is based on several observations. In many patients with acute myocardial infarction, plasma FFA are increased more than twofold.[4] Patients with plasma FFA levels of more than about 1200 μEq/1 (*i.e.* more than the 2:1 molar ratio) have a significantly increased incidence of serious ventricular arrhythmias during the first 48 hours after acute myocardial infarction[5 6] and also of deaths during their stay in hospital.[5] Elevation of plasma FFA in dogs with induced myocardial infarction by infusion of Intralipid and heparin is associated, in our experience, with the development of serious ventricular arrhythmias in the majority.[7] This has not been confirmed by Opie *et al.*[8]

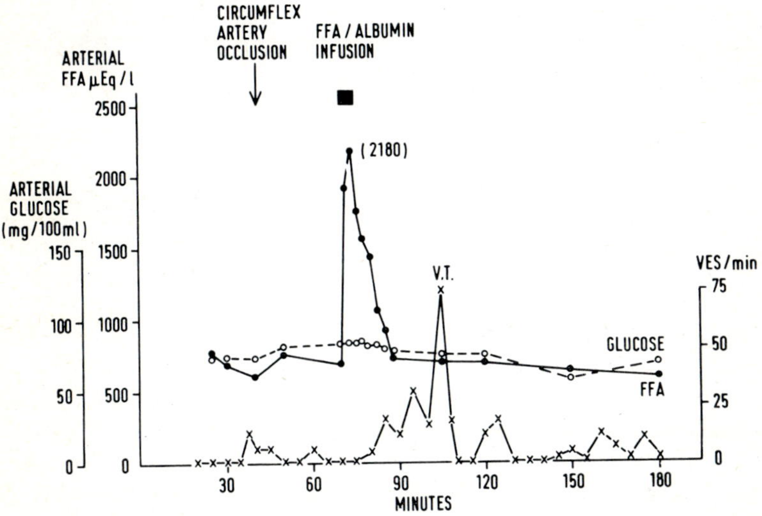

FIG. 23, 1. Effect on arterial FFA and glucose and on cardiac rhythm of infusing 135 ml of plasma containing 3,037 μEq of FFA into a 18·6 Kg dog. There was no change in pH, arterial potassium or albumin, pO_2 and pCo_2 in the recipient dog during the experiment. VT=Ventricular tachycardia.

but there are major differences between the experimental preparations which need further analysis and experiments.[9] Infusions of plasma with raised concentrations of FFA to dogs with acute infarction[10] has led to the development of ventricular arrhythmias in 12 out of 21 animals: while only 1 out of 18 dogs to which plasma alone was infused developed ventricular arrhythmias (Fig. 23, 1). Mjøs[11] has already emphasized that elevation of plasma FFA by Intralipid and heparin can increase $M\dot{V}O_2$ and decrease contractility. Kjekshus and Mjøs[12] have suggested that elevation of plasma

FFA by this means can also increase ST elevation and plasma creatine phosphokinase levels.

Blood glucose levels are usually increased by only about 50 per cent.[13] Since there is often very great suppression of insulin secretion, largely due to adrenaline activity,[14] there is probably little or no increased uptake of glucose by the ischaemic myocardial cells. Opie[15] has recently advanced a case for increasing circulating glucose concentrations in order to promote anaerobic glycolysis and ATP production. Approximate calculations show, however, that the maximal rates of glycolysis likely to be achieved in the infarcting myocardium during glucose and insulin administration could contribute significantly to the energy needs of ischaemic tissue only if at least one-third of the usual oxygen supply is still delivered by the collateral circulation and if ATP demand is halved.

Metabolic intervention might be possible therefore by lowering elevated plasma FFA levels and/or increasing myocardial cellular concentrations of glucose. The former might be achieved by the use of nicotinic acid[16] or by β-adrenergic blockade.[17] Glucose-insulin-potassium infusion or glucagon might achieve the latter.

Nicotinic acid analogues

Nicotinic acid reduces plasma FFA for a period of 3 hours after which there is rebound elevation of FFA[16]. Nicotinic acid influences adipose tissue metabolism by decreasing the available cyclic-AMP, thus reducing adipose tissue lipolysis and the release of FFA and glycerol into the plasma. Nicotinic acid itself produces marked peripheral vaso-dilatation and decreases cardiac work[18] and these haemodynamic effects are sufficiently marked to restrict its use as a means of reducing elevated FFA in patients with acute myocardial infarction. It has recently been shown that an analogue, 5-fluoro-Ronicol (β-pyridyl carbinol), has the metabolic action of nicotinic acid but few of the haemodynamic consequences: this substance is metabolized as 5-fluoro-nicotinic acid. It is effective in dogs in reducing plasma FFA elevation caused by catecholamine[7] and Figure 23, 2 illustrates that the action is also true for man. Following acute myocardial infarction (Fig. 23, 3) it has been shown that 5-fluoro-Ronicol produces a striking and sustained reduction of elevated FFA and this occurs with blood levels of 0·1 mg/Kgm. Evidence from other animal experiments indicates that there is a

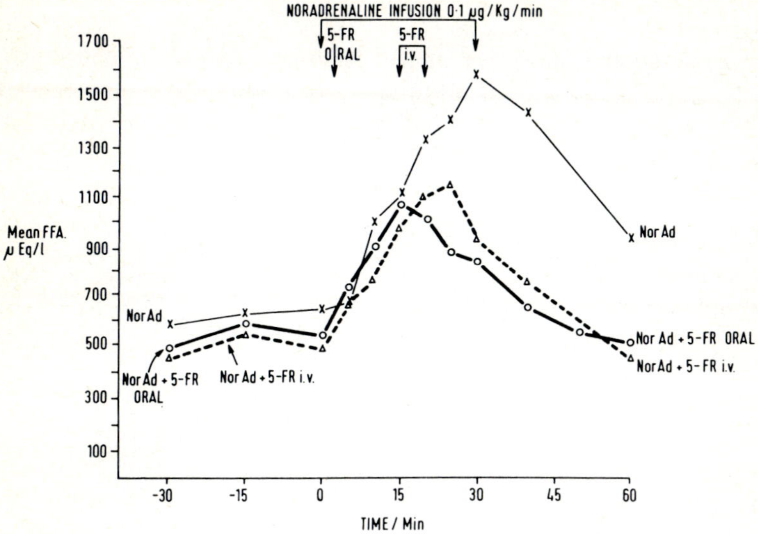

FIG. 23, 2. Effect of a nicotinic acid analogue, 5-fluoro-Ronicol (5-FR), given orally and intravenously on the noradrenaline induced elevation of plasma FFA. Each curve represents the mean results observed in three healthy men, and each of these men participated in each study.

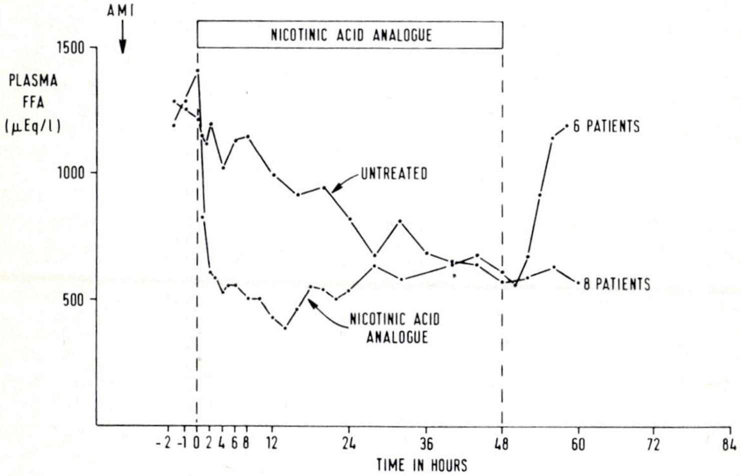

FIG. 23, 3. Effect of a nicotinic acid analogue, 5-fluoro-Ronicol, on plasma FFA levels in six patients with acute myocardial infarction (AMI).

significant correlation between reduction of elevated plasma FFA and decrease in ventricular ectopic rhythms when this drug is given.[19] This substance, and other related analogues, seem sufficiently promising to warrant a controlled trial in patients with acute myocardial infarction in order to determine whether reduction of elevated FFA by this means is associated with reduced incidence of serious ventricular arrhythmias.

Glucose-Insulin-Potassium (GIK)

It is desirable to give glucose with insulin in order to increase intracellular concentrations of glucose, to decrease potassium loss from the ischaemic area, to maintain the action potential in anoxic areas, to decrease circulating plasma FFA levels and to improve nutrition generally. This treatment has been advocated for many years as a 'polarizing solution' by Sodi-Pallares *et al.*[20] The theory of this treatment is that the damaged myocardium will remain polarized until a collateral circulation has developed. The transmembrane potential depends largely on the intra-extracellular gradient of potassium and, if adequate intracellular concentrations of potassium can be maintained, the cell should remain electrically stable.

The treatment schedule advocated by Sodi-Pallares *et al.*[21] is complicated but comprises the continuous intravenous infusion of glucose 10 to 50 per cent, insulin given into the infusate between 20 to 80 units per litre and potassium from 12 to 60 mEq/l together with a low sodium diet.

Unfortunately, no adequate controlled trial has been conducted of GIK as an early means of treating patients with acute myocardial infarction. All reported studies can be criticized. A Mexican study[22] of 25 treated and 25 control patients gave insufficient information concerning selection and randomization of patients and the majority received treatment beginning at the third day after acute myocardial infarction when the incidence of arrhythmias is low. Two Swedish studies differ in results: in the larger,[23] GIK was given only for a few hours a day and the results were negative; in the smaller,[24] continuous intravenous infusion for 72 hours reduced the incidence of arrhythmias but only 26 patients were studied in all. In another study the death rate and the incidence of ventricular fibrillation were lower in the group given GIK intravenously[25] but details are few and the study was uncontrolled. No difference was observed in the death rate or incidence of ventricular arrhythmias between 5 groups of 8 patients given GIK, GI, GK, G and no solution.[26] Malach[27] reported an increased death rate in 47 patients given intravenous GIK (45 per cent) compared with a control group of 54 patients (15 per cent) but also included heparin in the GIK infusion. Then, Mittra[28] reported a mortality rate of 11·7 per cent in the GIK treated group in contrast to 28·2 per cent in a control group. The GIK was not given as advocated by Sodi-Pallares *et al.*[21] but orally as a dose of 240 g glucose and 52 to 78 mEq of potassium in 24 hours and 10 units of soluble insulin subcutaneously twice daily. This study is open to further criticism since patients were not started with treatment until 18 to 20 hours after admission and comparison of the treated group depended on retrospective controls. Subsequently, the Medical Research Council in the U.K. established a comparable study in 13 centres with 430 patients as controls and 410 patients given oral glucose and potassium and subcutaneous insulin as described. There was no significant difference in mortality rates in the two groups.[29] This study was unsatisfactory, not only because of the routes of administration and concentrations of GIK, but because of unexplained unevenness of results between centres and the fact that more than half of all patients were admitted to the trial 7 or more hours after the onset of symptoms of acute myocardial infarction.

The place of GIK in the early management of acute myocardial infarction needs complete reappraisal. GIK has recently been shown to reduce the extent of necrosis as measured by ST elevation, creatine kinase release and ultrastructure changes in dogs with experimental myocardial infarction,[30] and G and GI have been shown to increase contractile function of the hypoxic myocardium.[31] It can be argued that GIK is particularly indicated in patients with marked elevation of plasma FFA; the effect of GIK solutions on such patients does not appear to have been previously reported. In Figure 23, 4 it can be seen that various concentrations of intravenous GIK effectively reduce the FFA blood level in patients with acute myocardial infarction. In Figure 23, 5 intravenous glucose is shown to have an effect independent of insulin. In Figure 23, 6 oral glucose is shown to be equally effective. Despite this effect of oral glucose, there are obvious difficulties in giving large concentrations orally for many hours to a patient after an acute myocardial infarct. Relatively large infusions of GIK are probably necessary for potassium transfer to have an effect in the prevention of ventricular tachycardia and fibrillation in dogs with experimental myocardial infarction.[32]

The most urgent need is a prospective controlled trial of the effect of the GIK régime close to that proposed by Sodi-Pallares *et al.*[21] on the monitored incidence of serious ventricular arrhythmias. This treatment should be begun as soon as possible after this onset of acute myocardial infarction. The main problem is the

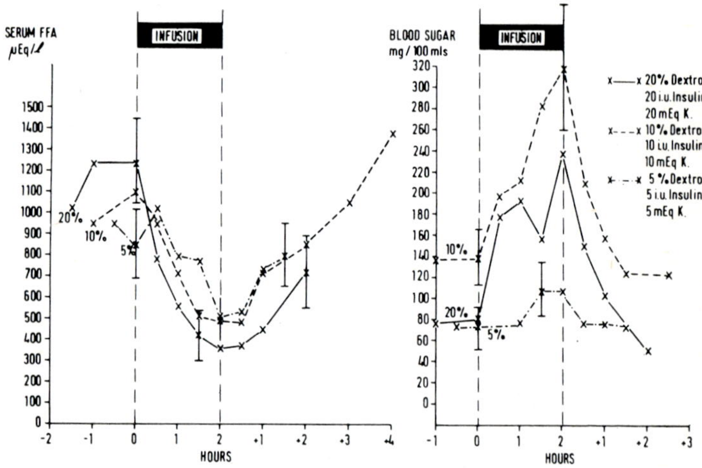

FIG. 23, 4. Effect on serum FFA and blood sugar levels of different concentrations of dextrose, insulin and potassium given intravenously to patients with acute myocardial infarction. Each curve represents the mean results found in three patients.

prevention of early death. If the myocardium is 'sensitized' in favour of the development of serious ventricular arrhythmias before the development of major ischaemia,[3] possibly by triglyceride accumulation, the maintenance of intracellular glucose and potassium concentrations may be crucial and a high intake of glucose, or of a sugar such as fructose which does not require insulin for entry into the cell, might theoretically be protective during this prodromal period.

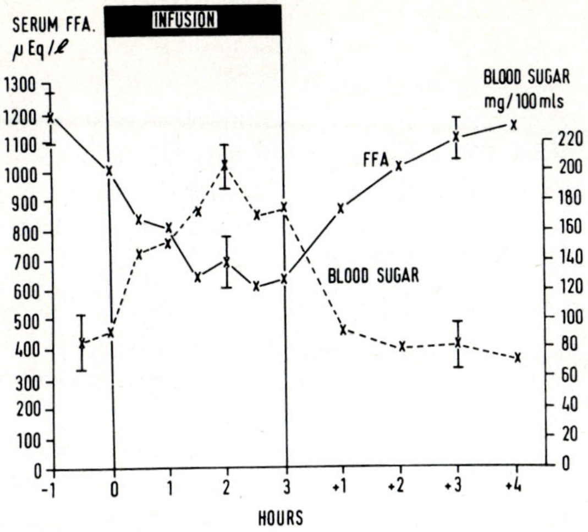

FIG. 23, 5. Effect of an intravenous infusion of 750 ml of 10 per cent glucose and 15 mEq potassium (no insulin given) on serum FFA and blood sugar levels in three patients with acute myocardial infarction.

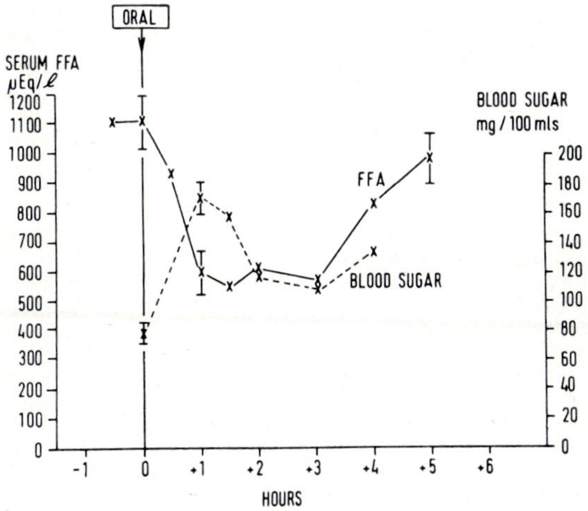

FIG. 23, 6. Effect of 75 g of glucose given orally with 24 mEq of potassium chloride on serum FFA and blood sugar levels in three patients with acute myocardial infarction.

Glucagon

Glucagon might promote the glucose uptake of the myocardium by increasing blood levels of insulin[33] but it also stimulates adenyl cyclase to produce cyclic-AMP and therefore has an action resembling that of catecholamines. It also has an inotropic effect probably by augmenting the movement of calcium ions into myocardial cells[34] but it does not, however, increase the 'electrical stability' of the heart after acute myocardial infarction.[35]

Potassium

Opie[36] has suggested that the effect of potassium infusions should be studied. Potassium and magnesium salts of dl-aspartic acid increase glucose utilization[37] and potassium aspartate and tri-aspartate have been reported to lower heparin-induced elevation of plasma FFA.[38]

Conclusion

Neither nicotinic acid analogues nor GIK solutions have been studied in sufficient detail, nor have their effects on morbidity and mortality been well enough delineated, to advise their use routinely in patients with acute myocardial infarction. Yet they both appear to be capable of providing ischaemic myocardial cells with substrates which may permit their survival. Their use appears rational and there is now a need to study systematically the potential of metabolic intervention.

REFERENCES

1 FULTON, P. M., JULIAN, D. G. & OLIVER, M. F. (1969). Sudden death and myocardial infarction. *Circulation* **39** *suppl. IV*, 182-191.
2 ARMSTRONG, A., DUNCAN, B., OLIVER, M. F., JULIAN, D. G., DONALD, K. W., FULTON, M., LUTZ, W. & MORRISON, S. L. (1972). Natural history of acute coronary heart attacks. *British Heart Journal* **34,** 67-80.
3 KURIEN, V. A. & OLIVER, M. F. (1970). A metabolic cause for arrhythmias during acute myocardial hypoxia. *Lancet* **I,** 813-815.
4 KURIEN, V. A. & OLIVER, M. F. (1966). Serum-free-fatty-acids after acute myocardial infarction and cerebral vascular occlusion. *Lancet* **II,** 122-127.
5 OLIVER, M. F., KURIEN, V. A. & GREENWOOD, T. W. (1968). Relation between serum-free-fatty-acids and arrhythmias and death after acute myocardial infarction. *Lancet* **I,** 710-714.
6 GUPTA, D. K., YOUNG, R., JEWITT, D. E., HARTOG, M. & OPIE, L. H. (1969). Increased plasma-free-fatty-acids concentration and their significance in patients with acute myocardial infarction. *Lancet* **II,** 1209-1213.
7 KURIEN, V. A., YATES, P. A. & OLIVER, M. F. (1971). The role of free fatty acids in the production of ventricular arrhythmias after acute

coronary artery occlusion. *European Journal of Clinical Investigation* **1,** 225-241.

8 Opie, L. H., Norris, R. M., Thomas, M., Holland, H. A., Owen, P. & Van Norden, A. (1971). Failure of high concentrations of circulating free fatty acids to provoke arrhythmias in experimental myocardial infarction. *Lancet* **I,** 818-822.

9. Oliver, M. F. (1972). Metabolic response during impending myocardial infarction. *Circulation* **45,** 491-500.

10 Oliver, M. F. & Yates, P. A. (1972). In *Metabolism of the Hypoxic and Ischaemic Heart,* p. 359. Edited by: P. Moret and Z. Fejfer. S. Karger.

11 Mjøs, O. D. (1971). Effect of free fatty acids on myocardial function and oxygen consumption in intact dogs. *Journal of Clinical Investigation* **50,** 1386-1389.

12 Kjekshus, J. K. & Mjøs, O. D. (1972). Effect of free fatty acids on myocardial infarction and metabolism in the ischemic dog heart. *Journal of Clinical Invesigaion* **51,** 1767-1777.

13 Logan, R. W. & Murdoch, W. R. (1966). Blood-levels of hydrocortisone transaminases, and cholesterol after myocardial infarction. *Lancet* **II,** 521-524.

14 Porte, D., Crabor, A. L., Kuzuya, T. & Williams, R. H. (1968). The effect of epinephrine on immunoreactive insulin levels in man. *Journal of Clinical Investigation* **45,** 228-236.

15 Opie, L. H. (1972). Metabolic response during impending myocardial infarction. *Circulation* **45,** 483-490.

16 Carlson, L. A. & Oro, L. (1962). The effect of nicotinic acid on the plasma free fatty acid; demonstration of a metabolic type of sympathicolysis. *Acta Medica Scandinavica* **172,** 641-645.

17 Fitzgerald, D. This symposium.

18 Ekström-Jodal, B., Harthon, L., Haggendal, E., Malmberg, R. & Svedmyr, N. (1970). Influence of nicotinic acid and pentaerythritoltetranicotinate on the cardiac output in man. *Pharmacologia Clinica* **2,** 86-89.

19 Smith, E. R. & Duce, B. R. (1972, in press). Antiarrhythmic and serum free fatty acid lowering effects of 5-fluoro-3-hydroxymethylpyridine hydrochloride following experimentally induced myocardial infarction in the dog.

20 Sodi-Pallares, D. (1966). Possibility of a therapy of cellular ion integration in cardiovascular diseases. *Archives International Cardiology. Mexico* **31,** 557-574.

21 Sodi-Pallares, D., Ponce de Leon, J., Bisteni, A. & Medrano, G. A. (1969). Potassium, glucose and insulin in myocardial infarction. *Lancet* **I,** 1315-1316.

22 Ponce de Leon, J. J., Oriol-Palon, A. & Sodi-Pallares, D. (1962). Clinical course of acute myocardial infarction treated with polarizing solution of glucose, insulin and potassium. *Abstract of the World Congress of Cardiology* Part IVB, 279-280.

23 Sievers, J., Lindh, J., Johansson, B. W. & Karnell, J. (1966). Acute myocardial infarction treated by glucose-insulin-potassium (GIK) infusion. *Cardiologia* **49,** 239-247.

24 Lundman, T. & Orinius, E. (1965). Insulin-glucose-potassium infusion in acute myocardial infarction. *Acta Medica Scandinavica* **178,** 525-528.

25 Day, H. W. & Averill, K. (1966). Recorded arrhythmias in an acute coronary care area. *Diseases of the Chest* **49,** 113-118.

26 Fletcher, G. F., Horset, J. W. & Schlant, R. C. (1966). Preliminary report of a double-blind controlled study of the use of 'polarizing' solution in acute myocardial infarction. *Circulation* **34 III,** 102.

27 Malach, M. (1967). Polarizing solution in acute myocardial infarction. *American Journal of Cardiology* **20,** 363-366.

28 MITTRA, B. (1965). Potassium, glucose and insulin in treatment of myocardial infarction. *Lancet* **II,** 607-609.
29 REPORT BY MEDICAL RESEARCH COUNCIL (1968). Potassium, glucose, and insulin treatment for acute myocardial infarction. *Lancet* **II,** 1355-1360.
30 MAROKO, P. R., LIBBY, P., SOBEL, B. E., BLOOR, C. M., SYBERS, H. D., SHELL, W. E., COVELL, J. W. & BRAUNWALD, E. (1972). Effect of glucose-insulin-potassium infusion on myocardial infarction following experimental coronary artery occlusion. *Circulation* **45,** 1160-1175.
31 AMSTERDAM, E. A., FOLEY, D., MASUMI, R. A., ZELIS, R. F., MASON, D. T. (1972). Enhancement of myocardial function during hypoxia by increased glucose availability. *American Journal of Cardiology* **29,** 251.
32 BURKE, W. M., ASOKAN, S. K., MOSCHOS, C. B., OLDEWURTEL, H. A. & REGAN. T. J. (1969). Effects of glucose and non-glucose infusions on myocardial potassium ion transfers and arrhythmias during ischaemia. *American Journal of Cardiology* **24,** 713-722.
33 FOA, P. P. (1968). Glucagon. *Ergebn. Physiology* **60,** 141-219.
34 NAYLER, W. G., MCINNES, I., CHIPPERFIELD, D., CARSON, V. & DAILE, P. (1970). The effect of glucagon on calcium exchangeability, coronary blood flow, myocardial function and high energy phosphate stores. *Journal of Pharmacology and Experimental Therapy* **171,** 265-275.
35 LVOFF, R. & WILCKEN, D. E. L. (1972). Glucagon in heart failure and in cardiogenic shock. *Circulation* **45,** 534-542.
36 OPIE, L. H. This symposium.
37 LABORIT, H. (1966). Sur le mécanisme d'action des sels potássigne et magnésien de l'acide aspartigine. *Agressologie* **7,** 515-527.
38 GRAVILESCO, S., DANCIU, T., FIAT, F. & POP, T. (1970). Effects of potassium and tri-aspartate on heparin-induced serum free-fatty-acids elevation, in man. *Agressologie* **6,** 501-505.

DISCUSSION

Barratt. I showed 7 or 8 years ago in rats and in dogs that clofibrate lowers free fatty acid levels in the resting state. The response of plasma FFA to the infusion of noradrenaline was modified by clofibrate in a very similar manner to that which you showed for 5-fluoro-Ronicol.

Wallace. What is the end point in these trials?

Oliver. Death is the main end point. We have two other major end points: one is the occurrence of ventricular tachycardia and the other ventricular fibrillation which we assume to rank as death even although it can be corrected in the coronary unit.

Opie. It is interesting to see just how far we have got in this dialogue by promoting both of these hypotheses—namely that ' glucose is good ' and ' fatty acid is bad ', while not entirely accepting all the points of view put forward for either hypothesis.

As far as the ' glucose is good ' hypothesis is concerned, it has suffered from the fact that there has been no careful clinical trial. Sodi-Pallares advised a complex dosage schedule, even more complex than you suggested, going up to 50 per cent glucose in some cases. When we used the doses in baboons, we found no better effect than with the lower dose schedule. In your glucose studies, the initial free fatty acid values were about 1000 μg/l indicating that these were not your most seriously ill patients. We really want to know what happened in the more seriously ill patients. Did their FFA fall? You showed a fall in plasma potassium in some of the studies using Intralipid and heparin. This is something we also noticed and, although the fall was not great, it might have contributed in some way to the arrhythmias.

Oliver. The fall in serum potassium is roughly correlated with the height to which free fatty acid rise and presumably is due to haemolysis. You are correct about the Sodi-Pallares régime. He attempts to titrate the concentration of his glucose infusion with the blood glucose levels produced.

Herbaczynska-Cedro. Using bioassy techniques, we detected increased blood adrenaline levels following coronary ligation. Glucose and insulin infusion abolished this increased adrenaline secretion and the blood adrenaline levels returned to normal or decreased. This was not confirmed by biochemical determination of catecholamine levels in blood. As increased adrenaline secretion after coronary ligation is induced reflexly by stimulation of cardiac receptors at the site and boundary of the infarct, it is probable that glucose and insulin solution has some local effect on the infarcted area and may decrease this reflex response.

Noble. Is Dr Oliver proposing a properly controlled clinical trial of GIK in which conventional anti-arrhythmic treatment like lignocaine is disallowed?

Oliver. No. At this stage we would have to give conventional anti-arrhythmic treatment in all cases.

Mjøs. Do you think that clofibrate is as good a blocker of catecholamine-induced lipolysis as nicotinic acid?

Carlson. Clofibrate is active *in vitro* on rat fat pads and on human fat in inhibiting lipolysis but you need quite high doses to see this effect; it may be dose dependent.

Opie. We have also found that a relatively small dose of glucose given intravenously without insulin will reduce elevated fatty acids. When we measured the circulating insulin concentration in patients with myocardial infarction who were not severely ill, there was sufficient circulating insulin to expect some effect from glucose.

Oliver. That is why we need to study the effect of glucose in patients who have no measurable circulating insulin.

Mjøs. You showed that infusion of glucose alone lowered elevated free fatty acids in patients with acute myocardial infarction. What is the mechanism involved? I ask because we would not expect there to be any rise in insulin in response to glucose under these conditions. Perhaps it is another action of glucose and not an antilipolytic effect?

Oliver. I was also surprised about this. Oral glucose has greater effect. In order to answer your question, we would need to know plasma insulin and adrenaline levels.

Mjøs. In dogs, intravenous glucose infusion without insulin lowers elevated free fatty acids. Similarly, a continuous infusion of noradrenaline with glucose restricts the rise in free fatty acid concentrations.

CLINICAL IMPLICATIONS

D. G. JULIAN

ACUTE myocardial ischaemia presents in many different ways. It may occur as exercise-induced ischaemia in stable angina pectoris, as a major clinical feature of unstable angina or acute coronary insufficiency, as the early phase of acute myocardial infarction and as sudden death without preceding symptoms. It must also be assumed to occur frequently without symptoms or catastrophic effects in view of the common finding of focal fibrosis of the myocardium in individuals dying of causes other than coronary disease.

It is a remarkable thing that acute ischaemia may occur in response to exercise many thousands of times in patients with stable angina pectoris without leading to serious ventricular arrhythmias or significant permanent cardiac damage. Many hundreds of thousands of exercise tests have been undertaken in such patients and only in a very few cases has ventricular fibrillation ensued. When it has done so, it seems to have occurred most commonly in patients who have been submitted to maximal or submaximal exercise tests and, under these circumstances, seems most prone to occur some minutes after the end of the test. Dr Maseri's concepts may be relevant here. With severe exercise, the patients may be getting a complete shutdown in the ischaemic area and ventricular fibrillation develops when reflow occurs.

Patients with unstable angina are certainly at risk from ventricular fibrillation, either after the onset of symptoms of classical infarction or without these symptoms, and present as sudden death. Dr Allison and Dr Oliver have both suggested that acute coronary insufficiency might give rise to metabolic changes which could predispose the patient for the production of arrhythmias. One might anticipate, therefore, that the patient with prodromal symptoms would be at a higher risk of developing arrhythmias when he sustains a heart attack than the patient without such symptoms. It is in fact difficult, if not impossible, to prove this but the evidence is rather against it. Several studies have shown that prodromal symptoms appear to be more common in those developing myocardial infarction than in those who die suddenly.[1 2] This difference might be accounted for by the fact that one is unable to get adequate ante-mortem information on those who die suddenly. However, in the study of Fulton *et al.*[2] it was found that of those who died suddenly, 10 per cent had previously consulted a general practitioner on account of prodromal symptoms compared with 30 per cent of those who subsequently sustained a myocardial infarction. It is also of interest that arrhythmias and sudden death were no commoner in those admitted to a coronary care unit with prodromal symptoms than those who had no such symptoms.[3]

Before considering the application to clinical medicine of some of the findings concerning the genesis of arrhythmias, it is worthwhile discussing the relevance to the human of some of the animal models. As Dr Jennings pointed out, it is essential that we select an animal which is appropriate to the subject we are discussing and a different model may apply to several different clinical situations which we encounter. It may well be that the phase III of the Harris preparation,[4] in which chaotic arrhythmias occur many hours after infarction, does not resemble the situation we see in man in the early hours after infarction. The drugs which are frequently effective in the Harris phase III are not those which are most effective in the clinical management of acute infarction. For example, diphenylhydantoin is very effective for the Harris phase III arrhythmias but is of comparatively little value in human myocardial infarction. On the other hand, the type of preparation that Lown[5] and others have used, that is, a conscious dog in whom a balloon can be inflated in a coronary artery, seems to be more clinically applicable to acute ischaemia. The results of anti-arrhythmic therapy in this preparation are, in general, similar to those that we find in clinical practice.

When ventricular fibrillation occurs in an acute heart attack, it does so under three rather different circumstances. First of all, it may occur as asymptomatic sudden death; secondly, it may occur within the first four or six hours of an acute infarction and, finally, it may develop some hours or days later. In the first two instances, it can be described as primary ventricular fibrillation. When it occurs later, it has usually been preceded by shock or cardiac failure and may be considered secondary.

Dr Wallace, Dr Han and Dr Reuter have described the electrophysiological mechanisms which adequately explain the occurrence of ventricular fibrillation at or soon after the onset of an acute heart attack. The changes in extracellular and intracellular potassium caused by focal ischaemia, potentiated by the local cellular depletion of catecholamines, will be sufficient to account for sudden death in these patients. One does not need to propose that there is any generalized metabolic disturbance. However, it is probably true that the onset of ventricular fibrillation would be facilitated by certain pre-existing situations. As Dr Oliver has suggested, this might be the accumulation of triglycerides. In order to curtail this and for other reasons that have been proposed by Dr Opie and Dr Allison, the use of glucose-insulin-potassium might diminish the risk of this fatal arrhythmia. The observations of Dr Wallace and Dr Shahab, amongst others, have shown the effect of sympathectomy or of catecholamine depletion in the prevention of ventricular fibrillation. Dr Wallace has told us about the actions of 6-hydroxydopamine which seems totally to protect animals against the ventricular fibrillation of acute coronary occlusion.

Unfortunately, even if we could devise a prophylactic regime on the basis of these observations we cannot yet clearly define the high risk group of patients for whom short or long term treatment could be given safely in the hope of preventing ventricular fibrillation when they get an acute heart attack. Only a minority of patients present to a doctor with prodromal symptoms[2] and, even with public and medical education, it is doubtful whether this number can be much increased.

There appears to be no animal model which closely mimics the situation which occurs in human infarction in its first three or four hours. There is none which suffers pain and fear, transport in an ambulance and subjection to the variety of drugs that the human does. Nor do animals resemble humans in regard to the anatomical variations in arrhythmic response that we see in man. We may learn more from human observations in this situation than we do from animals. The recent findings of Pantridge and his coworkers in Belfast are of particular interest.[6] They have now seen 77 patients within the first 30 minutes following the onset of symptoms. In this group, 14 per cent developed ventricular fibrillation in the first half hour, 4 per cent in the second half hour and 3 per cent in the following hour. There is therefore a high incidence of ventricular fibrillation throughout the first two hours but it is progressively diminishing.

Pantridge believes that one can, at this stage, categorize patients whose response is predominantly sympathetic and others whose response is predominantly parasympathetic. The clinical features of sympathetic response are those of sinus tachycardia and transient hypertension or a combination of the two. The features of a parasympathetic response are sinus bradycardia, hypotension or a combination of these two. In anterior infarction, the majority of patients show a sympathetic response, but a substantial minority show a parasympathetic predominance. In only a small proportion is neither response seen at an early stage. In the case of inferior infarction, the predominant characteristic is a parasympathetic response. Pantridge has found in patients presenting with an inferior infarction for the first time that only the parasympathetic response is encountered. As Dr Han and his colleagues have shown, the bradycardia which occurs as a response to vagal activity provides the opportunity for the dispersion of refractory periods that encourages the development of ventricular ectopic rhythms. In many of these patients in whom the parasympathetic response predominates, it is likely that a peripheral sympathetic response is also occurring. One can see this when the bradycardia is relieved by atropine and an excessive tachycardia may develop. This sympathetic response, whether in combination with or apart from the parasympathetic response, will also make ventricular ectopic rhythms more likely in the presence of ischaemia. These findings may be of value in determining the appropriate therapy. Dr Wallace has suggested that lignocaine is preferable to beta blockade in the presence of acute infarction for the treatment of ventricular arrhythmia. Whilst this is probably the case after the first hour or two, it is still uncertain whether practolol may not be more effective in the first few minutes when lignocaine appears to be relatively ineffective. The evidence that Dr Fitzgerald has put forward might also support the use of practolol at this early stage.

It is probable that the development of shock and failure and secondary arrhythmias that occur after four to six hours is largely determined by haemodynamic and metabolic responses during the first three hours. The observations of Maroko and his colleagues[7] have been frequently quoted during this symposium. These workers have shown that a variety of inotropic drugs, including isoprenaline and digitalis, can increase the size of an infarction whereas negatively inotropic drugs such as propranolol and practolol can decrease it. Dr. Mjøs has indicated that free fatty acids may contribute to increasing the size of the infarction. Methoxamine appears to diminish it. Glucose-insulin-potassium may also reduce the size of the infarct.[8] There is therefore a sound basis for assuming that if one intervenes during the first three hours of infarction, one may restrict the size of the infarction by appropriate treatment. Such a therapeutic regime could include pain-relieving drugs which would diminish the catecholamine response, the use of beta blockade, the employment of glucose, insulin and potassium, and of free fatty acid lowering drugs and, possibly, methoxamine.

Maroko and co-workers suggested that these interventions must take place within the first three hours to be effective.[8] Pantridge's observations[6] on the application of intensive care are of interest in this connection. He has shown that patients seen within one hour of the onset of infarction had a mortality of 9 per cent in the first four weeks. From the findings in our community study,[9] we would expect a mortality of 28 per cent at four weeks in patients seen at this stage. In Pantridge's experience, the mortality is also around 9 per cent in those seen within the second and third hours, but rises to twice this figure if the patient was seen after this time. Of particular interest is the mortality from shock in these different groups of patients. In those seen within the first three hours, death from shock was around 5 per cent rising to 13 per cent in those seen later. These observations clearly require confirmation to ensure that the groups studied were comparable in other respects. I would suggest, however, that early intervention, whether it be by conventional anti-arrhythmic therapy, by relieving pain or by metabolic means could have an important effect in preventing myocardial damage and subsequently arrhythmias.

In summary, our major concern as clinicians is the prevention of sudden death and myocardial damage in those of our patients who have ischaemic heart disease. As yet, our ability to prevent death from ventricular fibrillation is confined to a small group of patients who are under intensive care early in their course of myocardial infarction. The problem of reaching patients at an earlier stage is unresolved. Our most important immediate aim should be to find some regime which could be given over many months to patients with known medium or high risk of developing heart attacks. This could well be by sympathetic depletion, by use of prolonged metabolic manipulations or by employing long term anti-arrhythmic drugs. Unfortunately, all anti-arrhythmic drugs at present in use are unsuitable on the grounds of toxicity or ineffectiveness for this situation. None the less, research needs to be directed very intensively in this area.

Equally, research needs to be directed to find out whether in the human it is true that intervention during the first three hours after the onset of an acute infarction can determine the size and severity of that infarction. Certain observations suggests that this is so, but large scale trials of patients seen early in the illness are essential before this matter can be clarified.

In achieving these aims, it is clearly necessary to have animal models which will permit us to make deductions which are relevant to the human condition. Several preparations are now available which allow us to undertake experiments which appear to be more appropriate to the various clinical situations. Hopefully we may gain from these information which will enable us to make therapeutically valid conclusions.

REFERENCES

1 Kinlen, L. J. (1969). D.Phil. *Thesis.* Oxford University.
2 Fulton, M., Duncan, B., Lutz, W., Morrison, S. L., Donald, K. W., Kerr, F., Kirby, B. J., Julian, D. G. & Oliver, M. F. (1972). Natural history of unstable angina. *Lancet* **I,** 860-865.
3 Solomon, H. A., Edwards, A. L. & Killip, T. (1969). Prodromata in acute myocardial infarction. *Circulation* **40,** 463-471.
4 Harris, A. S. & Bisteni, A. (1955). Effects of sympathetic blockade drugs on ventricular tachycardia resulting from myocardial infarction. *American Journal of Physiology* **181,** 559-566.
5 Lown, B. & Wolf, M. (1971). Approaches to sudden death from coronary heart disease. *Circulation* **44,** 130-142.
6 Maroko, P. R., Kjekshus, J. K., Sobel, B. E. Watanabe, T., Covell, J. W., Ross, J. & Braunwald, E. (1971). Factors influencing infarct size following experimental coronary artery occlusions. *Circulation* **43,** 67-82.
7 Maroko, P. R., Libby, P., Sobel, B. E., Bloor, C. M., Sybers, H. D., Shell, W. E. & Braunwald, E. (1972). Reduction in experimental myocardial infarction size by glucose-insulin-potassium administration. *American Journal of Cardiology* **29 (abstr.)** 277-278.

8 Webb, S. W., Adgey, A. A. J. & Pantridge, J. F. (1972). Autonomic disturbance at onset of acute myocardial infarction. *British Medical Journal* **2,** 89-92.
9 Armstrong, A., Duncan, B., Oliver, M. F., Julian, D. G., Donald, K. W., Fulton, M. F., Lutz, W. & Morrison, S. L. (1972). Natural history of acute heart attacks. *British Heart Journal* **34,** 67-80.

Discussion

Kurien. With regard to the autonomic response in anterior and posterior infarction, could you give an analysis of the incidence of ventricular fibrillation in each category?

Julian. I am afraid that I cannot. Even if I could it would mean very little because these patients are being treated. Those who have bradycardia are given atropine. It is impossible to say what the natural history of the attack would have been in relation to the occurrence of ventricular fibrillation.

Donald. Could we ask you about further details of the 'shock' that Pantridge's early treatment is supposed to have prevented? Early hypotension is often transient and serious, severe cardiogenic shock is inclined to occur later. Has he significantly altered mortality from cardiogenic shock and, if so, how?

Julian. I believe he would claim that coronary perfusion would be improved by correcting hypotension and thereby limit the size of the infarct. The size of an infarct is probably an important factor in the development of shock. Presumably, reflex factors are also important in its genesis. I believe that pain plays an extremely important part; as it produces a sympathetic response, its relief may be effective in preventing shock.

Donald. Does Pantridge give drugs to relieve pain immediately and does he give drugs routinely to combat hypotension in the early phases?

Julian. He gives atropine if there is hypotension and bradycardia. Pain is relieved quickly by analgesics.

Oliver. What is the evidence for this categorization of patients with inferior infarcts as having a parasympathetic response and those with anterior infarcts as having a sympathetic response? Are there differences in the plasma concentrations of noradrenaline and adrenaline according to the position of the infarct?

Julian. I think the parasympathetic response is a reasonable presumption in that it is correctable by atropine. Furthermore, one cannot assume that because there is a parasympathetic response, the sympathetic response is not also increased in the same patient. In fact, when one blocks the parasympathetic response with atropine the tachycardia is greater than one would expect from the release of the parasympathetic response alone. Both factors operate but the parasympathetic may be overriding.

Kurien. In dogs, noradrenaline infusion produces bradycardia. This is due to reflex stimulation of the carotid sinus by elevation of the blood pressure. This can be abolished by atropine and it disappears when the catecholamine stimulation produces a tachycardia. So I do not think it is necessary to postulate that this is an entirely vagal response. It may be a vagal response secondary to elevation of sympathetic tone.

Julian. Would it continue when the blood pressure had fallen? If the patient is hypotensive, why should he respond in that way?

Kurien. In that situation vagal tone has not completely returned to normal, because as has been shown in some cases of posterior infarction you do get combined sympathetic and vagal response. You are postulating that there is no sympathetic tone but I do not think we can say that unless we have measurements of catecholamine levels.

Fitzgerald. Patients who suffer from a myocardial infarction are frequently in a state of enhanced autonomic tone. If a beta blocking drug is given, there will be an ‘ unmasking ’ of vagal activity. This may account for the development of severe bradycardia in some patients following beta blockade. The reduction in heart rate and subsequent fall in cardiac output can be prevented or reversed by the administration of atropine sulphate (1 to 2 mg i.v.). A considerable amount of the so-called ‘ cardiac depressant ’ effects of propranolol are due to its action in exposing the heart to unopposed vagal activity.

Julian. As you pointed out yourself, this can be blocked with atropine.

Fitzgerald. Sloman showed that atropine prevented the fall in cardiac output due to propranolol in subjects with myocardial infarction (*Medical Journal of Australia* (1968) **1,** 333-334). It is conceivable that pharmacological isolation of the heart, as proposed by Jose, may be useful in the early phase of infarction though such a suggestion may be too provocative. In considering the question of myocardial depression by beta blocking drugs, it is of practical importance to define our terms. Ventricular function is markedly influenced by catecholamine activity but the heart can function adequately without sympathetic activity except under maximal exercise. Since catecholamines increase ventricular function, blockade of their action will reduce that function in proportion to the degree of sympathetic tone. All the beta blocking drugs in clinical use can reduce ventricular function and it is not true to say that there are beta blocking drugs which do not have cardiac depressant activity, as I have defined it. The degree of reduction of ventricular function depends on a number of variables, one of which is vagal tone.

As an example, if I take a single dose of 600 mg of propranolol orally, my resting heart rate is reduced from 52 beats min to 44 beats min. If I then receive atropine 2·5 μg intravenously, my heart rate immediately rises to 90 beats min. One might then ask, does propranolol slow the heart? The answer is: it does, but the major slowing is due to the vagus. In a patient unable to increase his stroke volume, cardiac output is largely rate determined. It is then more accurate to say that propranolol permits the vagus to slow the heart.

One must be quite clear, therefore, as to the possible ways in which beta blockade can reduce cardiac output, (a) by removing catecholamine support to the heart, (b) by favouring unopposed vagal activity. It is equally important to remember that propranolol can ‘ depress ’ the activity of heart beating at 150 beats min to 90 beats min and subsequently increase cardiac output.

Wallace. Our experiments with the catecholamine-depleted animal which still has an intact vagal nerve supply are relevant here. When you produce right coronary occlusion in the pig that has been treated with 6-hydroxydopamine or if you give digitalis to a dog treated with this drug, ventricular extrasystoles do not develop. The animals have frequently periods of 10 to 12 seconds of asystole. This is a consequence of tremendous vagal activity occurring in a catecholamine depleted, sympathetically unsupported heart.

INDEX

Printed by The Central Press (Aberdeen) Limited, Aberdeen